Mask Makers and Their Craft

Also by Deborah Bell

Masquerade: Essays on Tradition and Innovation Worldwide, edited by Deborah Bell (McFarland, 2015)

Mask Makers and Their Craft

An Illustrated Worldwide Study

DEBORAH BELL

McFarland & Company, Inc., Publishers
Jefferson, North Carolina

The present work is a reprint of the library bound edition of Mask Makers and Their Craft: An Illustrated Worldwide Study, *first published in 2010 by McFarland.*

LIBRARY OF CONGRESS CATALOGUING-IN-PUBLICATION DATA

Bell, Deborah.
Mask makers and their craft : an illustrated worldwide study / Deborah Bell.
p. cm.
Includes bibliographical references and index.

ISBN 978-0-7864-9753-9 (softcover : acid free paper) ♾
ISBN 978-0-7864-5764-9 (ebook)

1. Masks. 2. Theater. 3. Performing arts. I. Title.

PN2071.M37.B45 2015 646.4'78—dc22 2010026202

BRITISH LIBRARY CATALOGUING DATA ARE AVAILABLE

Front cover: clockwise from top—20th century wood-carved *tigre* mask by an anonymous mask maker (www.casadelacuesta.com); Tsimshian masks created by Victor Reece, worn by Mariko Ohara and Melina Laboucan-Massimo in *Matriarchs of the Earth* (photograph by Ron Naversen, www.fullcircleperformance.ca); "Le Gourmand" mask created by Rob Faust (www.faustwork.com); "The Sage" mask created by Rob Faust (robfaustspeaker.com)

Printed in the United States of America

McFarland & Company, Inc., Publishers
Box 611, Jefferson, North Carolina 28640
www.mcfarlandpub.com

To the mask makers

Table of Contents

Acknowledgments

This book would not have been possible without the input of my husband, D. H. Lawrence scholar Keith Cushman. He wielded his remarkable editorial pen to improve my prose, and he also regularly functioned as a reality check for my ideas. As I shared my ideas with him, I grew more confident and articulate in expressing them. Over the years I have occasionally published scholarly articles, but for almost four decades I have been primarily engaged in designing costumes and teaching costume-related subjects. The satisfying experience of creating costumes and my interest in *commedia dell'arte,* as well as my long-standing admiration of the great Dario Fo, drew me to masks early on. Also, through the decades I've designed and created masks for theatre, opera, and dance and consequently have recognized the effort and skill it takes to make an exciting, dynamic mask that fits easily and performs well.

When I attended an international mask conference organized by Loyce Arthur and Ralph Hall at the University of Iowa in 2001, I realized the tremendous contributions of mask makers even though they remain "invisible" both collectively and as individual artists. I decided to interview and write about some of the mask makers I had met at this mask conference. They inspired me to seek out other mask makers, men and occasionally women who were usually well-known in their own regions but not necessarily known worldwide. It has been both humbling and exhilarating to meet and interview these mask makers and to see them at work. I deeply admire their astonishing artistry, which many of them achieve despite limited materials and tools. My explorations have also introduced me to some of the creative challenges of contemporary mask makers.

Ron Naversen graciously allowed me to reprint his article on mask making in Bali in chapter 2. Ron and I have presented several workshops on masks and mask making together, and he organized a highly successful international mask conference at Southern Illinois University Carbondale in 2005. I consider him to be the quintessential mask connoisseur, and I have valued our deepening friendship and mutual interest in this vast topic.

United States Institute for Theatre Technology pillars Alexandra Bonds, Marianne Custer, Tim Kelly, and David Roger have significantly helped me in this endeavor. Fellow costume designer Alexandra Bonds first advised me on how to prepare my work for publication. David Roger, editor of *Theatre Design & Technology* (USITT's professional journal), along with Lance Brockman, Tim Kelly, and anonymous *TD&T* readers, have given me very helpful advice and encouragement concerning articles I've written on this topic. Marianne Custer has kindly read numerous proposals for funding requests and served as a referee along with Alexandra Bonds.

I have admired Joan Schirle at Dell'Arte International School of Physical Theatre for years. When I first interviewed her in 1986, I was struck by her professional tenacity and her performer's artistry. Later when I took a summer *commedia* improvisational workshop with her, I recognized her to be a master teacher. She became a crucial source of information concerning Carlo Mazzoni-Clementi's connection with major *commedia* artists in mid-twentieth-century Europe and with Dell'Arte International. Joan put me in touch with Arne Zaslove and other Dell'Arte International artists who recounted the remarkable story of this American institution's early years. Dell'Arte International has produced more international mask makers and masked performers than any other such school.

I thank Paola Piizzi and translator Alexandra Speirs at *Museo Internazionale della Maschera Amleto e Donato Sartori* for their careful reading and editorial comments regarding the Sartoris' influence on *commedia* mask making.

Extraordinary mask makers Torbjörn Alström, Donvieve, Rob Faust, Bruce Marrs, and Michael Meyer were especially indispensable in advising me on how to approach the world of mask making. With the exception of Meyer, all of these artists perform in their own masks. They offered practical insight and suggested nuanced, discerning approaches. Samuel Abrantes, Kiyomatsu Akira, Ivete Dibo, Antonio Fava, Ralph Lee, Newman, Leonard Pitt, and Jeff Semmerling are other innovative mask makers whom I interviewed but did not profile in the book. Space limitations and an effort to strive for balance prevented me from including them.

I am especially indebted to those translators who also served as expert cultural advisors and often were in-country organizers as well: Samuel Abrantes, Adigun Ajani, Gerard Besson, Fr. Claude Boucher, Sharon Jinkerson-Brass, Jimoh Buraimoh, I. Made Kíchen, Anabelle Lassalle, Sangdae Lee, Bill LeVasseur, and Ago Mauriello. Maureen and Guy Pickering at Kumbali Country Lodge in Lilongwe, Malawi, and Douglas Curran helped me establish important contacts with Fr. Boucher and helped me schedule interviews. Thanks too to translators Aluwatoyosi A. Adekeye, Priscila Bergamasco, Takeo Iida, and Douglas Shimizu.

In my travels during the past decade I have met more wonderfully hospitable people than I could possibly acknowledge here. I fondly recall Karima and Kena Muyaes' Sunday dinner invitation at their lovely home in Mexico City, where I had the opportunity to meet mask maker Antonio Cervantes Delgado and to take many photos of masks in Karima and Kena's collection. Alicia Martínez Álvarez celebrated our interview and a special masked performance by members of her theatre company with a delicious lunch that she specially prepared. Anabelle Lassalle served as a tour guide and drove me around Port of Spain, Trinidad, one memorable afternoon. Taxi driver Romulo drove me around Rio de Janeiro for several days — forgoing his usual higher fares. Adigun Ajani taught me so much about Yoruba cosmology, the annual Osun Festival in Osogobo, and divination practices that continue to influence Nigerian mask makers. His family's many kindnesses — including having me to their home for dinner and showing me how to drape native clothing — were life-transforming memories.

I quickly realized that the creators of Carnival in Rio de Janeiro required their own separate book — because Carnival is an immense undertaking, requiring at least the effort that goes into making a movie. Milton Cunha of G.R.E.S. (*Gremio Recreativo Escola de Samba* or Recreation Group School of Samba) Viradouro gave me a tour of Viradouro's huge Carnival parade factory in Rio and discussed his challenges as a *carnevalesqua* — a conceptualist/designer for the costumes and parade floats. Another *carnevalesqua* who serves as a newscaster for the Rio de Janeiro Carnival celebrations, Alexandre Louzada, discussed his work in detail with me. Representatives of G.R.E.S. Vila Isabel invited me to attend a thrilling, spectacular performance "rehearsal" at midnight, with music, dancing, and hundreds of community participants.

A number of my university colleagues — Walter Beale, Jim Evans, Hope Hodgkins, and Jim Wren — contributed their skills and knowledge. Dan Smith's expert photography skills significantly enhanced my photos, and he helped me to organize them and prepare them for delivery to McFarland. Reference librarian Nancy Fogarty gave me good advice about seeking a publisher, and my department head, Jim Fisher, pointed me to McFarland. Religious studies professor Charles Orzech suggested invaluable sources for my explorations into myth. The exemplary careers of emeriti Theatre professors Alan Cook and Marsha Paludan helped inspire me to take on this vast topic. Cook's expertise and contacts in Nigerian theatre in Osogbo helped me prepare for travel there. Margo Bender, Veronica Grossi, Anelise Z. Hofmann, and Norma Valazquez translated important documents. Hofmann and Valazquez also worked tirelessly in assisting and arranging my trips to Brazil and Mexico to locate and schedule interviews with mask makers.

Jerry Cushman generously gave me his collection of classic books on masks, which I have savored and put to good use. I have appreciated his encouragement as well as the encouragement from friends Cynthia Anthony, Sara Johnson Lassalle, Charlotte Hurwitz, John Lee Jellicorse, Linda Jones, Marna King, and Diane Mumford. I also wish to thank Takeo Iida, Iwasaki Mitsuko, and Kiyomatsu Akira for their great effort in making sure that I could include a description of the beautiful masks of the late Iwasaki Kyoun.

I am deeply grateful to the United States Institute for Theatre Technology for a $7,000 grant to interview mask makers in Nigeria and Malawi and a $4,000 fellowship for interviews with mask makers in Mexico. I also want to thank The University of North Carolina at Greensboro's International Programs Center for two Kohler grants ($2,000 total) to interview mask makers in Italy. I thank the University for granting me two research assignments to complete this work.

I am indebted to a number of authors, photographers, and artists whose work in related fields has profoundly inspired me in my own endeavor. Laurel Aguilar, Adigun Ajani, Gerard Besson, Jimoh Buraimoh, Douglas Curran, Sidney Kasfir, Barbara Mauldin, Peter Minshall, John Nunley, and Judy Slattum have set standards of excellence to which I can only aspire.

Introduction

Masks have always fascinated us. Consider the masks showcased in the popular Broadway productions *Phantom of the Opera, The Lion King, Beauty and the Beast,* and *Wicked.* Two shows that opened on Broadway late in 2004, *Gem of the Ocean* and *Pacific Overtures,* made significant use of masks. *Shrek The Musical* was nominated for a 2009 Tony Award in Costume Design. Julie Taymor's masked designs for *The Magic Flute* have graced the stage of the Metropolitan Opera. *Avenue Q* presented puppets that resemble mask performance. Film and television versions of *Spider-Man, Batman, Planet of the Apes, WALL-E,* and *Star Trek* all embrace the medium of mask performance. Bayreuth's 2010 *Lohengrin* has rat masks for the male chorus. Prominent theatre festivals regularly produce plays with masked characters large and small in the forms of dragons, demons, angels, and mythic heroes. Across the United States and all over the world, annual masked characters from *The Nutcracker* entertain our families at holiday time. Depending on how one defines the mask, even rock performers like Elton John, and Cher have used masked performance effects. Some current rock bands such as Kiss, Slipknot, Buckethead, Insane Clown Posse, and Daft Punk are easily identified by the masks they wear.[1] Rapper MFDoom wears a plastic mask and hat.

Any good bookstore offers a book or two on the topic of masks, yet little information exists about the mask makers themselves. How odd since the theatre world devotes substantial attention to directors, designers, playwrights, and performers. Somehow the mask maker remains invisible, or at least anonymous, partly because the masked performer takes precedence.

The quality of the "traditional" masked performance invariably demands the impressive skills and magic of one individual, the mask maker. While musicians, a lighting designer, and set designer occasionally assist, the "traditional" mask maker often serves as the masked performer as well as his/her own playwright, choreographer, director, and costume designer, unlike so much of today's commercial theatre where masked performance results from the efforts of a variety of specialized artists and artisans.

I use the term "traditional" to help distinguish between the popular and commercial masked effects of film and Broadway and the masked performance work of those artists/artisans worldwide who have kept the ancient traditions of mask work alive with the efforts of single masked performers or small groups of masked performers in intimately staged community presentations or rituals. These traditional masked presentations have strongly influenced much of today's popular masked effects (those directed toward mass audience appeal). For instance, Julie Taymor spent her earlier years observing and participating in community masked performances in Bali, India, and Sri Lanka as well as studying at *L'École Internationale de Théâtre Jacques Lecoq* (Jacques Lecoq's International School of Theatre) in Paris.[2]

I have visited and interviewed notable traditional mask makers from Brazil, Trinidad, South Korea, Japan, Mexico, Canada, Bali, Nigeria, Italy, Sweden, and the east and west coasts of the United States. I have observed many of these mask makers at work in their studios and I have come to appreciate the impressive contributions of these individuals. Their masks in performance, like music, have the potential to transcend language.

Some of the traditionally influenced mask makers I have visited make classical masks for contemporary performances and ritual presentations while others are avant-garde performance artists with a decidedly more experimental dimension to their work. Mask makers who concentrate on creating time-honored classical masks, such as the Balinese masks used in *Topeng* dance, Japanese *Noh* masks, and Italian *commedia*-styled character masks (or their Korean *Hahoe* counterparts), concentrate much of their efforts on perfecting the technical qualities of their masks, while others explore new characters and performance styles and concentrate their efforts more on the expressive qualities of masks.

Of course every successful mask maker combines elements of both artistry and craftsmanship. Even when the mask maker replicates a traditional mask, s/he uses a personal carving or sculpting technique that makes each mask an original in its unique hand craftsmanship. A number of mask makers I interviewed commented on how their own technical expertise, combined with the qualities of the actual wood, clay, or leather, directly influenced their vision for the mask. Others admitted rejecting their masks after the rehearsal process commenced in order to create ones better suited for the performance project at hand. Yet after creating a seemingly highly expressive mask, a performer cannot always make it appear effectively on stage. Regardless of the technical and expressive virtuosity at work, all of these individuals explore ways to create the most evocative masks for dynamic masked performances.

In this context, mask makers are not unlike performers and playwrights who often describe their artistic processes in terms of combining art and craft. They speak about the craft and technique of performing and writing even as they try to identify the unique artistic element of their work. The spirit of artistry varies for the performer with each new performance in the same way that the quality or spirit of artistry varies for the mask maker with the creation of each new mask.

Dario Fo, Italian playwright, comic performer, director, designer, and Nobel Prize Laureate for Literature, describes this blurring of technique and art within his own creative process: "Manual labor is important and I like to construct and invent along with the technicians. I spend time with them, talk with them, I want to know everything about the lights, about the various possibilities of actual stage construction. I'm not interested in a single solution, an act of repetition. This is true in general of my artistic activity. I'm always ready to change. I've also made many mistakes because I've tried to break out of a fixed pattern. A performance can't be repeated forever if it functions well. I prefer to throw myself into the search for renewed expression as an artisan, not as a demigod."[3]

I began to examine the creative processes of mask makers by asking each of them a series of questions, with a particular emphasis on how he/she focuses, reflects, or meditates when first beginning a mask project:

1. Mask making doesn't typically generate a large income. Why do you make masks when you and most other mask makers do not generally receive adequate compensation?
2. How did you get into mask making? Did you have a mentor?
3. Specifically how and why are myth and archetypal images important to your masks?

4. How do you inter-relate with the mask performer in creating the mask and how extensive is your collaboration with other members of the company such as director, lighting/scenic designer?
5. How do you "meditate" or "pray" or "center and focus" on how to begin your beautiful masks? How do you clarify objectives for yourself for making the masks?
6. How do you go about gathering/ordering/preparing the materials that will be used in your masks?
7. How does your sense of honesty relate to your sense of theatricality? Do you know in advance what will be the mask's essence — or does it usually evolve during the construction of it? What is a successful mask for you?
8. What are your biggest challenges in creating masks?

Theatre practitioners, whatever their area of expertise, can all learn from the versatility possessed by the traditional mask maker who integrates dramatic objectives with mask making and masked performance. They often combine storytelling, music/rhythm, and dance with remarkable directness. The typical playwright, designer and artisan, as well as performer, can gain substantial insight for their work on stage and screen by reflecting on the range of spiritual and cultural motivations held by mask makers worldwide as they synthesize storytelling, design, and performance.

The immediacy of the integrated creative act of masking strikes at the heart of all dramatic endeavors. The mask maker and masked performer elegantly condense the primary artistic agendas of theatre production, invariably transcending language. The creative processes and techniques of traditional mask makers vividly remind us of how we have traditionally defined the essential theatre experience. Yet even as they collectively offer broad insights into the essential theatre experience, their highlighted responses, including photographs of their masks either in performance, in their studios, or in museums document unique approaches and reflect a range of global perspectives and skills.

We've never attempted to examine the mask maker's story and how his/her story might compare to those of other mask makers worldwide. Their collective stories can generate relevant questions regarding how masked performance is evolving. At this critical juncture when globalization can dramatically shrink the most obscure, isolated communities, many of these traditional mask makers increasingly find that their efforts collide with outside influences. New stage and film adaptations use traditional mask work, but in new ways, frequently distorting the specific time-honored cultural and spiritual motivations of the traditional mask maker. Consequently, while traditional masks interface and synthesize with contemporary performance presentations in exciting new ways for stage and screen, the traditional mask maker blends vaguely into the background, often with limited financial support and very little recognition.

We live in an age of instant communication and information. World traditions dramatically blend and evolve with increased outside influences. At the dawn of the new millennium, we should not forget the original motivations behind the centuries-old practices of the traditional mask makers. We should record as many of their insights and unique perspectives before they are gone. These artists offer a broad foundation of ancient insights even as they are disappearing as quickly as our glaciers. The traditional mask maker typically relies on training or inspiration handed down by earlier generations and can still perpetuate the ancient call of his community's mask in its diverse forms. Future generations of mask makers and performance artists for stage and screen should take advantage of the collective wisdom of the ancestors which traditional mask makers manage to represent with such clarity.

Few researchers have written detailed accounts about these artists and artisans. Hailing from Minneapolis, artist and artisan Donald Cordry came to Taxco in the region of Guerrero, Mexico, in 1931. Although he had no formal training, he soon became a prominent Mesoamerican scholar and lover of the arts and crafts of Indian Mexico, particularly Mexican masks. He spent over forty years traveling around Mexico on horseback, getting to know the local mask makers in several areas of Mexico. He and his wife, Dorothy Mann, documented this work and in 1981 published one of the definitive books on masks, *Mexican Masks*. Three decades later it is considered a classic. Cordry is one of only a handful of writers who have documented and analyzed masks of a certain area. He also interviewed the local makers of the masks. His interviews provided much attention and insight (if not total accuracy, according to Mexican mask museum curator, Bill LeVasseur[4]) into the creative challenges and processes of these mask makers. He also carefully described the materials used in making the indigenous masks and tried to demonstrate pre–Hispanic as well as Hispanic influences.[5]

Peter Furst, in his foreword to Cordry's book, explains that Cordry would visit "remote Indian villages where masked dances were still practiced or remembered. He found more than one old mask whose meaning had been forgotten by all but the oldest villagers." The ephemeral quality of wooden masks (they can usually survive the harsh climate and insects for only a few years or decades) makes them especially precious. Cordry's book is filled with wonderful photographs of Mexican masks, ensuring that we will always be able to see glimpses of their power.

Laurel Birch Aguilar spent almost a decade with communities in Malawi, getting to know their masked performance rites and rituals. She eventually became one of the few women allowed membership in the *Nyau* Secret Society, where masks are created during puberty rites as an acknowledgment of accepting greater community responsibility. Using these masks, members of this secret society learn the ways of guiding the community's dead souls peacefully to their graves. Other society members create and perform in masks that teach important lessons and traditions in rites and rituals via mask performance. Aguilar's book, *Inscribing the Mask*, describes aspects of interviews she had with *nyau* mask makers, though secrecy demanded that she not actually identify them by name.

Except for Cordry and Aguilar, I know of no others who have extensively described the work and creative agendas of individual mask makers. *Mask Makers and Their Craft: An Illustrated Worldwide Study,* though not exhaustive, offers a detailed inquiry based on interviews of thirty-one contemporary, notable mask makers from wide-ranging areas in the world where we can still see traditional masks and mask performance. This inquiry documents the work of these traditional artists as they confront the changing Internet-induced landscape of dissolving traditions and evolving multi-cultural perspectives.

Chapter 1 examines ways that traditional masks and mask performance (regardless of locale) maintain a sense of universality and consequently demonstrate ways in which global mask makers share common agendas even when their local beliefs and customs vary considerably.

In an attempt to identify and describe widely differing viewpoints on how to define a mask, chapter 2 introduces examples of contrasting agendas between mask makers in parts of Africa with some others in the Western hemisphere. It also explores characteristic aspects of traditional mask making that promote healing. Finally, it examines the range of considerations coming from academic and artistic communities as they present varied ways of how to describe functions of the mask by how it is exhibited. These interpretations take advantage of unique exhibition sites such as a seventeenth-century Italian villa, a Malawian mission museum, a South Korean tourist site museum, a Midwestern United States university museum, and a museum housed at a Mexican bed and breakfast. These sites demonstrate the range of multi-cultural diversity that international masks communicate to contemporary audiences, regardless of language, gender, age, societal, or ethnic differences. They also exemplify the difficulty in precisely defining the mask. Huge walking mobiles, operated by one "masked" performer become monumental masks similar to those of Bread and Puppet Theatre while Italian *commedia dell'arte* mask specialist Donato Sartori has created sculptured leather "body masks" as well as gigantic fabric draped masks for buildings. As both stage and screen adopt new video and animation techniques, cannot WALL-E be considered a "masked" character, complete with human voice, gestures, and facial features? (Later in chapter 3 German mask maker Michael Meyer describes how prosthetic appliances become masks to transform the performer.)

Chapter 3 introduces techniques in mask making while chapter 4 identifies a panoramic view of mask makers worldwide with brief descriptions that profile each artist's distinctive approach to the work.

Chapter 5 summarizes the major legacies of Italian mask makers Amleto and Donato Sartori (as well as Donato's annual *commedia* mask workshop) with that of several master mask makers who have taught at California-based Dell'Arte International School of Physical Theatre. Additionally Dell'Arte International has substantially led the world stage in maintaining masked performance as a major global art form. The legacies of these two mask-making centers on two continents continue to generate a significant number of contemporary mask makers worldwide.

Finally, chapters 6 and 7 examine ways in which traditional approaches in mask making and mask performance continue to influence contemporary commercial mask performance ventures in film, on Broadway, and in touring masked performances. Mask maker Rob Faust, along with other contemporary mask makers, confronts a critical juncture in utilizing traditional approaches while simultaneously responding to the changing mythic and cultural landscape of our twenty-first century.

1

The Traditional Mask in Performance

Mythic Influences on Archetypal Exaggeration

Masked performance and its stories have revealed the figurative rhythms of birth, celebration, and death since primitive times. The illusion of masking to imply, evoke, or become another character/spirit invariably requires a state of pretending. In pretending, the masked performer/storyteller and viewer/listener can share an experience as an exaggerated state where reality becomes more real than real. This heightened quality of the successful masked performance transports the viewer into a more universal, eternal, divine level of reality. Some compare this heightened level of reality to the reality evoked in dreams and unconscious states, allowing the viewer to experience a sense of the sublime.

How does a mask function? This question is worth exploring before identifying general considerations confronted by mask makers as they contemplate each creation of a mask. As we explore a multitude of ways in which each mask functions, we become increasingly cognizant of the difficult challenge in defining the mask. Is it only worn on the face? Is it worn on the head? Does the costume actually serve as an extension of the mask? Can a mask literally be a deity or an ancestor, and even if it is not worn? When does a mask become an idol? Do puppets have masks (or are they "faces")? Is WALL-E a film-animated character who wears a mask? Does Gollum in *The Lord of the Rings* wear a "motion capture" mask? If a mask hides the performer's face, is not George Clooney wearing a mask when he performs as Mr. Fox in Wes Anderson's *Fantastic Mr. Fox* (2009)? If a Trinidadian performer for Carnival wears several masks simultaneously, does the performer artistically wear only one mask? We can describe how the mask functions far more easily than we can define the mask.

Masks have existed at least since the ancient beginnings of mythology. The elemental forces of our unconscious (subliminal) desires and fears found in masks and mythic stories are the basis of all art. Masks, like myths, use the illusion of metaphor/imagery as a primary way of expressing and examining ultimate mysteries inherent in the human condition.

Cave paintings spanning far back into the Paleolithic era depict the first "recorded" masks — animal heads probably worn by hunters. Some contemporary traditional mask makers still conjure essential appearances of ancient primitive masks and attempt to present versions of them in their own mask making. For example, Swedish mask maker Torbjörn Alström has researched Paleolithic masks in cave paintings in Sweden, and the Swedish government has commissioned him to experiment with a wide range of materials such as fish skin, furs, bark, and leather, which he thinks might have been used by the earliest mask makers in his country. Consequently he has incorporated a variety of skins as well as leather in his masks. His Pulcinella mask utilizes fish skin for an especially primitive textured effect. Mexican mask maker Juan Horta Castillo (who died in 2006) regularly incorporated ancient Mayan animal imagery into his masks.

Joseph Campbell states that myths (which he refers to as the primal "masks" of god) initially developed as primitive man confronted his impending death. Campbell says that the early mythic stories attempted to understand the consequences of death, particularly humanity's yearnings to maintain some sort of spiritual connection with the dead. Mythic stories also assisted humanity in its need to cope with its conflicted duty to kill in order to live.[1] The confrontation and fear of death demanded some sort of spiritual/eternal level of reality to transcend the limitations of life on earth. Remnants of weapons, special clothing, and jewelry have been found in burial caves dating back to Neanderthal man, who placed the regalia alongside the dead person to serve him in the spirit/afterlife world of the dead.[2] Campbell suggests that a similar spiritual identification occurred when the hunter somehow possessed the animal's eternal spirit while wearing the animal head during the hunt or in preparation for the hunt.[3]

No one really knows whether the Paleolithic "literal" masks of animal spirits came before or after the earliest mythic stories of the gods in the spiritual realm, the focus of Campbell's detailed life-long comparative study. But at some point masks helped to identify the earliest mythic gods and ancestors as well as animal spirits. Indeed some of the animal spirits were treated as gods. Masks ushered in some of the earliest known ancient artistic renderings of these entities. The successful mask and mythic story, utilizing exaggerated physical illusion and metaphor, had the power to become more real than real on a spiritual, eternal level.

Consider how a totem mask resembles a real tiger. It renders a spiritual/eternal idea of the tiger, not an actual tiger. And, depending on how the mask maker focuses on emotive qualities of the tiger — its ferociousness, its feminine feline qualities, its authoritativeness — the mask will reveal various levels of the tiger's spiritual/eternal reality. The spiritual reality of the mask comes from the frozen yet vitally expressive state of the mask. Peter Brook succinctly describes this concept when he talks about the traditional mask as a portrait of a man without a mask, or "a soul portrait," which is the ultimate metaphysical (spiritual) quality of the mask.[4]

Most traditional mask makers still consider (either consciously or subliminally) metaphorical aspects of myth, the mask's earliest sister art form, as a way of evoking the spirit of the mask. Almost all of the mask makers I interviewed incorporate mythic stories and characters related to their own cultures. These stories invariably balance such dualities as good and evil, power and vulnerability, love and hate, the old and the young. The mythic stories of any culture dramatize a struggle to understand our basic fears and desires as they relate to these dualities.

While the myths used by the mask makers I interviewed usually come from legendary stories such as those found in the *Mahabharata*, Mexican *Pastorela* celebrations, Japanese *Noh* dramas, Greek dramas, or even the classic Italian Roman/Renaissance *commedia*-styled skits, some of the mask makers take exception to this general format by also exploring contemporary situations with contemporary characters. For instance, Balinese mask maker I. Bagus Anom and the late Mexican mask maker Juan Horta Castillo have taken great delight in spoofing tourists with their masked versions of tourists with blank gazes. These tourist masks occasionally blend with legendary characters in the stories of local comic masked performances. American mask maker Bruce Marrs, in addition to his delightful versions of *commedia* characters looking like today's drinking buddies and misfits, also creates original masks for the contemporary satires of Dell'Arte International School of Physical Theatre (where he's taught for over two decades), which take aim at current political and economic situations. Swedish mask maker Torbjörn Alström rarely works with mythic stories, preferring to create contemporary characters in contemporary situations. He says, "Somehow I believe that if my mask work really succeeds, you will not see the myth behind it. You will perhaps feel something familiar. I believe that the mask creates an atmosphere of myth around the performance. In this way, myth will always be present, modern or old."

Even if myth is not totally evident in the mask maker's work, s/he inevitably explores archetypal qualities such as those seen in mythic characters. These archetypal character qualities most often show up in the forms of demons/villains, heroes, gods, and protectors, such as animal totems—but also in the form of Everyman figures. They can range from heroic figures on a major quest to flippant slaves/servants outwitting their masters, or nonchalant gods conquered by trickster figures who force the gods to accept a truthful idea. We see masked characters as archetypal figures found in historical mythic dramas or in contemporary productions because they have the power to resonate at eternal, universal levels. Torbjörn Alström creates a contemporary version of this universality when he presents his *commedia*-esque Pulcinella character as an Everyman figure (not specifically as a Renaissance version of Pulcinella) who depicts humankind's potential malaise regardless of time or place. Masks seem particularly effective for presenting archetypal characters in a performance, perhaps because of their obviously exaggerated qualities. Bruce Marrs' *commedia*-inspired misfit masks, Kyoun Iwasaki's "despairing woman mask," and Joyce Radtke's spiritual guide masks depict timeless characters and transcend cultural influence.

Canadian mask maker and performer Xstine Cook notes that "the mask and puppetry are three-dimensional forms that transcend into the magical arena of performance. They speak to a very deep and ancient part of our humanness. They can sail across all kinds of barriers and are not limited by language, age, or culture. Artists sensitive to symbols and non-scientific information interpret those visions through the art of mask making. They imagine the future, recognize societal patterns, and interpret history. Successful artists who create masks or puppets help people understand their emotions and spirituality. These artists function as interpreters, reporters, commentators, and divining rods."[5]

Skilled performers energize contemporary versions of traditional archetypal protector masks that were created by primitive cultures in such masked characters as Mufasa (*The Lion King*), Elphaba (*Wicked*), Batman, Yoda, Gandalf, Albus Dumbledore, or Ari, the Eleanor Roosevelt of *Planet of the Apes*. The contemporary commercial masked performers, like the ancient masked performers, can generate tremendous power by imaginatively connecting the literal world of audiences to the divine or eternal aspects of protection, using masks to conjure characters, gods, heroes, protective warriors, animal totems, and tutelary spirits that we recognize as universal, but also as aspects of these spiritual assistants within ourselves.

Ultimately, however, we see masks beyond those we regularly observe in performance venues. Walter Sorell asserts that we live with masks (even figurative masks) more often than we acknowledge. "What is mask and what is face when a pilot returns from a bombing mission during which he has executed thousands of people and, taking off his mask, shows his smiling face with the gratified expression 'mission fulfilled'? Or, is not the astronaut divorced from reality when, in his space suit, he dances on the moon?"[6]

Taking Sorell's assertion even further, is not each of us a mask maker at some level? We masquerade as personalities not quite our own to avoid conflict or to evoke a more favorable response within social contexts. A person does not need a theatrical setting, a costume, or an actual mask to engage in this type of masquerade. We are all familiar with the typical socially accepted (even socially demanded) form of masquerade seen in the job interview process, where the job candidate "dresses" for the part and attempts to visually and verbally "blend" with the ideals of the employer in order to receive a job offer. Many of us can relate to the ritual of dressing to please our parents long after we have become independent adults. The persona that one creates in order to masquerade in this way requires an intentional manipulation of appearance in order to fulfill the objectives of the masquerader. Such masking can project an entire personality through facial expression and makeup, but it also includes a total body stance complete with gesture and appropriate clothing. We can most easily see these mask effects in photographs where the personality has become frozen and thus seems exaggerated.

If one considers a mask as an entire embodiment of character consisting not only of a facial covering but also "a visual exaggerated framework" surrounding the face and including hair, dress, and physical gesture (as many mask makers do), then young women are perhaps the ultimate mask makers in the way that they manipulate and follow fashion trends to project their overt as well as subliminal gender-related identities and goals. Young people of both genders in many cultures have traditionally created and defied fashion trends with blatant exaggeration as a way of expressing their rapidly changing awareness of self-image. Even when they follow trends, they often seem especially enthusiastic about their personal choices. But women, more frequently than men, dictate and control their appearance with more sophisticated exaggeration, in order to more effectively communicate non-verbally. And one could make a persuasive case that girls, more often than boys, demonstrate a higher level of sophistication in utilizing superficial appearances.

How ironic that while traditional masks have historically been made by men for millennia, females spanning cultures and historical periods (when allowed to appear on stage) until very recently seldom wore actual three-dimensional masks. This tendency is underscored in a punch line delivered by an Italian actress I once interviewed who specializes in contemporary *commedia dell'arte* performances. Sixteenth-century Italian *commedia* developed a series of masked characters that presented comic and satiric skits primarily based on local issues in the towns in which they performed. All the male characters except for the rather effete young lover wore leather masks, while the female characters almost never appeared on stage masked. "Why weren't the female characters masked?" I asked. "My dear, which mask would a female character choose?" she responded. "A woman wears a thousand masks."

This book does not focus upon the typical daily "masqueraders" (regardless their gender or range of superficial facial expressions) found in most societies nor the frozen fashion photographs of *Vogue* and *GQ*. Instead this book focuses on contemporary traditional mask makers. Across continents, these artists continue to incorporate (or consciously defy) profound cultural and mythic associations with centuries past. When successful, the masks they create for performances and rites-of-passage tell marvelous stories in formal settings and demonstrate glimpses of eternity and wisdom.

Equally fascinating is the issue of how traditional mask makers compare and contrast with contemporary commercial mask makers and special-effects makeup artists found in internationally known adventure films and touring *Cirque du Soleil* productions, Broadway theatre productions, and urban street masked performance art. Can we afford to forget the historic significance and technical triumphs of traditional mask makers still found in many local communities across the globe today? What can these mask makers still teach us?

The Sacred Quest

Who among us does not occasionally require, or at least desire, the protection of another person or force beyond ourselves? The masked protector character such as Batman or Yoda conjures such figures in the successful performance. The masked performer's sacred quest to present a protective figure promotes vitality and security for its audience.

We use the term "romantic" in a variety of ways but when the word is not capitalized, we tend to think of it as indicating particularly amorous relationships. And surely, at its most basic level, the masked performer of the protector embarks upon a sacred quest that operates much like the romantic lover. The truths generated by the personality and skills of the performer (masker) as well as those generated by the romantic lover demand the illusionary sublime guise of harmony, guided more by instinct than reason. Romantic love songs invariably evoke the fragile state of "pretend play" created by the lovers focusing on exaggerated truths that promise integrity, balance, and wholeness. A performance of the masked protector, like the courting rituals of the lover, somehow artfully suspends the imperfections of living into a larger context which offers resolution at a sublime (unconscious) level. When this state is successfully reached, the mask maker assists the viewer's entrance into the realm of the sacred, offering a sense of divine protection.

Webster's Dictionary more specifically defines "Romantic" as "having no basis in fact, imaginary" and also "marked by the imaginative or emotional appeal of the heroic, adventurous, remote, mysterious, or idealized." It adds that the term is "characterized by an emphasis on subjective emotional qualities and freedom of form."[7] The Romantic's search for heroes is often a search for mythical or legendary figures, frequently of divine descent and endowed with great strength or ability, such as an illustrious warrior. Sacred heroes are consummate protectors in a similar way to that of magnificent, magical ancestral totems and tutelaries which protected primitive communities. (These sacred protectors — like amorous lovers — are not necessarily appealing in the "light" of rational reality, as Shakespeare's Titania realizes when she awakes lying next to an ass.)

Contemporary playwrights like Tony Kushner continue the Romantic sacred quest for divine guidance in spite of the cynicism of the twentieth century. Kushner's *Angels in America* (1992) dramatically incorporates protector ghost and angel characters. Just as romantic love songs often beckon dancing lovers in the soft shadows of moonlight, Prior's ghosts (protectors/lovers) Romantically insist on dancing with him in the night as he approaches his death accompanied by the music of a lone oboe playing in the background, evoking a dream-like, illusionary state. At the end of the dance, the messenger Angel comes to aid Prior on "The Great Work" of his final journey. While these ghost and angel characters do not wear actual masks, they must appear as "real" apparitions. The spreading great opalescent gray-silver wings framing the Angel's face (and arguably serving as a mask as do a devil's horns) suspended in the air, theatrically and Romantically evoke a protector/guide more real than any human.

Additionally, traditional masked protector performance assumes a level of divine protection for its audience that compares closely with Romantic utilizations of conscious states. (In this case, the term "Romantic" when capitalized refers to the early nineteenth-century aesthetic sense of the word, used to identify the dominant literary and painterly style of the period.) *The Oxford Anthology of British Literature*, Volume II, describes "High Romantic consciousness as a search or quest for the Sublime, a realization that internalizes the quest-pattern of the ancient literary form of the romance, or marvelous tale, suspended in its context halfway between natural and supernatural realms."[8]

Traditional masked protector performance Romantically appeals to our elemental urges to remain in harmony with nature. This "illusionary pretend state" often has accompanying animal spirits that have the ability to evoke a closer connection to the life force in nature.

Not surprisingly, animals frequently serve as ancient protectors/guides or inspire such guides. Ted Andrews notes, "There was a time when humanity recognized itself as part of nature, and nature as part of itself. Dreaming and waking were inseparable realities; the natural and the supernatural merged and blended. People used images of nature to express this unity and to instill a transpersonal kind of experience."[9] Because primitive societies often believed they were descendents of animals, they owed their existence to these omniscient totems.[10] Occasionally the powerful animal ancestor totem (considered to be father of the fathers) is worn as a mask on top of the human protector mask, suggesting even more strength. We see a version of this concept in Broadway's *The Lion King*.

We also find Romantic conventions in traditional masked performance when the masked performer and spirit literally become "one." Mask makers in secret societies in Nigeria and Malawi describe the effects of the mask performer literally becoming the spirit intended by the mask. Walter Sorrell describes this suspended event as "blotting out the self in order to become possessed" and points toward the "ancient Germans dancing themselves into a state of ecstasy by putting on animal skins and masks" as a way of citing vivid examples of "the magic power of the mask ... which on a higher plane, conjured up the spirit of the gods [or ancestors], who were thought of as becoming flesh with the dancer."[11]

Masked performances (those indicating masked protectors or the antithesis of masked protectors) can also offer "sacred humor," as the Balinese clowns have recognized for centuries. In his book, *Subversive Laughter*, Ron Jenkins describes their propensity to publicly engage in open satirical dialogue, debating with their gods about issues relating to such topics as lifestyle and threatening forces.

Modernists like Edward Gordon Craig, Meyerhold, Reinhardt, and Copeau consistently favored potent masked performances that projected a sense of the divine (as protector) within the context of the human condition. For three decades in New York at St. John the Divine and in surrounding towns, mythic mask maker/performer extraordinaire Ralph Lee has continued in the Bread and Puppet Theatre tradition with huge masked mythic forces representing cultural myths worldwide.

Above all else, the traditional mask maker inherently understands our fundamental yearnings for sacred states. We see protector and demon masks most frequently as dreamlike guises in the night (or in a darkened movie theatre)—not just because a mask seems more theatrically vivid in the night with the technical aids of focused campfire or stage light—but because the background or backdrop of darkness accentuates the greatest sense of unease, abandonment, and death. Romantically, the masked protector and its audience (as well as the lover and the beloved) can most dramatically experience each other in the shadows of the real world combined with the imaginary world of sacred states. Furthermore, the Romantic tale often incorporates a sense of the grotesque. In her book *The Secret Life of Puppets* Victoria Nelson describes the [sacred] grotesque encounter as

> the gateway to the underworld "through which enters the world to be swallowed up" [the primary *modus operandi* for Romantic realizations]. It is first and foremost about crossing into a different and transformative order of reality, and second about the unexpected recombinations of events, objects, species we encounter once we are inside. And for centuries it has been a secular society's only path back to the transcendent. We crawl into the hole — the grotto, the Symmes Hole, the black hole of the cosmos, the hole in our own heads — in the unspoken and often unconscious hope of undergoing deep change. The words used in the English language to describe this alteration — *metamorphosis* from the Greek, *transformation* from the Latin — describe this same experience.[12]

Nelson then reminds us that "The contemporary realm of popular entertainment is our main subterranean entry, the grotto entry, to the boarded-up mansion of sacred awe, where we conduct our primitive discourse on religious subjects — a discourse whose crudeness would horrify our pious ancestors, but nonetheless a discourse — behind our own backs."[13]

Forbidden Knowledge

Ancient cultural myths describe the capabilities within us to tap into the creative powers of unification with the sublime (in this case, referring to the subliminal powers/urges/desires/fears of the collective unconscious). These myths took place in the realm of the dream state to indicate this occurrence. For example, Persephone goes to the underworld of a magical place and is richly rewarded after meeting the challenges of the underworld. Northwest Coastal First Peoples describe another character called Kumugwé, chief of the undersea world, who lives in a great house:

> He had similar powers to those of shamans, including the ability to see into the future, heal the sick or injured, and bestow privileges to whomever he wished. His treasures included woven blankets, copper, songs, and dances. If one entered the realm of Kumugwé one could learn the ways of the undersea world [the state of the sublime] and return home with many magical treasures.
>
> The loon is often displayed atop Kumugwé as a reference to his great size: The loon mistook him for an island and landed on his head. On the chest of the loon is the figure of a person who has been to the world of Kumugwé and returned with treasures, one of them being a mask that the loon wears.[14]

This bountiful Romantic state of bliss — a sort of balanced, harmonious union with nature, along with animal and human community, as well as the ego and the id — can be induced by the required state of pretend play in storytelling or performance, but particularly in masked performance. Accordingly, this Romantic state makes a significant demand on the viewer who must recognize and support the premise that looking beyond the illusion might threaten the fragile state of this blissful consciousness. (Likewise, the romantic lover avoids looking too closely at the beloved, lest s/he be disillusioned.)

The demon Bak'was (recognized by several Northwest Pacific Coast First Peoples as the one responsible for loss of sanity and keeper of drowned souls) reflects another vivid mythic example that expresses this struggle to maintain the illusion of pretend play. "With his green hairy body, he enticed victims seeking escape into the night woods with faint firelight. If they reach for the fire, they lose all reason. They could rarely be brought back to sanity except with the aid of menstrual blood."[15] The menstrual blood could "protect" the endangered, alienated soul with the promise of the natural and figurative cycles of birth, death, and regeneration.

The illusion of the masked performance cannot be too specific; neither can it exaggerate too much. Its reality must connote invisible, unconscious states of reality. The viewer must accept the illusory presentation as a fragile lie, suspended between stark reality and subliminal truths. The masker forbids the viewer to look too closely at the actual illusion of the story or the mask. The artful guise insists on hiding realities even as it reveals others. Some realities are too painful to accept or witness, such as the reality of change, making difficult choices, or death. Some stories promise a semblance of constancy and predictability as a way of avoiding the ultimate uncertainties inherent in the human condition.

Mythic stories such as these, especially those involving protectors, make other Romantic demands with admonishments about flying too high and getting burned by the sun. Psyche is forbidden to actually see her lover, Eros. Eve is forbidden to eat (experience) the apple which will give her the experience of choosing, making her God-like and accountable for her choices. The traditional protector guise typically maintains some sort of Romantic insistence on forbidden knowledge in order to function as a protector.

Walter Sorell identifies early twentieth-century playwright Arthur Schnitzler's struggle with these same issues of forbidden truth by describing his major focus as "love and death, dream and reality." Sorell points out that Schnitzler acknowledges our inability to hide behind Romantic illusions. "[Schnitzler] saw man in his unrealized fear of death throwing himself into love to prove and find himself; he [as he said in *Paracelsus*] realized ... that: 'Dream and waking flow into one another. /truth and lie. Certainty is nowhere. / We know nothing of the other, nothing of ourselves. / We always play-act; he who knows it, is clever.'"[16]

One hundred years later, our twenty-first century intelligentsia might very well concur with Schnitzler, but popular film and stage productions still embrace age-old Romantic agendas found in protector masks, and Pixar's film animation (masked) character WALL-E still finds solace in friendship, even if it is with a (masked) cockroach. The current global stage and screen continue to beguile us with the subliminal guise of a world order striving for harmony and balance by invoking contemporary protectors as vivid as any "Romantically" evoked by the primitive shamans (those early protectors found in many cultures who harnessed the powers of unseen spirits). I will examine this concept more fully in chapter 6 as an essential theory regarding the way traditional masks significantly influence contemporary commercial masked performance.

Postmodern Agendas

Like many children's nursery rhymes and songs, *Row row row your boat gently down the stream, merrily merrily merrily merrily life is but a dream* is more profound than one might initially assume. The Paleolithic shaman could have sung such a tune easily, albeit with a more aggressive delivery as he carried vulnerable audiences artfully through an imaginary journey in space and time with carefully orchestrated metaphorical rituals.

Admittedly, postmodern style, a consequence of twentieth-century existential thought, avoids using such illusionary "dreams" for "pretend play" and ritual as the primary way of indicating eternal, divine states of reality. Postmodern style instead "plays" with the "act of play." It manipulates ritual in unexpected ways. It uses "identity assumptions" in order to speculate more than to substantiate.

The postmodern mask, rather than traditionally evoking another character, typically masks another mask. The postmodern mask deconstructs the process of illusionary masking (however methodically or haphazardly) rather than constructing answers regarding life's dilemmas. Yet a postmodern agenda for masked performance is not simply a twentieth-century phenomenon.

For example, maskers performing in spontaneous street activity of Carnival in many Catholic countries have functioned in this postmodern fashion for centuries. Their masks experiment with masked presentational roles as layers of superficial identities signifying roles as labels. The Carnival mask maker's agenda during the street celebrations does not treat the masked performance as a magical illusionary story, capable of transporting the viewer into a more profound level of reality. Rather, in most cases, the Carnival masker comments on the world as s/he sees it by presenting figures as symbolic identities or situations. An example of this would be Geraldo Vieira Jr.'s gigantic parade mask for *Trouble in de Bamboo* (chapter 2). Vieira's character does not live within a mythic story but serves instead as a pageant symbol. Also, a few of Juan Horta Castillo's devil masks for *Pastorela* celebrations (chapter 2) serve as something like signifiers and do not interact within an actual performance story. (Of course, Carnival maskers can and do present Romantic versions of myths, stories, and role playing when desired, but certainly with much less frequency during street masquerade activity.)

A number of archetypal masks, such as those evoking the contemporary protector, seem particularly well-suited to navigate between both the postmodern and Romantic realms of expression. They can appear effectively as signifiers/labels. They can also work well as illusionary characters that ultimately transport the viewer into the pretend world of the performer. The traditional protector masks and hero masks as well as the demonic masks have the capacity to utilize "postmodern" theatrical conventions of labeling. They can even synchronize this type of labeling with other aspects of Romantically conjured illusionary characters within some types of performance narration. Occasionally we can see this blend of postmodern and Romantic theatrical convention on the contemporary stage.

Playwright Sam Shepard often incorporates these postmodern conventions into his staged storytelling. He imaginatively explores such postmodern topics as the loss of identity regarding gender, nationality, parental/childhood/sibling relationships, and skewed mythical perspectives in stark theatrical ways. He rarely requires actual masks, and yet his exaggerated characters frequently appear mask-like. His characters are deranged fathers with exaggerated bloody bald heads, or rock stars with flamboyant hair and makeup, or beat-up, bruised female victims whose mummy-like versions of the semi-deaf and dumb express truths in a manner similar to Shakespeare's theatrical fools. In *A Lie of the Mind*, Shepard uses protective animal imagery as did the ancient shamans, but reverses its significance from that of tutelary imagery to death imagery, such as the bloodied, frozen stag in the middle of Baylor's living room or the references of Jake as the caricature of a hapless dog. Shepard even uses inanimate objects as mask-functioning ironic protective devices, such as the mobile of World War II fighter bombers in Jake's bedroom that swirl like Greek furies above his head, reminding him of his father's (and his own) lost ideals. Leslie Kane describes Shepard's characters and events as "literal and figurative snapshots abounding and prominently displayed."[17] These snapshots suggest frozen eternal states of being in a way that masks do.

Walter Sorell describes Lorca's characters as similarly figurative masked versions of theatrical presentation:

> How about the *personae* of Lorca's characters? They never deny their puppet origin. Their faces are masks for a reality that does not dare to be, or on the contrary, spills all over the stage. His characters are stereotypes of Spanish folklore, and they are types rather than

> characters. They wear the masks of feminine martyrdom, emasculated Don Juanism, or the brutal rigor of matriarchal ideas. These masks hide passion, sex, and honor, the three propelling forces in Lorca's characters. They are predetermined traps, prisons, and strait-jackets for his heroes and heroines. I have never seen a Lorca production in which his characters wore masks, but they could very well do so. On second thought, they do not have to. They all have the characteristics of a puppet that is a type.[18]

Natural and Ritualistic Harmony between the Mask, Music, and Dance

Mask makers (unless making masks for tourists) rarely intend for masks to hang on walls. They create masks to be part of a more elaborate artistic presentation and purpose. The mask brings life to the wearer and the wearer brings life to the mask. The mask maker must create a mask that is relatively easy to wear: one that allows for adequate visibility and that also helps to accentuate the rhythmic gestures of the performer.

Whatever his/her cultural background, the mask maker recognizes the value of incorporating masked performance with music, dance, and theatrical performances that emerge from the rhythmic dramatic states of tension found in storytelling. The shaman strove for subliminal dream/illusionary states with masks using the aid of rhythmic music much like a contemporary composer such as Andrew Lloyd Webber (and creator of Broadway's *Phantom of the Opera*). But the shaman used a drum rather than Webber's pulsating organ to accompany ancient sacred rituals. The creation of new myths, heroes, and protectors will perhaps require the aid of new theatrical devices (film animation versions of masked characters such as WALL-E could be considered one such innovative theatrical device), but inevitably these stories require selective use of music (if only drums) on stage and screen.

Why the necessity for music? Cycles of beats and harmonies suggest intense regenerative metaphors within the realm of time, in the same way as heartbeats or breathing indicate essential themes of birth, death, and rebirth. Christopher Bigsby describes the musical rhythms found in the dialogue of Sam Shepard in the following manner: "Rhythm is the delineation of time in space but it only makes sense with silences on either side of it."[19]Rhythmic qualities of dialogue or singing can resonate in the same way that music does, creating regenerative images/experiences and consequent dualistic themes. These issues demand aspects of protection in more expressively accessible ways for audiences of any era.

Regardless of how playwrights develop such obvious rhythmic dialogue, the musicality of dialogue as a theatrical device ultimately compares with that involving the drum beats and rattling used in the primitive protector masked dances. What is Carnival masked street performance without the rhythmic force of drums and trumpets? Balinese gamelan, drums, tinkling bells, gongs, and bamboo flutes conjure the *Topeng* heroes. Shepard presents his percussive dialogue with Red Clay Ramblers music while John Williams' music triumphantly announces and underscores the archetypal adventures of *Star Wars*. All theatrical presentations, primitive or contemporary, use rhythmic beats in some way to tempt and cajole the arrival of larger-than-life protectors, heroes, demons, villains, and beloveds. Masked characters rely even more on rhythmic dialogue and music, because the mask accentuates and intensifies their physicality and rhythmic gestures in our time-dominated universe.

2

Describing and Displaying the Work of Traditional Mask Makers

Defining and Identifying the Range of Characteristics

Mask collector Bill LeVasseur has had a long-standing interest in Mexican masks and masked performances. (The private mask museum he has designed in San Miguel de Allende in Mexico is described later in this chapter.) He credits Lévi-Strauss with a particularly important insight into the nature of masked performance saying, "A mask [or at least a face with superficial applications of makeup] needs at least one audience member who interprets the transformation of the wearer of the mask into another persona." LeVasseur acknowledges that only humans have the capability for pretending with masks. Animals perhaps transform themselves during mating season or camouflage themselves, but do so instinctually rather than intentionally as humans do. "A mask requires one audience member even if that audience member is a reflection in the mirror of a kid posing with eyeliner or sunglasses," he continues. "The kid transforms himself in the mirror using his sunglasses and gestures and that transformation is reflected back to him as both the wearer of the mask and the audience member."[1] At that elemental level a theatrical event occurs with masking.

A mask does not have to be a three-dimensional covering over the face. In traditional versions of the *Dance of the Moors and Christians,* Mexican performers playing the conquering soldiers of Santiago sport Spanish hats, swords, and *burroquites* (wooden versions of horses) around their waists. Their faces are uncovered, but the entire ensemble (particularly the frozen gesture of the *burroquites*) indicates something more in the realm of masks and puppets rather than simply costume. Charlie Chaplin's distinctive moustache and eyebrows generate an internationally recognizable mask. Gloria Swanson's eyelashes and long face as she appears in *Sunset Blvd.* evoke the ultimate *femme fatale* mask. Indiana Jones' bullwhip and hat complete the masquerade of his persona and without these masking devices, he is no longer the iconic image of Indiana Jones. At some point Zsa Zsa Gabor's blond bouffant wig becomes a mask. At some point the huge walking sculptures created by Trinidadian Peter Minshall become multiple masks when a (masked) performer struts across the stage supporting his larger-than-life (masked) mythic figures. Many ancient cultures recognized the power of a mask on top of a bare-faced performer, such as the masks seen in *The Lion King.* Surely at some level, the sunglasses worn by the evil pinstriped suited agents in *The Matrix* become masks.

As I demonstrate in chapter 7, there are as many ways to define masks as to define myths. This premise does not downplay the obvious significance of actual facial coverings as masks. But to ignore other versions of the mask risks dogmatic labels better left to the academics than to the artists who create them.

Determining the Mask's Style and Maintaining Consistent Integrity

An especially important consideration for the mask maker lies in determining the style of the mask. Of course, the mask maker's style invariably comes directly from personal cultural images and icons. The mask maker cannot consciously or subconsciously escape the assimilated range of influential, culturally specific visual images.

Does this subliminal collection of images necessarily benefit the artistry of the mask maker? While there are no easy answers to that question, mask makers I interviewed obviously enjoy learning about the work of other mask makers beyond their own cultural boundaries. Most of them already had knowledge of the work of the other mask makers I was interviewing. Donato Sartori has visited I. Bagus Anom's studio and other mask makers worldwide. Torbjörn Alström and Venicio Fonseca took Donato Sartori's mask workshop in their earlier years. Juan Horta Castillo admitted his strong interest in African masks. I. Bagus Anom has experimented with Japanese mask effects in his Balinese work, incorporating black teeth and other Japanese facial characteristics. Dong-Pyo Kim has traveled extensively to collect masks from other countries. I. Made Suryasa studied at UCLA and has an American wife; consequently he has an abiding awareness of Western masked performances. Donato Sartori, Juan Horta Castillo and his son Manuel, Victor Reece, Donvieve, Xstine Cook, Marlon Griffith, Alicia Martínez Álvarez, and Torbjörn Alström have offered mask-making workshops abroad. Nevertheless, even though the mask makers I interviewed had impressive knowledge about the international trends of mask making, they each tended to present work that strongly reflects the aesthetic of their own culture.

A great deal of rich and varied visual imagery from the Internet and cinema has the potential to significantly influence even the most provincial mask makers. All of the mask makers I interviewed, even those living in rural areas, had access to the Internet if not immediate access to new movies. While this information highway might threaten to dilute the unique qualities of each mask maker's style as well as individual aspects of a cultural aesthetic, none of the mask makers I interviewed seemed to be drastically changing the style of his/her masks as a result of such international Internet influence. I found this surprising, since one would assume that only the exceptional mask maker could escape the influence of the sea of images continually pervading our current Internet-based shrinking world. Probably they have kept their autonomy partly due to the fact that one cannot easily observe actual masked performances on the Internet. Without seeing the mask in performance, much of the mask's power is lost. Consequently the mask makers I interviewed tend to stay within the parameters of their own cultural aesthetic though as the cultural and spiritual values of their communities rapidly evolve, their traditional masks can remain relevant for only so long.

Another stylistic consideration involves the decorative aspects of the mask. To some extent the distance between the masked performer and its audience determines the level of decoration. For example, costume historian James Laver points out that the ancient Greek mask makers, whose masks were seen from great distances, believed that their primary goal was to amplify the characters literally and figuratively.[2] Consequently the ancient bold Greek masks lacked intricate detail. (Torbjörn Alström has experimented with types of carved wood to create contemporary versions of ancient Greek masks. *The Drama*

Review has published his findings entitled "The Voice in the Mask" in the summer 2004 issue.)

The masked medieval performer, unlike the Greek masked performer, performed relatively close to the street audiences. Therefore he required more elaborate artifice, often including highly detailed iconic decoration such as heavily textured "evil goat or ram horns" for the devil or intricately feathered bird imagery for the angels as well as dove imagery signifying the Holy Spirit.

On the other hand, distance has not always been the primary issue in selecting decorative and detailed touches of the mask. Tseëlon in his introduction to *Masquerade and Identities* describes how mask makers have changed their goals regarding style throughout history, citing Napier's examples of medieval performances as "antithetical to true identity. From medieval times onwards, the mask acquired evil and sinister connotations and (contrary to the ancient Greek mask) it has come to connote disengenuity, artifice, and pretence in contrast to original identity, which connotes truth and authenticity."[3]

The mask makers I interviewed all create masks that range from highly decorative to very bold, depending on each mask's function. Of course, one of the reasons for the success of these mask makers might have to do with their ability to astutely and sensitively assess just how much style and decoration evokes the appropriate expressive effect. They each strike just the right level of exaggeration, keeping in mind the type of performance where the mask will appear. Exaggerated stylistic and decorative elements can overpower the mask's characterization and message. The mask can become too abstract and detract from the mask's vitality in the same way that a dancer's overly complicated and abstract gestures can diminish the audience's attention.

Distinctive Aesthetic and Cultural Qualities

Nigerian Egungun and Epa Mask Makers

It was only a matter of time before my quest would lead to Africa, where mask makers have contributed greatly to the power of masked performance for millennia. Collectively, for example, African mask makers have influenced vital modern artistic achievements in the twentieth century. Bihalji-Merin in his book *Great Masks* quotes Picasso's breakthrough in understanding the concept of profound "wealth in form, power, and emotional tension" when applying the conceptual perspective of African mask qualities to the work of modern artists: "Men had made those masks and other objects for a sacred purpose, a magic purpose, as a kind of mediation between themselves and the unknown hostile forces that surrounded them, in order to overcome their fear and horror by giving them form and an image. At that moment I realized that this was what painting was all about. Painting is not an aesthetic operation: it is a form of magic designed as a mediator between this strange, hostile world and us, a way of seizing the power by giving form to our terrors as well as our desires. When I came to that realization, I knew I had found my way."[4]

Later Bihalji-Merin refers to the "central regions important in the world of masks; those of the West African cultural groupings, from Ghana to Angola" and to "African masked dancers who take part in funeral, fertility and initiation festivities, representing punitive and regulating powers." Traditional African conceptualizations used in creating masks for African performance have influenced numerous other twentieth-century Western artists such as Modigliani, Paul Klee, Eduardo Paolozzi, and Henry Moore.[5] Plays recently produced in the United States such as August Wilson's *Gem of the Ocean* and Julie Taymor's *The Lion King* have continued to incorporate significant aspects of African masked performance.

But are contemporary, traditionally based African mask makers still incorporating traditional values and techniques? African communities have been influenced by industrialized Western countries in terms of education and Western (as well as Islamic) myths. Today, Nigerian citizens encounter Western aesthetic and value systems more often than they did one hundred years ago. How does this situation influence their traditional masked performance festivals? Ultimately, what challenges do mask makers confront in the midst of such dramatic cultural change and what insights into traditional African mask making can contemporary Nigerian mask makers teach us?

I first decided to visit and interview mask makers in Nigeria after seeing Ojetunji Ojeyemi's magnificent *Egungun* masquerade at the 2005 International Mask Conference at Southern Illinois University Carbondale. My review of that event described him as a Nigerian performer who "held the audience spellbound with the rhythmic drumming, music, and masked dance of a typical Yoruba ancestral (*Egungun*) masquerade. Ojetunji (or Tunji as he calls himself) paraded onto the University's stage to prophesize, pontificate, admonish, and inspire the surrounding village people. Some were members of the audience who came on stage to participate."[6] Apart from his extensive experience as a masked performer, Tunji also designs and makes masks, though he focuses primarily on performance. A professor at Obafemi Awolowo University, he teaches performance techniques, dance, and choreography. He is also artistic director of a professional dance troupe, located in the city of Ile-Ife, the cradle of Yoruba culture.

MASQUERADE — YORUBA STYLE IN NIGERIA

We Westerners usually think of masquerade as a rather shallow event, recalling amateur audience participation during Carnival or Halloween; slow, stately-moving parade personalities on floats; or blandly waving cartoon characters at Disney World. Conversely, the *Egungun* masquerade, like the one Tunji presented in Illinois, involves serious spiritual emphasis on the realm of the dead. Unlike Western presentational forms of staged expression, some African rituals (while not as predominant as originally assumed) require the mask to take on the spirit/character that it evokes during the performance rite.[7] At this point, the mask becomes "alive" not symbolically, but literally. The *Egungun* masks conjure ancestral spirits and *Egungun* performers talk about the spirit of the dead literally inhabiting their bodies when masked. While *Eguguns* are rarely sinister, they carry such profound secrets that audience members maintain respectful distances. Traditionally, women are forbidden to either create or touch such forms, either in the act of making the mask or in performance, although some women, if they belong to the appropriate cult, can attend ceremonial performances.

Tunji and several other Nigerians I interviewed insisted that this concept does not denigrate women. After all, Yoruba women have their own masked spectacle in the form of the *Gèlèdé* masquerades which acknowledge their own impressive powers. (Even so, the masquerades are performed by male masqueraders.) The Yoruba communities consider women essentially separate but equal in terms of their own capabilities.[8] Pernet in his book *Ritual Masks* describes the *Gèlèdé* Festival as "honoring [Yoruba] mothers. It publicly recognizes the power of women (old women, ancestresses, or deified women), not only their creative power but also their secret and destructive power which expresses itself in witchcraft. The participants aim then at conciliation between [Yoruba] mothers and the witches (*àjé*) so that they will use their powers for good rather than the destruction of the community."[9] Beckwith and Fisher describe this ritual more specifically as one where "the objective is to identify and eliminate the negative aspects of female power and replace them with the more benevolent themes of fecundity, maternity, and well-being."[10] Certainly there is a respectful salute, along with a wary eye toward women during the *Gèlèdé* celebrations. John Nunley underscores this concept by describing the historic fascination that men have in masquerading as women spanning many cultures, yet he also notes that whenever men mask themselves as women, it involves "a complex act of appropriation and representation. Men often masquerade as women in rituals to ensure a good harvest and numerous descendants. Thus fertility — both agricultural and human — becomes the 'male' responsibility."[11]

However one interprets the *Gèlèdé* celebrations, the annual Osun Festival in Osogbo most certainly celebrates and empowers the feminine, fertile, and creative powers of Osun, an important Yoruba *òrìsà*. This concept brings certain stature to womanhood and motherhood in a manner unlike any other in Yoruba society. The term, *òrìsà*, helps to explain the essential purpose and functions of Yoruba masks. Occasionally considered a god, an *òrìsà* more specifically refers to a spiritual aid who serves to promote better understanding of the omniscient god, Olodumare. This is similar to the way spiritual aids such as the Virgin Mary or Christ help to reveal the Christian god.[12]

My excellent and resourceful Nigerian guide, Adigun Ajani (an authority on Yoruba myth, former museum curator, and esteemed artist in the Osogbo community), proceeded to underscore this idea of an abiding Yoruba respect for female capacities with a legendary story. He explained that "Orunmila (*òrìsà* of divination) once reported to Olodumare (God) that several of the major male *òrìsàs* such as Sango (*òrìsà* of thunder), Esu (trickster *òrìsà* of checks and balances), Obaluaye (*òrìsà* responsible for disease), Oro (*òrìsà* of secrets) and especially Ogun (*òrìsà* of iron and war) could not create wealth. Olodumare asked why they did not bring along Osun (the female *òrìsà* of fertility and creation). Olodumare, in his wisdom knew that unless she was involved as a primary female force, they could never be successful."[13]

Ojetunji (Tunji) Ojeyemi's Perspective on *Egungun* Masquerade and Its Reflection of Yoruba Spirituality

Ojeyemi participated extensively with *Egungun* masquerades as a young audience member and later as a mask maker and *Egungun* performer. The son of a Nigerian chief and born into the lineage of the Oje (traditional Yoruba cult of masquerades), Ojeyemi was initiated into the guild of mask dancers and acrobatic performers at the age of six. He has since been a pivotal presence in annual Nigerian *Egungun* festivals.

Yet other mask makers I had interviewed in Osogbo expressed anxiety regarding how they might continue to create such elaborately detailed and specifically relevant masks for masqueraders like Ojeyemi when Yoruba values and style are increasingly diluted in the midst of encroaching Christian and Muslim influences. West African masks require specialized skill even as they demand significant understanding of ancient spiritual beliefs; spiritual beliefs that have unified the Yoruba community during centuries of economic, social, and political challenges.

Ironically, cultural leaders throughout Southwestern Nigerian communities strive to maintain the sanctity of their spiritual rituals and masked performances associated with

Yoruba traditions by also allowing tourism to help support their continuation. This struggle continues anywhere in the world where ethnic traditions increasingly confront the invading, diluting effects of the vast global information highway. Consequently, traditional Yoruba masked performance tradition seems at risk, unless the Yoruba spiritual foundations are maintained and perpetuated. Currently these foundations confront a critical shift in the history of Yoruba culture.

Ojeyemi poignantly described his contemporary Nigerian yearning to maintain Yoruba myth and ritual as he introduced me to the world of *Egungun* masks and insisted that we cannot take masks for granted; they function only when people hold great spiritual beliefs, allowing the masks to harness significant power.[14] "An *Egungun* in a traditional performance can project humorous admonishments while also teaching important wisdom from the ancestors," Ojeyemi explained. "Yet some masqueraders today are very old and fearful. We call this kind of masquerader *Alagbo* who can also perform miraculous healing as a *babalàwo* (an herbalist/diviner with powers similar to those possessed by shamans or medicine men.) These performers are so powerful they sometimes have bees around them! Traditional *Egungun* masqueraders such as these can use chanting and medicine to test each other in a competitive way."

He described a typical *Egungun* ceremony which occurs between the third and seventh days before the actual burial:

> Several days after death, the *Egungun* as the spirit of the deceased will come to visit. [The *Egungun* masquerade does not allow any visible skin of the masquerader. Gloves and leggings complete a hugely proportioned masked figure.] During this grieving period, the deceased's children will pray and ask the *Egungun* for blessings. Traditionally *Egunguns* speak incoherently but the elders understand what they say. After visiting, the *Egungun* will disappear, leaving the deceased's family members and friends crying.
>
> My father would take me to these rituals and we would hear the voice of the deceased coming from a calabash after it was hit three times. People would run and scatter. The cloth used for burying the deceased would fly and disappear on the third day. I experienced this ritual three times in my childhood. On the seventh day, the elders would prepare sacrifices and feasts early in the morning and then would meet the *Egungun* who came dressed in fabric worn by the deceased as well as other fabric pieces worn by close relatives or fabrics specially imported because of their beauty. Afterwards the elders would tell the small children to go away. The elders proceeded to hold a cock behind the *Egungun*, close their eyes when presenting the gift and the *Egungun* would take it and disappear.
>
> Nigerian women understand that when they hear the sound of an approaching *Egungun*, they should look downward at least until the *Egungun* changes into a female character. Once in 1993 when I was performing the *Egungun* ceremony with women in the audience, I felt very strange both physically and emotionally. Suddenly I remembered that before he died my father had warned me that one of the charms I would inherit for the *Egungun* costume was especially potent and I should not use it in the presence of women. While I was performing in this *Egungun* disguise, I was linked to the ancestral god and I realized that I had neglected to remove the charm which was placed inside the costume. Something very serious happened to me, especially after I became a female version of the ancestral god. In the presence of the dancing women around me I could not focus and became physically drained. I walked away briefly from the performance site to remove the charm — and then I felt okay, but I am convinced I could have been seriously harmed if I had continued to wear it in front of the women.

Ojeyemi's close relationship with his father expresses much of the underlying rationale for the Yoruba propensity to maintain and champion the art and rituals associated with

Egungun masquerade. Ancestor worship runs deep in the undercurrents of the religion and social structure. "Early on as a child, my father foretold that I would make my career as a dancer and as a teacher. He often stated it to my family and directly to me. He was highly disciplined and during my training as a dancer he would have me do the same technique repeatedly to perfect it to the point that I would cry. My father was a great dancer and I inherited his skills and improved on them. He is dead since 1999," Ojeyemi explained.

> But when I want to talk with him I put on his cap when I sleep and by 2 A.M. I am connected to him. If I perform in his *Egungun* mask and costume and make some rituals, I talk to him and I hear his voice.
>
> My last performance with him was broadcast by the London BBC at the *Egungun* Festival in Gbongan. I involved my father in this event, and we went in front of the old palace. As we arrived, the weather changed into rain. My father stepped out and conjured the sun to return. During this particular part of the event, my masquerade had evolved into a tiger, and I went to the top of the palace roof which was two stories high. I knew I needed to complete the performance by "flying" down from the building but I had lost courage. My father got up and raised his hand with the drummers. My ears were blocked and I couldn't hear the drums; I heard only my father's voice chanting that I would be light like cotton wool. I found myself suddenly safely on the ground, and people were shouting in amazement. On that day, my wife exclaimed that she had married a spirit. But it was my father's spirit that sustained me.
>
> You don't joke with this profession. Some of our masquerades are fake, but when you encounter the power of your ancestors you seriously need to be prepared. I am an educated professional in the modern world and I am a political activist like my father. I lead a contemporary human rights organization called Campaign for Democracy and Human Rights. Yet, I still respect and believe in our traditions. I still sacrifice to my father. I know my father still loves me and is always behind me. Every year I kill the goat and commune with him. If I am confused or if someone is sick, I cover that person with the *Egungun* mask and the person will be healed quickly. No one can steal my most valued possessions in my bedroom because I keep the *Egungun* mask high in my wardrobe closet. No thief dares to enter.[15]

Michael Harris underscores Ojeyemi's vivid description of the fundamental intersections of contemporary Yoruba culture and its "moral imperatives" with artistic effort in his 1991 interview with another professor, Moyosore Okediji, also at Obafemi Awolowo University. In this interview, Okediji states that "I am trying to do exactly what the traditional carver is trying to do.... [T]he secularization of society has shifted the role of the artist in one sense, likening it to the work of a psychiatrist ... and in another sense the artist has some of the obligations of a priest, because if you consider any religion, the vehicle has always been art, whether poetry, or very good prose, or music, or visual art." Harris adds, "In Yoruba culture, this would also include the drama of ritual performance."[16]

Agbede Adebisi's Brass *Egungun* Masks

Another mask maker, Agbede Adebisi, specializes in the creation of masks rather than in masked performance. Adebisi's brass *Egungun* masks are renowned throughout the region. His grandfather's masks found their way into major European collections.

Like many mask makers worldwide, Adebisi learned his craft from his father, beginning at the age of twelve. He creates his brass sculptures utilizing the traditional "lost wax" process with nineteenth-century bellows and kilns. Special red clay from Benin called *amo pupe* takes three days to harden as a negative image covering the positive beeswax image of the mask underneath. After the clay dries, it is placed over a very hot fire sustained with charcoal.

The wax melts and he pours the melted brass inside the clay mold. When it cools, Adebisi breaks the clay to retrieve the brass form. It can take as long as three weeks to create an *Egungun* mask using brass features. His family usually helps to build the accompanying costume created out of strips of cloth worn by the deceased and his ancestors.

Adebisi's masks are in high demand. "Occasionally," he laments, "they are stolen to sell to Europeans or other foreigners," though the need to make replacements keeps him active and financially solvent. (I was surprised to learn that *Egungun* masks actually could be stolen, in spite of Ojeyemi's belief that *Egungun* masks served as protection for all other valuables nearby.)

His own family *Egungun* mask incorporates strips of his late father's wearing apparel as well as metallic cloth previously worn by his late mother. In accordance with tradition, his *Egungun* mask is reverently stored in the attic of his home or resides in the highest place within the highest room in his home. His greatest challenge comes when attempting to acquire appropriate materials. The brass is very expensive and sometimes he must compromise by mixing lead with it. Only the clay from Benin works best to create the molds.[17]

KOLAWOLE ADEOLA'S MASKS FOR *EPA* MASQUERADE AND CORONATION CEREMONIES

The gregarious and quick-witted Kolawole Adeola, who calls himself Kola, specializes in *Epa* masks for the Yam festivals, *owi* masks that appear at night during funerals, and *Gèlèdé* masks honoring women in *Gèlèdé* celebrations, as well as *Egungun* masks. He belongs to the *Ògbóni* Secret Society, which pays special homage to *Obegi*, the spirits representing twins, who are believed to have the power to create good fortune and health. Often the masks for this secret society are metal and not necessarily worn on the head. They can serve as a heraldic device, carried or worn in front of the torso. Participants can bang on them (like a gong). Masks used by this secret society feature arms folded across the chest with fists aligned.

The *Obegi* twin figures frequently adorn the *Epa* masks for use during masquerades at the Yam festivals. The *Epa* masks help to promote the male/female *òrìsà* spirit for agriculture, ensuring a good harvest and commercial success. The masks often combine male/female components, such as a high mask of a woman with a male face, and they are frequently worn over the head, or on top of the head over a cloth roll. "When I create an *Epa* mask, I usually follow the instructions of my clients while striving to achieve a sense of Yoruba style," Adeola says. "My masks

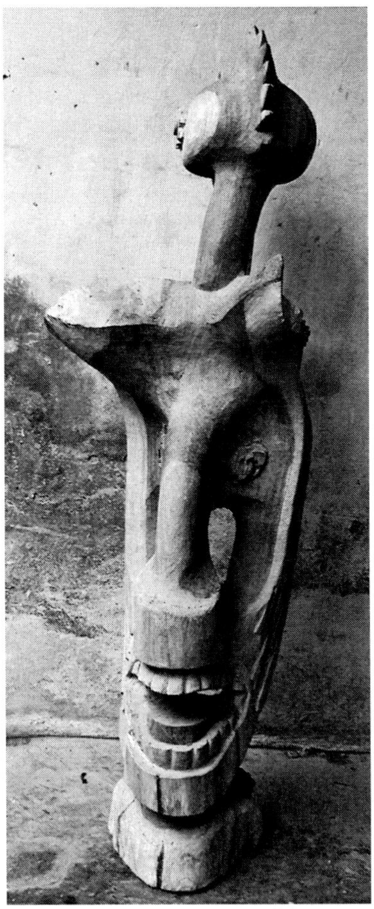

This mask, created by Adigun Ajani, is worn on the head of the masquerader. The front depicts the *òrisà* Orunmila (wisdom) while the back, depicting the *òrisà* Obatala (supreme god), protects the back of the masquerader. The carved-out portion at the bottom has the head shape of the masquerader, who both wears the mask and carries it while dancing.

have both spiritual and commercial dimensions, and my non-commissioned masks sell very quickly. It is difficult to maintain a supply of new masks for sale."

Adeola believes that his great-grandfather inspired him in his training, even though his father actually taught him how to carve.

> Early on, I had no job, and poverty encouraged me to seriously train for this profession. But my great-grandfather's masks were beautiful and famous. Often people would ask me to replace them after termites had destroyed them. So I learned at an early age how to appreciate the act of copying fine work to the best of my ability, and this training provided a solid foundation for excellence as I developed my own abilities to create more original work that comes from my heart. Now I rarely work for money. I can afford to work for God because my successful masks create sufficient income to care for my family. But if I need inspiration, I don't go to books or pictures. I have all the inspiration I need when I remember the masks of my father, my grandfather, and great-grandfather. Then I go directly to the wood to be carved, and I see my head [mask] in the bush [forest].

Adeola described important considerations for his masks, such as the necessity to use appropriately aged wood: hard enough but not dead. The wood must cure for three months

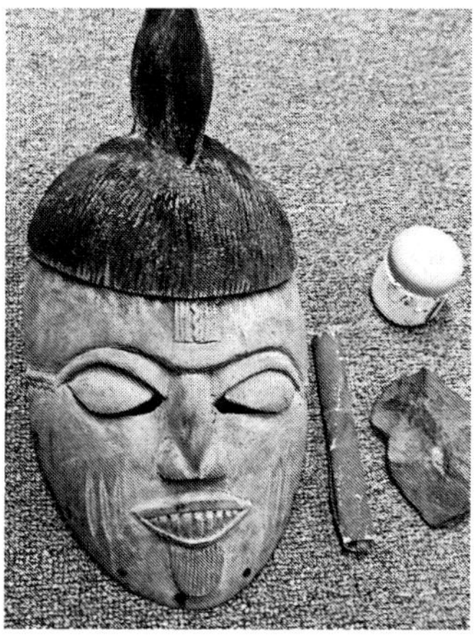

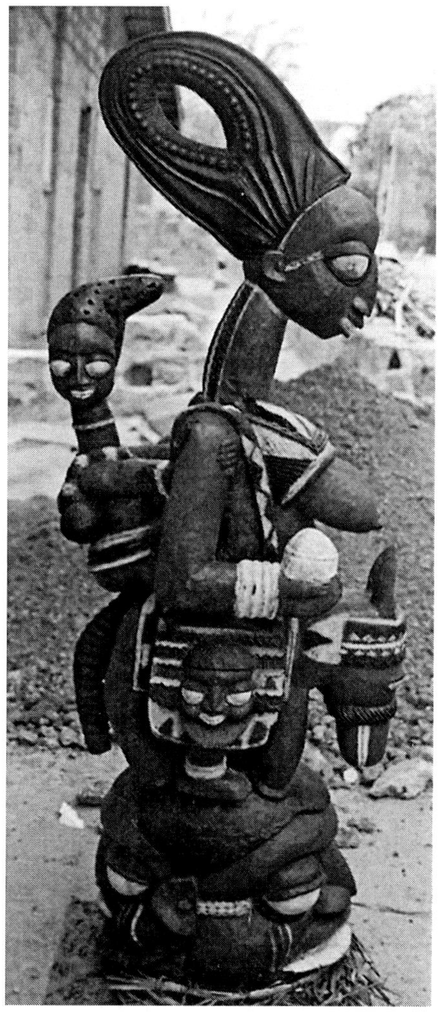

Left: **Another carved wood royal mask created by Kolawole Adeola. A new chief wears a mask such as this one during the coronation ceremony when he takes on his new responsibilities in the community. The ceremony celebrates the wisdom of the departing chief while also celebrating the potential of the new chief. The mask would eventually have indigo blue hair, beard, scarring, white teeth, and deep red lips and cheeks (created by scraping powder from red rock in Benin, mixing it with glue, and applying the mixture).** ***Right:*** **An example of Kolawole Adeola's carved wood *Epa* masks. The *Epa* masks accompany the *Epa* or Yam Festivals which celebrate good harvest and commerce. Adeola's copy of an *Epa* mask is called an *Ejio* mask originally created by his grandfather ninety years ago. The mask comes from the area known as Aree Afao Ekiti in the Ekiti Kingdom. Adeola's grandfather worked alongside prominent carvers like Obembe Ologunde from Ilesa, Agbonbiofe, from Efon Alaye and Oyemolatiran Olayanju from Owo in Ondo State. The original had been damaged by ants. The king of Aree Afao Ekiti asked Adeola to repair it. He has replicated several masks like this one for important royal members of the Yoruba community. Photographer: Kolawole Adeola.**

or the mask may eventually crack. He always guarantees his work by using appropriate wood. Adeola also prefers symmetry in his masks and spends time standing above them and looking at them upside down to help achieve that symmetry. Nigerian masks can occasionally have a double series of four "beads" on the forehead area (although the number of beads and the pattern of them vary significantly with any in-depth exploration of these masks). He explained that his beads signify power at the head (mask), with the fourth row signifying a "fourth dimension" which aims for balance in the midst of power. I found myself wondering why the world's military uniforms or government and corporate business regalia have not yet adopted versions of this symbol.

Adeola thinks that he does his best work in the early morning hours. "I need to get up early and drive far away into the bush, away from noisy cars and away from my children demanding biscuits!" he laughs. "For me, 8 to 10 A.M. is the ideal time to carve the head. My brain is cold and fresh and I can fully concentrate. I also prefer to do important finishing work at this time."

The challenges he faces as a mask maker seem daunting. "Too often we are forgotten in the bush," he says. "Too often our ancestors are forgotten. There is very little patronage nowadays. I make a decent living but many do not. Nigeria does not generally promote the carver as an artist and is not inclined to promote African heritage to the extent that it needs promoting. Prominent mask makers from the past are in museums, but the world seems to show little interest in the current generation, which seems less likely to stand on accomplishments of our ancestors. Our children don't see the value of carving without proper promotion. Also we mask makers generally lack appropriate documentation. We generally lack good cameras to protect and record what we are doing."[18]

Behalji-Merin reminds us that earlier cultures worldwide supported the mask maker with dignity and privileges. "[T]he creator of the masks belonged to an elite [group] and did not have to go to war or to the hunt. Thus gods protected those who gave them form. The mask maker worked in secret, in the tranquility of the forest. He was given much time in order to create in deep concentration figures of ancestors, fetishes, and masks. His work served the good of the community."[19] Today most people view the contemporary traditional mask maker's work with a curious sense of ambivalence, not only in Adeola's West African region but also in most regions of the world.

AJIBIKE OGUNYEMI'S IRON MASKS

Ajibike Ogunyemi, a blacksmith in the community, has specialized in metal masks, though not as frequently as he used to. He has created metal masks from very thick concentrations of iron as well as from light weights of iron. "I have my health (a blacksmith needs strength), appropriate tools, and an abundance of iron, but my greatest challenge is accepting the need to stop working when the sun goes down. I lack electricity, you see, so everything must stop. I have been a blacksmith for over fifty years. My forefathers were all blacksmiths. I've created many iron masks as a blacksmith. Yet none of my children seems interested in pursuing a career in my profession. They seem too impatient to tolerate the heat from the fire and the physical endurance required for a fine finished product."

Ogunyemi uses the nineteenth-century bellows to maintain high heat for his fires and always pounds the metal in the manner of talking-drum praises (*oríkì*) for Ogun (*òrìṣà* of iron and war) when he works. "That way, Ogun will come down and support the job," he says. "I take a lot of time to get it exactly right. But I never chant negatively or curse. When I'm finished I call another person to see it. If the person can say exactly which

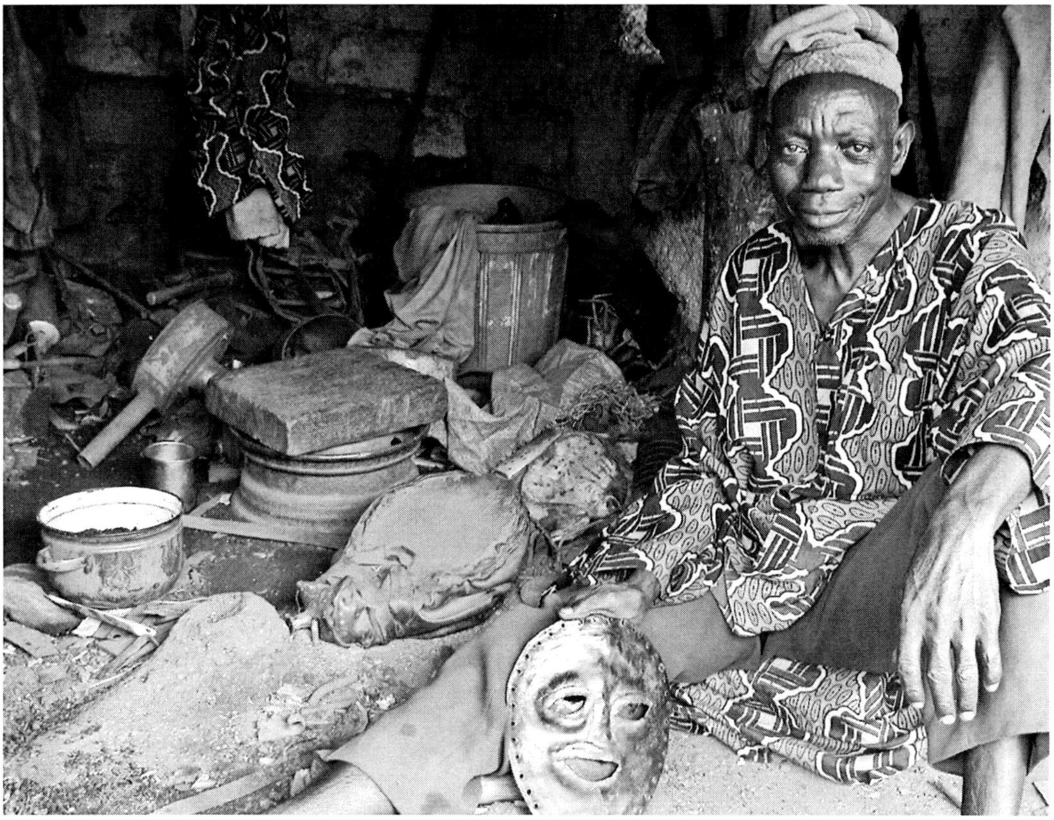

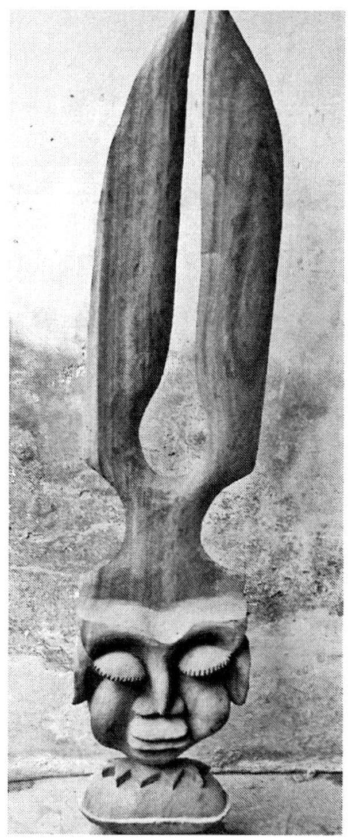

Above: **Ajibike Ogunyemi with his nineteenth-century blacksmith tools, shown here at his studio in Osogbo, Nigeria.** ***Right:*** **Adigun Ajani's sculpture of the *òrìsà* Ogun with machete-like horns. (Mask maker Ogunyemi is a devotee of Ogun.)**

òrìsà the mask signifies, I know that it is successful. For me, that is the ultimate test." He considers himself an Ogun devotee, and he reminded me that during a crisis, Ogun devotees meditate on the machete symbol in order to discover the truth. "If the mask is wrong, it needs to be destroyed and re-created," he concluded.[20]

Kasali Akangbe Ogun's Mask Carvings

I met Kasali Akangbe Ogun (not an Ogun devotee though his late father was a committed Ogun worshiper) at his studio near the Osun grove. Of all the mask makers I interviewed in Osogbo, he probably has the most extensive international reputation. He has exhibited his masks and other wood carvings in London and the Edinburgh Festival; Hamburg and Bayreuth, Germany; the National Black Theatre in Harlem; the University of Iowa; institutions in Austria and France; and numerous sites in Lagos and Osogbo. He also represented Africa at an international symposium in Germany with other renowned wood carvers from New Zealand, Indonesia, Canada, and Italy.[21]

Akangbe Ogun acknowledged that he first received strong encouragement from the European Suzanne Wenger, who came to Osogbo in the early 1950s. She has been a cultural advocate for Yoruba art and artists since her arrival and has attracted international interest in the sacred Osun grove by encouraging a wide range of talented blacksmiths, stone cutters, and wood carvers in the Osogbo area to create numerous impressive shrines dedicated to the *òrìsàs*, particularly Osun. These shrines and sculptures evoke exceptional archaic power and feeling. Akangbe Ogun thinks that perhaps some of the international attention his mask work has received evolved from the attention brought from abroad in response to Wenger's artistic revitalization of traditional arts at the Osun grove. No doubt Akangbe Ogun's iron work there — particularly his stunning roofs and pillars — received recognition. He created similar architectural pieces in other areas of Nigeria.

Akangbe Ogun's wood carving emphasizes ancestral symbols or figures of Yoruba *òrìsàs*. He allowed me to spend a Sunday morning at his studio, watching him begin a huge mask, starting with an old, fully cured tree trunk. His carved *òrìsà* masks reveal the physical prowess necessary to achieve work on such a grand scale.

During Akangbe Ogun's demonstration, he pointed to three cut trunks of trees near his studio and said, "I use *omo* wood (similar to mahogany) and prefer to have the trunks

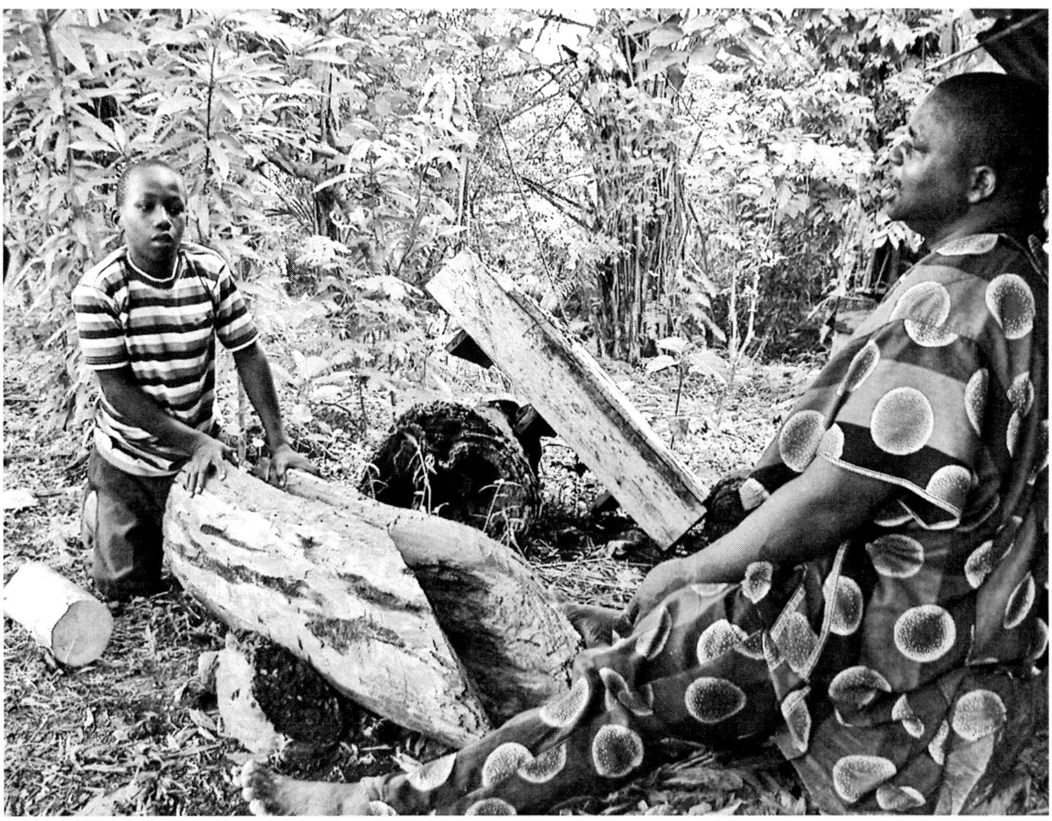

Kasali Akangbe Ogun and son, Adekunle Abduljeleel, at his outdoor studio, in Osogbo, Nigeria.

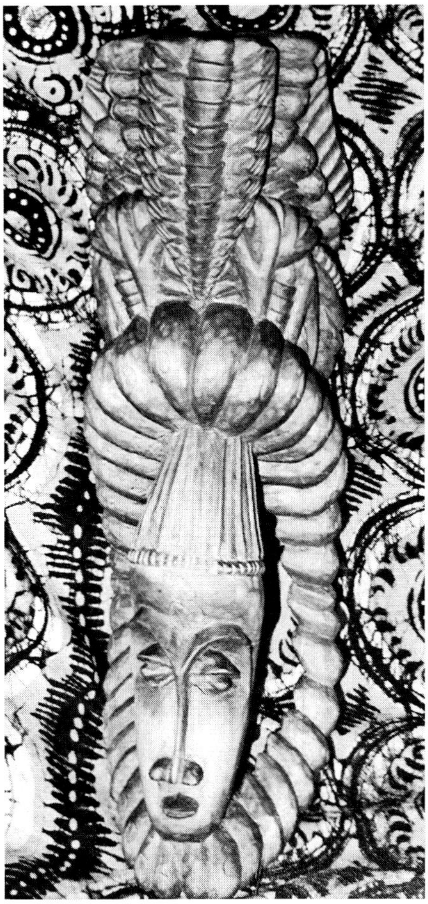

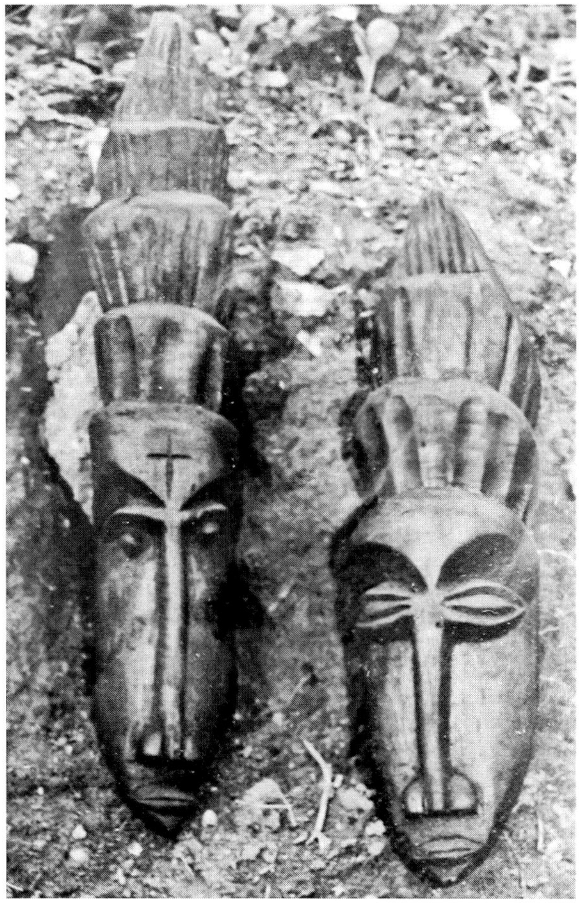

Left: **A mask of Osun (*òrìsà* of fertility and prosperity) created by Kasali Akangbe Ogun. *Right: top*—These carved wood masks are versions of Esu (*òrìsà* of connections between the human and divine realms), created by Kasali Akangbe Ogun in Osogbo, Nigeria. *Bottom*—A carved wood mask created by Abesu Rabiu, in Osogbo, Nigeria.**

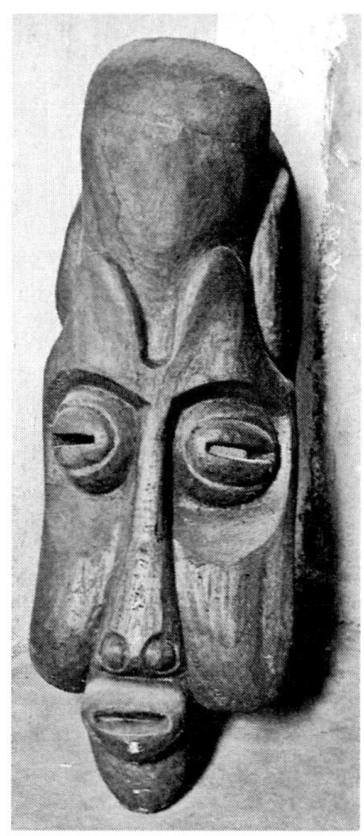

cure for seven years. I then take away the bad bark and work with wood that may have lived for several centuries under the right conditions." He cuts the trunk vertically in half. He began his carving by paying homage to his ancestors and other divinities. The completed carving (which I did not see in such a brief time period) would eventually take an oil polish that darkens the color and makes it termite-proof. "I look forward to the future when my masks will inspire one of my children to do the kind of work I leave behind. I dislike selling my work and only do it to feed my children," he said.

"A successful mask must show strength, and the elements within and around the mask must tell stories," he continued. "The work needs integrity combined with beauty suitable for showing

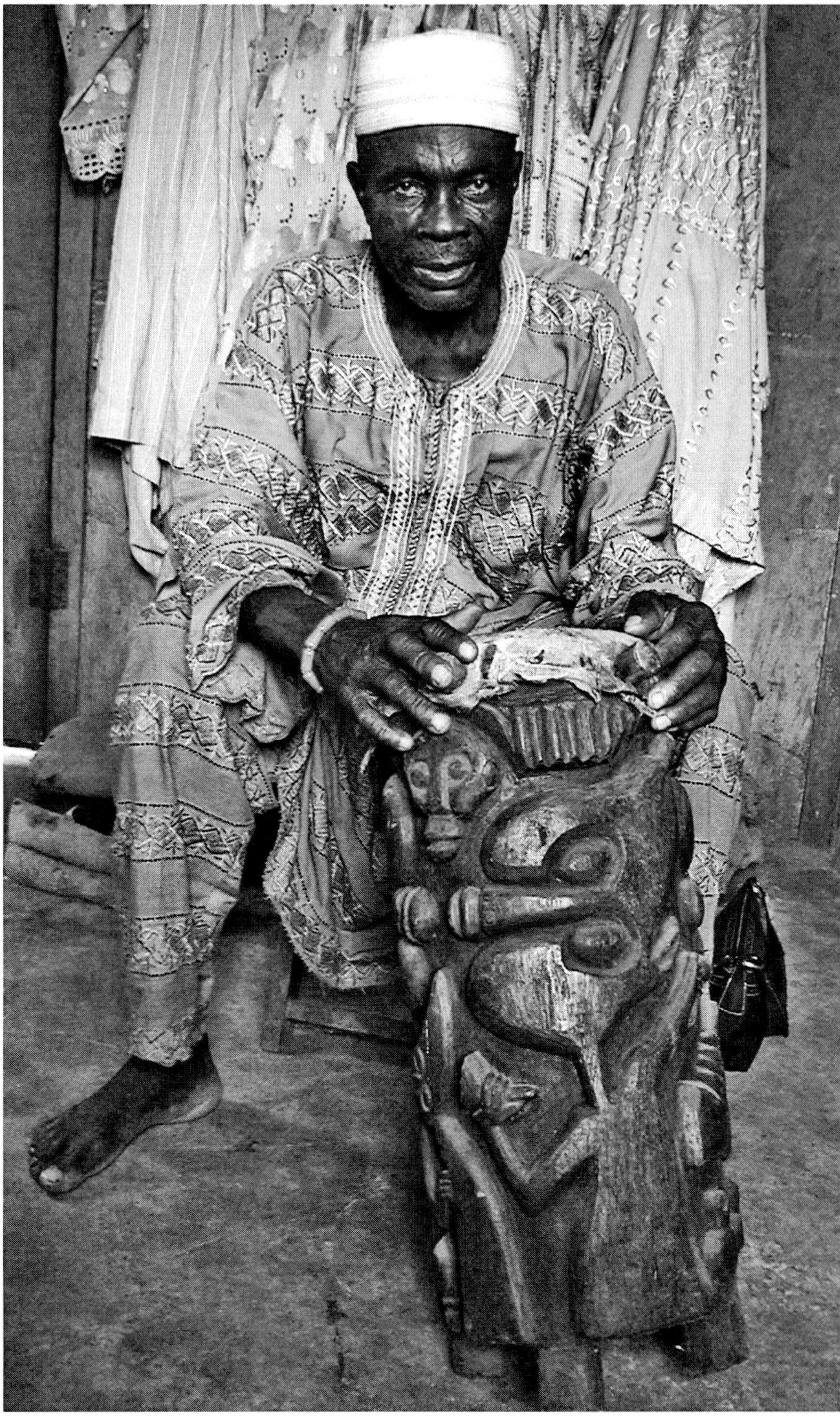

Like so many Nigerian mask carvers, Abesu Rabiu prepares to work by first paying homage to those who have done the work before him. "I then produce the work in my imagination. When I see the wood before me, something tells me how to continue. The more I do the work, the more imagination and inspiration come." Abesu carved the faces on these drums; they reflect his style.

its *odu* or ideal spirit. The mask must be frank and yet dynamic. I'm not talking necessarily about scale, but it must have a strong, dynamic face. The carving must be led by Olodumare just as one's life is led by Olodumare."[22] (Robert Pirsig has similar advice for achieving high-quality artistic effort in *Zen and the Art of Motorcycle Maintenance*: "You've got to live right too. It's the way you live that predisposes you to avoid the traps and see the right facts. You want to know how to paint a perfect painting? It's easy. Make yourself perfect and then just paint naturally."[23])

Yoruba Inspiration for Masks from Nature and the *Òrìsàs*

My guide Adigun Ajani explained that the *òrìsàs* demand worship since they aid mankind in understanding the ultimate divinity in all aspects of life on earth. To worship them is to worship the heads *(ibori)* in ritual. "To worship the heads" is the same as worshiping *òrìsàs*. The heads are often symbolized by "masks" that represent each *òrìsà*, who then inhabits the head/mask and makes it come to life. "*Òrìsà* wants his devotees to visit him but he can't be seen, so he prefers to put on the masks to relate better to each other," he said. "Each *òrìsà* touches the hem of the garment of eternity."[24]

Ajani introduced me to a revered *babalàwo* (herbalist/shaman) named Sangodare Gbadegesin Ajala who added that because of his extensive training during his childhood he can identify 256 faces that appear in nature in trees, rivers, mountains, etc. He suggested that these natural states of being (as well as *òrìsàs*) become the inspiration for the Yoruba masks.[25]

All masks are sacred, but perhaps the most sacred are the *otonporo* masks used to protect Osun in her grove by the river. Ajani explained that the masks are very old, created by the ancestors, and annually washed with spiritual leaves and herbs in preparation for the Osun Festival. "You can't make a god without shedding blood [that is, one cannot experience the concept of eternal divinity without the experience of loss and death], so during the annual purification process, the masks are also cleansed with the blood of animal sacrifices," Ajani added. "These masks are so sacred, only an intimate circle of priests ever see them."[26]

Ajani introduced me to an Osun priestess, Oyabo Osunyemi, who annually helps to prepare the Osun shrines for the Festival. She acknowledged that only priests can cleanse the *otonporo* masks. "I don't mind that I'm not allowed to see the masks," she said. "Women must not see God. I have natural, intuitive feelings toward my obligations as a priestess of Osun, and that is sufficient for me. Osun reveals herself to me when I divine truths as I carry out my rituals."[27]

On the final day of the Osun Festival a virgin carries the *otonporo* masks to the river bank inside a covered calabash to protect Osun and her creative spirit. The covered calabash of sacred unseen masks rests on the river bank during the culmination of the Festival while a variety of non-sacred, commercially based masqueraders celebrate the benefits of Osun's constant restorative powers in a more raucous, carnivalesque way.

Ajani explained that Osun's feminine powers are universal and magnificent. "Osun is always accompanied by water, and water can overcome fire. The fiery, angry spirits are subdued by Osun. She is sensitive and is always ready to marry any other *òrìsà*. She has many husbands, including potentially threatening *òrìsàs* such as Sango (thunder and lightning), Obatala (intelligence and destiny), and Ogun (iron and war). This explains why many other *òrìsà* carvings surround her in her grove and why she often serves to balance the other *òrìsàs*' deep-seated urges to control. Consequently anyone wishing to understand Yoruba myth and masks should come to the Osun grove first."[28]

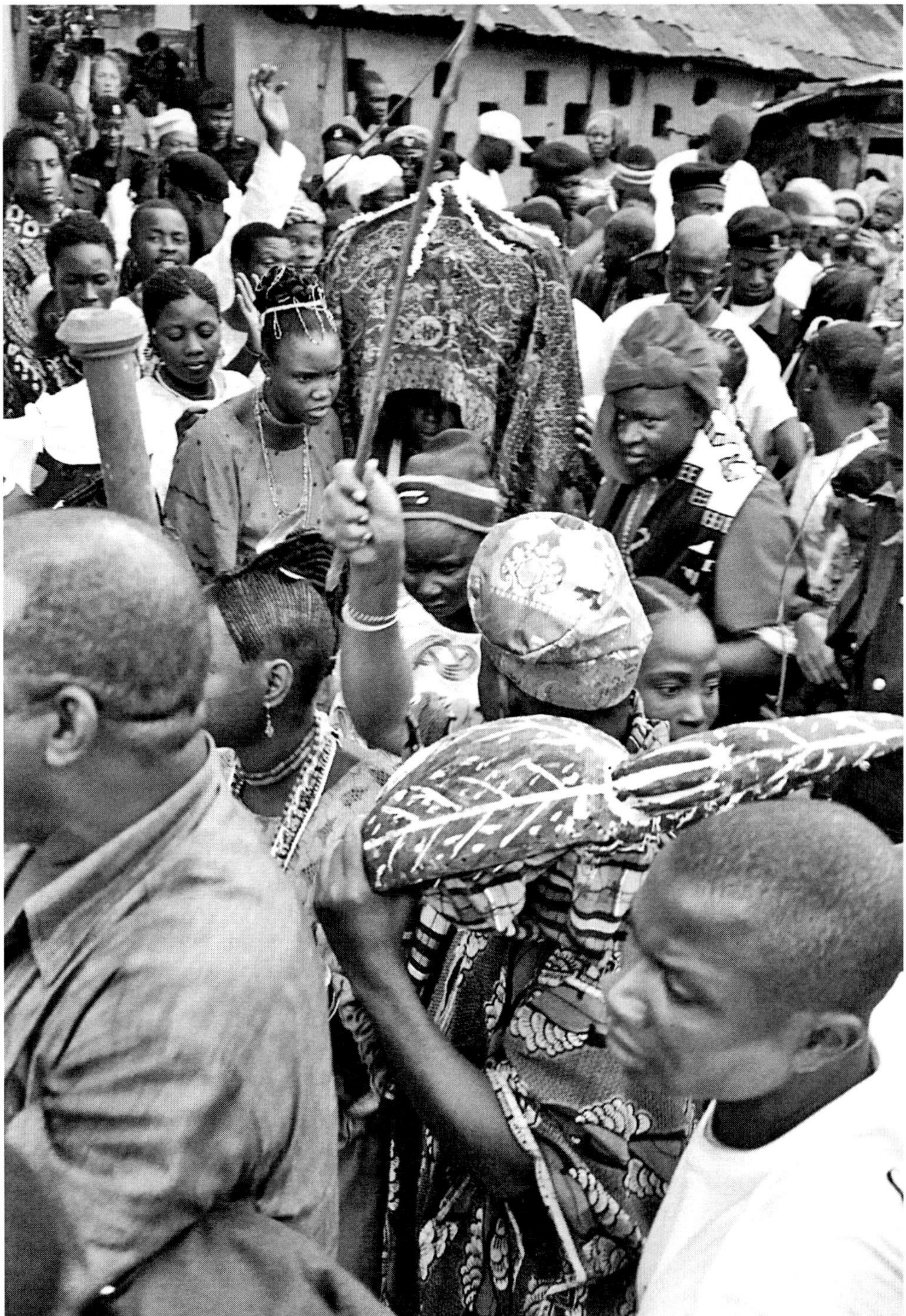

A virgin Osun devotee slowly carries a covered calabash of sacred *otonporo* masks from the center of town down to the river bank for the 2006 Osun Festival, in Osogbo, Nigeria. Photographer: Adigun Ajani.

Contemporary Yoruba theatrical masked ritual celebrations involving the ancestors, women, commerce, or rebirth continue not only in Nigeria, but also in areas of Brazil, Cuba, and Haiti where Yoruba slaves were brought in earlier centuries. Even after an extensive passage of time, the masks and celebrations beyond Nigeria uncannily resemble those of the motherland. And Yoruba mask makers in Osogbo and Ile-Ife, Nigeria (at least a select minority), still beckon and cajole the *Egungun*, *Gèlèdé*, *Epa*, Osun, and other *òrìsà* spirits to life. Only Olodumare knows how long future mask makers will continue in the Yoruba tradition when confronted by so many contemporary daily distractions from abroad as well as from within.

Chewan Secret Society Mask Makers for the Nyau Gule Wamkulu (Great Dance) *in Malawi*

While mask makers I've interviewed worldwide are usually forthcoming about their artistic effort, some belong to secret societies that forbid discussions about the craftsmanship, form, and substance of their masks. These secret societies invariably support and protect religious rituals, and are not restricted to the African continent. (Freemasons in the United States come to mind, though their secret society does not involve masks, and the Hopi in New Mexico are reticent to reveal the underpinnings of their masked ritual performances.) There are several secret societies in Africa.

I had heard of an extensive collection of masks exhibited at the Mua Mission's *Chamare*

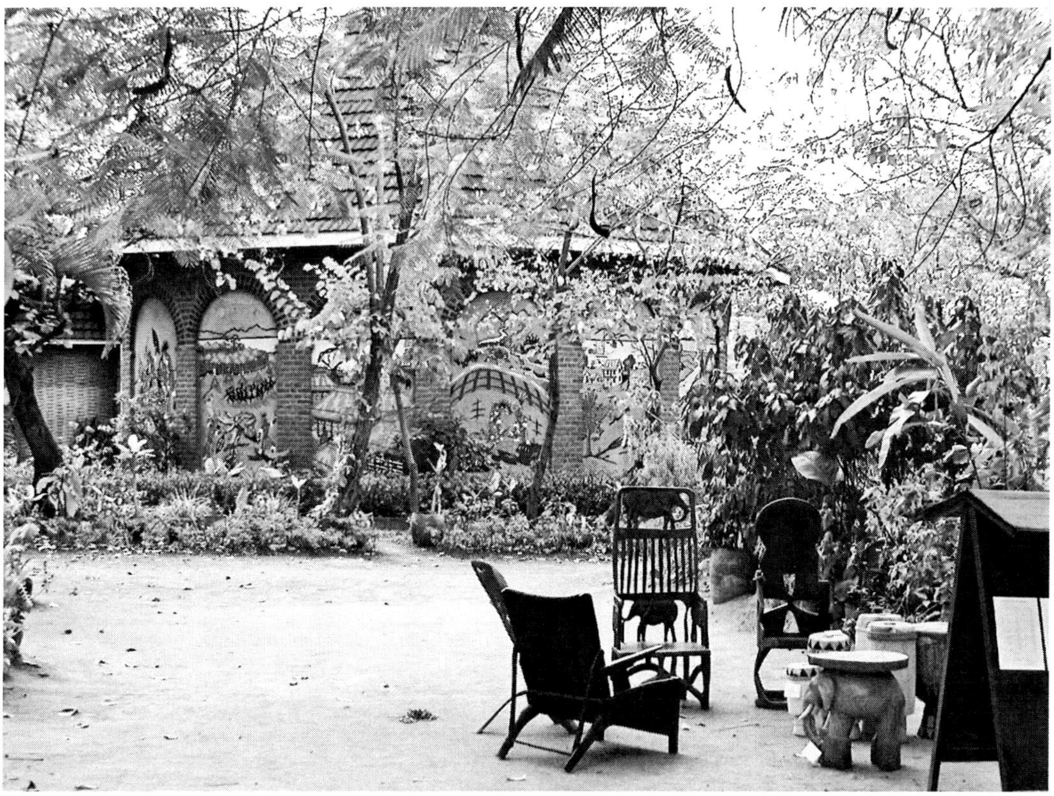

The *Chamare* Museum at *KuNgoni* Center of Culture and Art at the Mua Mission near Dedza, Malawi.

Museum in Malawi. After learning that these masks were created by Chewa mask carvers belonging to the *Nyau* Secret Society, I decided to visit the area to see examples of the masks and to learn more about the process of these mask makers; fully cognizant that I would not be eligible to interview them. Fr. Claude Boucher, a *Nyau* Secret Society member who has lived among a Chewa community as a Catholic priest at the Mua Mission outside Dedza since the late sixties, agreed to meet with me. He established the KuNgoni Center of Culture and Art in 1976 to promote the art and skills of the region's citizens and by 1999 he completed the construction and layout of the *Chamare* Museum, which exhibits over four hundred masks associated with the *Nyau* Secret Society and its *Gule wamkulu* rituals. He also has a substantial private collection of *nyau* masks.

Chewa predecessors probably came into the Mozambique, Zambia, and Malawi areas during the first millennium B.C.E. Bantu migrations from what is now Nigeria and Cameroon. A Zaire cave painting depicts a type of *nyau* (*Kayisa Maliro*) mask dating as far back as 992 C.E.[29] Recent interpretations of cave paintings combined with oral traditional stories suggest that the various groups who claim Chewa ancestors (and their immediate Phiri predecessors) date back only to the most recent millennium. Ngoni invasions in the nineteenth century led to domination of the Chewa and yet the Chewa religion and culture ultimately usurped those of the conquerors.[30]

The Chewa mask makers perform in the *gule wamkulu* (the great dance) also referred to as *pemphero lalikulu* (the great prayer) ritual ceremonies which honor the ancestors as part of puberty initiations (male and female), chief coronations, and funeral rites.[31] Chewa boys between the age of twelve and fifteen are initiated into the *Nyau* Secret Society by leaving their mothers and joining the men (from area villages) in the bush where they are tutored in the ways of village law and Chewa cultural values. They participate in these masked ceremonies by creating masks for themselves that represent aspects of what they have learned during the initiation. While participating in the initiation rites, they improvise the creation of temporary masks using available natural materials. Their elders can also commission masks created by very skilled carvers in the area. Only after the boys have completed the initiation can they assume membership within the *Nyau* Secret Society and the mantle of manhood. This graduation allows them to participate in the sacred masked funeral rites that ensure safe passage of the deceased members of the community into the ancestor spirit world. Without these rites, the Chewa believe that the dead spirits would roam the village and haunt family members.[32]

Douglas Curran, a Canadian photographer and film maker who lived within Chewa communities for several years (ultimately as a *Nyau* Secret Society initiate), points out that the *nyau* mask makers appropriately create *nyau* masks in the *dambwe*, a secluded section of the community graveyard. The *dambwe* serves as both a workshop for constructing the large zoomorphic mask structures and an entry point into the spirit world.[33]

The *nyau* wooden and feather masks represent the spirits of the ancestor world and include important animal spirits that are revered as ancestors of humans. The distinctive basketry mask structures (enveloping the entire body) most notably evoke the wild antelope spirit known as *Kasiya Maliro* which leads souls into the world beyond death.[34] Masked spirits such as *Mkango* (the fierce prancing lion), *Woiepa Sakwea* (Born Ugly Must Not Be Sad), and *Kasiya Maliro* (the supreme antelope figure of Mother Earth[35]) come to life as the initiates respond to the teachings of their male elders. A mask of the Portuguese slaver *Apatakasi*, reminiscent of the slave trade practices centuries ago, can still be found in the masquerades. The primordial masked spirits, particularly those representing the wild animals such as the elephant (*Njobvu*), the supreme antelope (*Kasiya Maliro*), and the python (*Ndondo*), continue as traditionally dominant figures in the *gule wamkulu* celebrations. The number of the masked spirits slowly increases with time as recently dead spirits join the ancestral world. Some evolve over time with embellishment and others fade away as the collective group memory of them fades.

Other *nyau* masked spirits project satirical or demonic dimensions to help educate the younger community in maintaining social and cultural behavior codes, particularly regarding sexual guidelines and taboos. The mask of *Pedegu*, the hapless and impotent orphan who ignored his parents' admonishments to plan for the future, is a favorite. As new social issues and tensions arise, *nyau* mask makers create masks that help draw attention to problems such as the need to confront the AIDS epidemic.[36]

Similar spontaneous satirical masked events have been seen in traditional *commedia* performances, Carnival street performances, or *Hahoe* masked performances in South Korea as humorous, witty responses that identify topical community concerns and frustrations. The satirical *nyau* masks, wherever they show up, invariably function as a release for social tensions. *Gule wamkulu* rituals and celebrations avoid humorless, didactic presentations, yet their overriding agenda seriously emphasizes parameters for appropriate living. The masked ritual performances demonstrate reverence for the dead along with ancestral community values, lead newly deceased spirits beyond the grave, and request that the ancestors encourage God (*Chauta*) to send rain.

I asked Fr. Boucher why the Chewa feel compelled to subscribe to a masked secret society, especially since this group summarizes and promotes time-honored cultural and religious traditions of the community. Why would a society want to hide its cherished values rather than share them with others beyond its immediate community? Conversely, how might a secret society benefit the group at large when a substantial number of members within it (most of the opposite gender) are excluded from membership? His response reflects the wisdom of his own perspective as a priest, artist, historian, and businessman.

> Historically, the concept of taboo [forbidden knowledge] has served societies well. Some forms of knowledge are not readily accessible to certain groups. Some groups need protection from certain areas of knowledge. Gender roles are very specific in Chewa society. Women restrict issues of feminine fertility to themselves. Men balance women's mysterious power to procreate with their own separate, exclusive power to organize and create the *gule wamkuu* masquerades. A taboo culture can be very delicate. By limiting access to knowledge about the *gule wamkulu* process, the *Nyau* masquerades serve a larger purpose. Like any theatrical accessory, if you know how it is created the fun is gone. You lose the illusion. They [the Chewa community members] understand that the masked characters come from another world as a way of virtually projecting the Chewa cosmology.[37]

He references a key component of any successful artistic effort. Art functions as an illusion in order to reveal a more complex level of reality.

I am reminded of Victoria Nelson's similar statement regarding the experience of artistic effort in her book *The Secret Life of Puppets*: "To go higher, you must first go lower. But *caveat lector:* those in the know view the process as irreversible. What comes out of the hole, the hole of this book that you must crawl into [i.e. experience], will not be the same as what went in."[38] Clearly the transformative potential in a *nyau* masked performance demands a level of secrecy in order for the artistic magic to function. Yet the Chewa also recognize the protocol of secrecy as another way to establish more crucial understanding at a higher level and not immediately accessible to the passerby. The complexities of this understanding

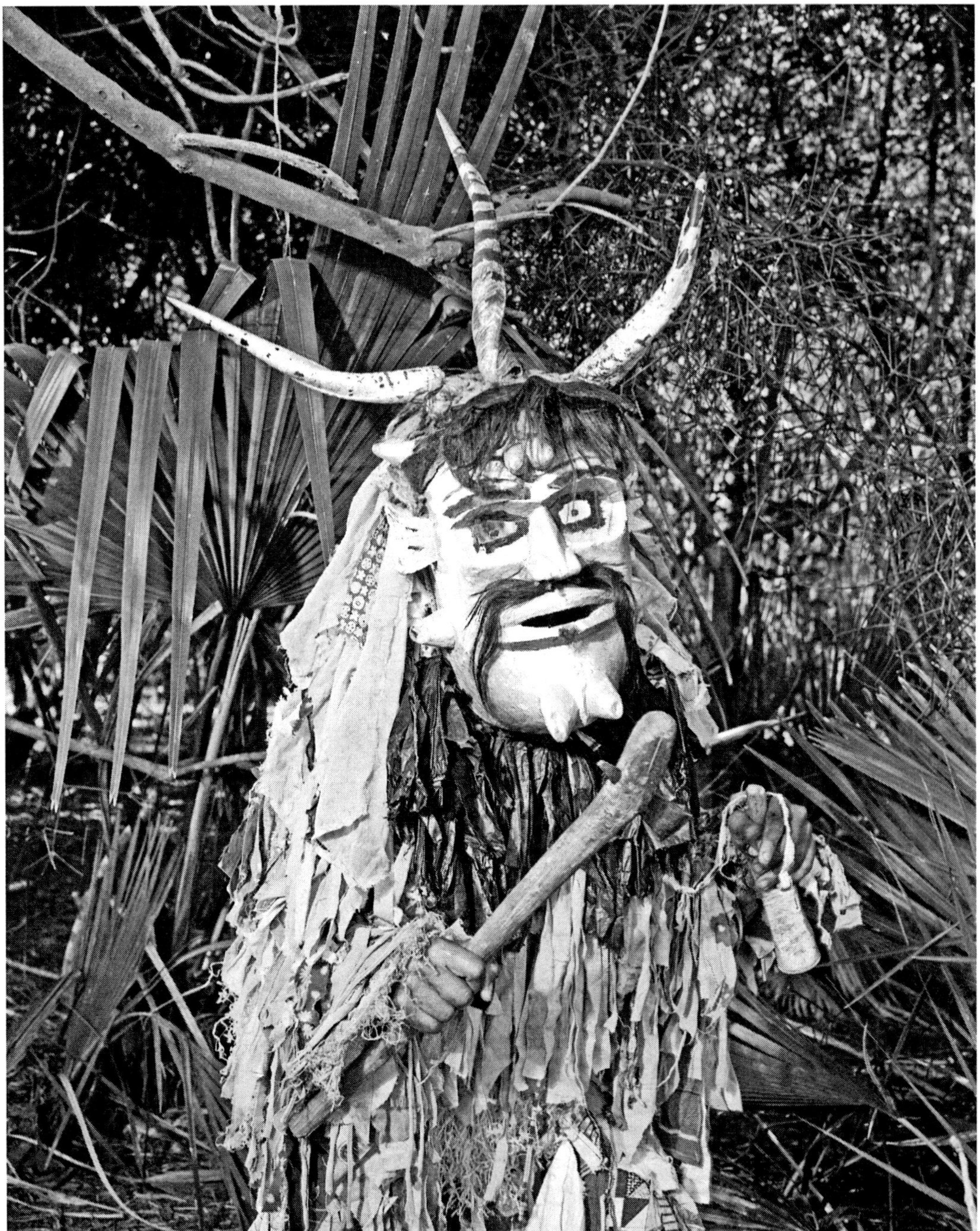

Example of *Nyau* Secret Society Mask called *Kondola.* According to Douglas Curran, as Chewa culture undergoes changing pressures and influences, the mask also transforms to reflect and engage new paradigms. *Kondola* originated as *Msakambewa* (the Mouse Hunter), later became *To Ndola* (a man employed in the Zambian copper mining town of the same name), and ultimately—due to the evils of urban living—became a woman chaser known as *Chizonono* (one who is contaminated with gonorrhea). Photographer: Douglas Curran.

demand a higher level of commitment. Only *Nyau* Secret Society initiates who have expended exceptional commitment are capable of more fully appreciating their world order.

Of course the uninitiated can appreciate fragmentary aspects of *gule wamkulu* celebrations, but at a reduced level of understanding. Masked characters such as the *Kasiya Maliro* have such multi-dimensional meanings that each member of the community will understand it and experience it according to the maturity level of the viewer. In fact, Laurel Birch Aguilar asserts that the most intrinsic element of the Chewa culture, the *Kasiya Maliro* mask, is a "triumphant work of art that discloses a totality of *Nyau* cosmology within one single form." She goes on to describe the *Kasiya Maliro* as revealing "a grasping of the understanding of life behind death, of life behind the spirit of the deceased, of man behind the mask."[39] I would add that the concept of *Kasiya Maliro* triumphs precisely because it can be grasped at varying degrees of understanding for the initiates and non-initiates alike.

Primary Research on *Nyau* Mask Makers from *Nyau* Secret Society Initiates

I have tried to get a sense of the creative process of the *nyau* mask makers by exploring the socio-religious fabric that inspires them and by studying finely detailed samples from the *Chamare* Museum's masks in addition to those found in Father Boucher's vast private collection of *gule wamkulu* masks. Ultimately my Western sensibility does not allow for an integrated appreciation of the *nyau* mask creation process. I can only conjecture, though interviews with Boucher and correspondence with Douglas Curran, who have intimate understanding of the motivations and challenges confronting these contemporary mask makers. Aguilar also spent several years with Chewa communities and participated in the female *Chinamwali* initiation rites. Despite her gender, she eventually acquired initiation into the predominantly male *Nyau* Secret Society. (Older, esteemed Chewa women also occasionally qualify for initiation.) Her book, *Inscribing the Mask*, provides an in-depth description and analysis of *nyau* masks. Her detailed descriptions, as well as my interviews with Boucher, have helped to substantially increase my appreciation of the complexities of *nyau* mask preparation. Those who have spent years with the Chewa can more extensively translate complex concepts of Chewa mask making without divulging trusted secrets. At one point, Chewa Chief Chitule who guided Curran through the mysteries of *nyau*, assured him that as a foreigner, Curran had the potential to draw more respectful worldwide attention to *nyau* cosmology than many Chewa, and Chitule actually encouraged Curran to film and photograph the masked celebrations.[40] Kenji Yoshida and Aguilar also have published a number of exciting photos of the masks in action at *gule wamkulu* events.

Curran acknowledges particular considerations of the *nyau* mask makers and carvers:

> The language of Chichewa is not abstract in itself and the Chewa don't think in the same manner about things as Westerners do. Many will create a mask out of a dream and if you ask what considerations caused them to make a mask in a particular way they will simply state that they dreamed it. One should not expect to look for direct answers to conceptual or hypothetical positions of decision-making on the part of the carver.
>
> Additionally, mask carving is changing for one of the most immediate and practical reasons: there is no money in it! The amount that a dancer can pay for a mask, given his ability to generate money in the form of dance gratuities (*kafupa*), is very little. Consequently the [financial] return for everyone in the economic structure is negligible. Never make the assumption that the guys don't go where the money is. It is no longer to be found in *gule wamkulu* as a means of income redistribution.[41]

Curran suggests avoiding conclusions about the creative processes of *nyau* mask makers within a metaphysical context. He believes that the Chewa, as well as most Africans, tend to be less direct than Westerners, that is, less objective in their way of referring to sensibilities.

Curran's premise summarizes the challenge of my inquiry. I have personally interviewed and written about mask makers in several countries and I have presented concise personal accounts of their approaches to mask making while comparing and contrasting their creative challenges from a global perspective. Until coming to the Mua Mission in Malawi, I had maintained a consistent format in my interviews with these mask makers but those belonging to the *Nyau* Secret Society could not meet with me. Both Curran and Boucher assured me in advance that I would not be able to actually speak to Chewa *nyau* mask makers out-of-hand.

No doubt, without actual interviews I have a less complete perspective as to plausible motivations and challenges behind the creation of their masks. But Fr. Boucher has lived with the Chewa community at the Mua Mission since the late sixties and his interview added substantial insight. I have also examined the spiritual context associated with *nyau* mask making events at the initiation rites, as well as by highlighting colors, characterization, and materials of these masks based on informed accounts of how they function within Chewa rituals. I have relied largely on research by (non–Chewa) *Nyau* Secret Society members Boucher, Curran, Ott, Aguilar, and Yoshida to gather important background on motivations for the *nyau* mask maker's work in order to suggest potentially distinct challenges for traditional mask makers in this part of the world, as compared to findings based on interviews with other mask makers.

CHEWA CREATION MYTH AND RELATED SPIRITUALITY AS SEMINAL INSPIRATION FOR *NYAU* MASK MAKERS

Nyau masks in *gule wamkulu* rites and celebrations reflect elemental communal values *(mwambo)* by referencing the clans' tribal creation myth. This myth, briefly summarized, hearkens back to a primordial time when God split open the sky and came down with the first humans and animals [even though the animals are considered to be ancestors of humans] to the top of Kaphirinthiwa mountain accompanied by pouring rain. All enjoyed prosperity and peace until humans discovered fire (some say sorcery) which when consequently misused, caused much destruction and fear. Aided by a spider's silken thread, God returned to the sky in exasperation and decreed that humans must die. Only after death would he allow them to join him in spiritual forms. Separation from God eventually caused the rain to stop, the earth to dry up, and humans to regularly (seasonally) beg for a return of rain and a renewal of life.

The Chewa creation story assumes elements of a typical agrarian myth with its focus on life, death, and regeneration cycles as well as adherence to community values, while the Chewa religion still supports elements of an older era as a hunter/gatherer society by incorporating animal and ancestor worship; also relying on shamans/herbalists (each village has its community *Sing'anga*) for the well being of each community. This masked shamanic figure interrogates and heals sick people as well as interprets dreams.[42]

Though not part of the *gule wamkulu* ancestral world of *nyau* masked figures, the *sing'anga* regularly communicates with divine forces including the ancestors. He does not participate in actual theatrical styled presentations, but the *Sing'anga* artfully organizes and performs rituals. The *Sing'anga* promotes healing based on the assumption that creation as a whole, including man, trees, and animals all go back to the same cosmic origin: finally to God.[43]

Water and Fertility Imagery Used with Dreams as Inspiration for *Nyau* Masks

Curran states that the *nyau* mask makers derive much of their inspiration during a dreaming event. Boucher confirms that this part of the mask-making process involves "fishing for spiritual ancestors seen in an upside down reflection of the sacred pool"[44] in order to create the masks in the bush during the initiation rites. Yoshida also describes this event similarly: "Women are told that men 'fish up' *nyau* out of the water there."[45] Curran notes that [masked] wild animals are "fished up from water at the center of a deep pool at the center of the sacred grove using eggs as bait,"[46] bearing subliminal association with feminine creative powers.

While women bear responsibility for creating life, the *nyau* masked performances (particularly during the funereal rites) empower men to perform divinely appropriate spiritual action. Men virtually direct the deceased member into the ancestral spirit world with the aid of the masked *Kasiya Maliro*. Or they conjure ancestral spirits via masked figures to advise and admonish the community. Men create their masks using female aquatic images to "give birth" to their masked spirits. (Aquatic images are also prevalent in the Chewa creation myth involving rain and rain ritual foundations.)

The water and egg imagery also calls to mind not only literal physical states of creation but also dream-like states that induce unconscious metaphorical desires for vitality and transformation. How appropriate for a *nyau* mask maker to initiate his work in this way. Could this "Chewa fishing dream process" used to create *nyau* masks have a corresponding resemblance to creative processes used by some Western mask making and masked performances? I explore this premise further in chapter 7.

Susan Smith in her book, *Masks in the Modern Drama*, believes that "the urge to understand and reconcile the parts of oneself through the mask is an ancient one" and cites Carl Jung who "observed that primitive man [assuming that his 'bush soul' was incarnate in a wild animal with which he had a psychic identity] practiced 'mystical participation' by wearing the mask of the animal." She compares this ancient practice with contemporary theatrical presentations, referring to the "externalizing of the inner self as a masked figure [that] characterizes many dream plays." Later she concludes, "As the masked projection served O'Neill, MacLeish, and other playwrights who dramatized spiritual conflicts, so it served the surrealists, who also used the dream image as a link between the material and spiritual worlds, between the private and the universal."[47]

The *nyau* masks consistently refer to those representing spirits of the dead. However, Aguilar identifies some *nyau* masks (*Chadzunda* and *Maliya*) signifying status relationships in the land of the dead that also mirror the same relationships in the living Chewa community.[48] This seems especially pertinent as the reversed masked characters are dragged up from the sacred graveyard with its mystical and metaphorical "pool of water" where they are birthed. These masked characters can represent positive, negative, and neutral forces that appear as ancestors not only in initiation rituals but during funeral rites and chief coronation events. They can also represent archetypal family groupings in everyday life.

Contrasting Tensions of Life and Death; Desire and Fear; and Ritual Role Reversals Related to Chewa Mask Imagery

As with any agrarian myth, the Chewa religion affirms a spiritual basis for the life, death, birth cycle, by believing that this cycle ultimately reflects an eternal world order.

The state of corporal existence, however, regularly confronts the duality of fear and desire. And this is universally recognized as the fundamental tension inherent in the human condition. We invariably rationalize our motivations in life based on either our inherent desires to perpetuate vitality or our inherent fears of losing vitality. Joseph Campbell succinctly refers to this state of human existence as "a wonderful, wonderful opera, except that it hurts." Central to his lifelong exploration of myths lies his summation that the myth (illustrated by the mask) as a metaphor of God artfully allows for an awareness of eternity beyond states of fear and desire.[49] Susan Smith, takes this concept even further when she asserts that the mask frequently functions as a release. When a man masks himself as aspects of an angel or a demon she argues, "He expresses first his desire to believe in the other world and, second, his fear that it may not exist. The mask is at once emblematic of his hope and his anxiety."[50]

With these elemental mask agendas in mind, consider the Chewa mask maker's reliance on two of his own mythic images: the chameleon (connoting life/birth) and the lizard (connoting death.) The chameleon not only changes its color in response to its surroundings, but also seems "lizard-like" except for its head, which looks like the head of a lizard wearing a mask! (I refer to the contrasting images that are reflected on the (Mua) Missio Banner, created in 1985 by Boucher and Tambala Mponyani and currently exhibited in Munich.[51]Martin Ott describes these figures as "always depicted together and in tension with one another."[52])

During my visit with Boucher, he recounted a related Chewa myth. "God sent the chameleon to a funeral to demonstrate to the mourners that there is life after death. The lizard overtook the chameleon in the race to get to the funeral, declaring that the chameleon and all the mourners would eventually die. But the chameleon won the virtual competition. With its independently movable eyeballs that allow it to look backward and forward simultaneously and also with its ability to change colors, the chameleon symbolized immortality and could demonstrate the triumph over death."[53]

Similarly, a full-bodied basket-woven mask of the *Kasiya Maliro* signifies these crucial aspects of Chewa cosmology most associated with the issue of death and immortality. This mask serves as the "consoler of the souls, the mask of transition, [who] dances in front of the deceased's home, and circles the grave." In the same way that the boy is reborn into the womb of this large-scale ancient mask during initiation rites, the deceased will likewise be reborn during the luminal period which follows death, led to the spirit world by the same *Kasiya Maliro* that originally gave birth to the initiate.[54] Ott compares the *Kasiya Maliro* to the dove imagery of Christianity's Holy Spirit; describing it as "the ego's integration with the subconscious; the messenger of secret wisdom."[55]

Yet this large-scale "supreme *Kasiya Maliro* messenger" takes on the look of an earth-bound horned antelope. How odd, since as a messenger spirit, this figure might have greater reason to resemble a bird. Ott's reference to the *Kasiya Maliro* as similar to Christianity's dove (as the Holy Spirit) easily relates to African totemism. Bird imagery used to suggest spiritual messengers is traditionally prevalent in many African as well as North and South American Indian communities. The *Kasiya Maliro*'s primary "earthly" function, however, as symbolic of both the womb and the tomb, justifies its animal appearance. The horns and the dramatic crescent-shape arcs of the back of the *Kasiya Maliro* mask magnify the universal dualities of this spirit that embodies qualities of angelic and demonic imagery, desire and fear, and life and death.

Surely the Chewa mask maker experiences the intense visceral fear of this mask during his initial encounter as an initiate when climbing into this great mask in the dead of night at the graveyard. Conversely he experiences the divine pleasure (as the masked *Kasiya Maliro*) of leading (or witnessing the entity leading) the deceased spirit's passage beyond the grave. Yoshida describes this masked messenger as "that which abandons the deceased" and the *Kasiya Maliro* is immediately burned after returning from the grave for a final dance. The smoke from the giant mask disappears into the air, signaling that the deceased has become an ancestral spirit.[56] On some level, subliminal or otherwise, Chewa undoubtedly recognize the dualistic aspects of this mask's horns and back crescents as compounding the *Kasiya Maliro*'s reflection of such contrasting powers. Aguilar, in interviews with *Nyau* Secret Society members, quotes several, stating that the two crescent curves at the *Kayisa Maliro*'s back are arcs that can be likened to "the rising and the setting sun."[57] The highly curved back of *Kasiya Maliro* also represents a stylized womb, confirming its status as the "mother of life."

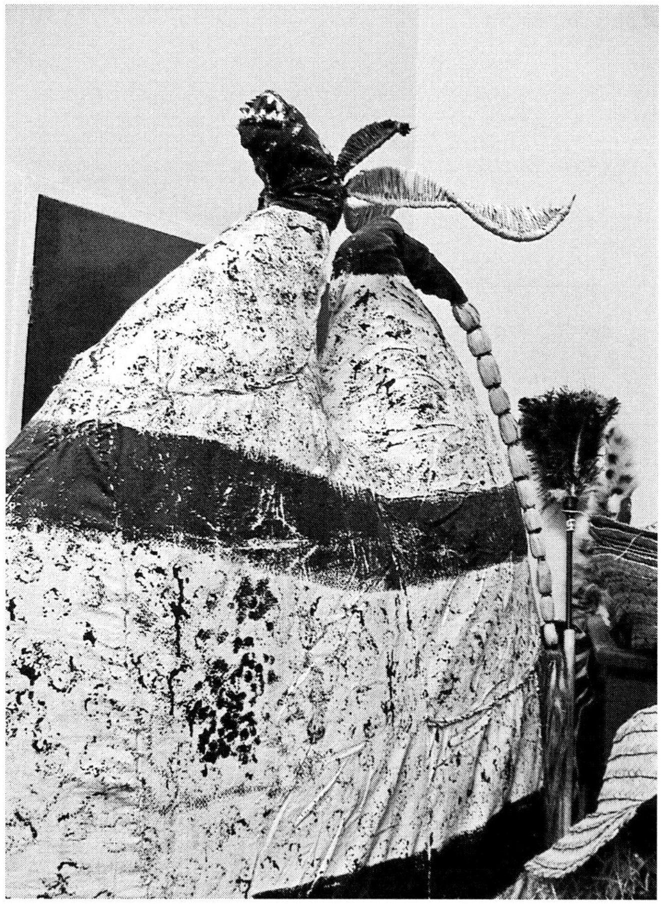

A *Kasiya Maliro* body mask that uses woven dried grasses. A fabric cloth adheres to the top of the basket-like mask that is then painted. This mask, over five feet high, is part of Fr. Boucher's private collection at the Mua Mission in Malawi.

Other indications of the duality of desire and fear in the *gule wamkulu* performances include the frequent introduction of negative *nyau* personalities or spirits to demonstrate spirits which the community members want to avoid. Such masked role reversals can take many forms in the world of *nyau*. *Makanja* dances on stilts, elevating himself to enhance his reputation and reflecting arrogance; Pedegu becomes ineffectual due to his own laziness but hopelessly desires respect;[58] and "Modern Maria," derived from the Virgin Mary (always played by a male) can occasionally appear a bit too comely to evoke reverence.[59]

Boucher describes the men in a Chewa village as feeling like "strangers" in a matriarchal society that allows them little authority. They are able to reverse "feelings of oppression" by participating in the creative state of making masks. He describes rigid codes of behavior in the culture that inhibit a relaxed frame of mind. The *gule wamkulu* celebrations allow them the chance to let off steam,[60] and provide a forum for ultimate role reversals.

CURRENT CHALLENGES FOR THE *NYAU* MASK MAKER

Curran describes the *Kasiya Maliro* mask as one made with long slender branches of bamboo soaked in water to become rounded ribs. Palm leaves are wetted to be woven into jaws and the head, while thick mud is smeared over the covering of corn husks to accentuate the eyes and decorative patterning.[61]

Boucher acknowledges remarkably improvised creativity that current versions of the *Kasiya Maliro* demonstrate. In addition to this mask's traditional use of wood, palm oil, sisal, rags, domestic animal skins, and corn husk leaves, some current versions use a synthetic woven jute material made out of plastic. One version in Boucher's private collection is covered in painted cloth glued onto the basketry.

Traditional masks have always used locally available materials, and Boucher does not object to the incorporation of plastic today for a revered *nyau* mask. But he thinks that readily purchased, mass-produced plastic masks from South Africa that project contemporary global personalities such as Charlie Chaplin or George Bush destroy the integrity and relevancy of the hand-crafted *gule wamkulu* mask celebrations. He prefers not to see them in this context and, according to Aguilar, some Chewa citizens agree with Boucher. She mentions that during *gule wamkulu* celebrations, audience members repeatedly pointed out that sacks used as costumes have more prestige than dancers who use Western clothing with additional strips of cloth. Older masqueraders automatically receive more respect. Animal hides indicate more rank and respect and indeed animal figures always outrank the other masked figures because animals are considered the ancestors of humans.[62] Curran describes this use of fur from wild animals as cementing the connection between the masked dancer called *Chirombo* (singular) or *Zilombo* (plural) with the image of a wild animal. Furthermore, the image allows that dancer to ignore traditional community standards of behavior.[63]

Boucher acknowledges other significant challenges for the contemporary mask makers. Back at the turn of the twentieth century, *nyau* masks tended to be larger in scale than they are now. Nowadays the masks tend to be similar in scale to the masquerader's head and face, requiring more intricate detail. He also mentioned that whereas the costume can be simple for the night performances, the day costumes can require more elaborately painted cloth.

The price of the carved mask, even if created by a professional, tends to be rather low and the dancer always paints his own body. The non-commercial religious performances have traditionally relied on modest support from audience members who spontaneously offered a few coins to the dancer who then shared that stipend with the mask maker. But during recent droughts and weak economy, mask makers are tempted to commercialize their work and to take short cuts. (I saw tourist versions of *gule wamkulu* masks for sale in Mtakataka.) Also the younger generation still participates but the generation gap between the youth and the elders increasingly results in more superfluous tricks and shallow events. Boucher can remember earlier times when local materials such as ash and charcoal substituted for paints, giving a more traditionally authentic appearance. But in recent decades purchased paints make the mask coverings glossy and vivid.[64] Aguilar noted that blue *nyau* masks started to appear during the '80s and I noticed one such blue mask in front of a shop outside Dedza. Masks are continually evolving into new characters such as one with black hair, full beard, and moustache that currently indicates a Near-Eastern Muslim teacher (*Malimu*). Consequently, the style of the masks continues to change in spite of the emphasis to maintain traditional effects.

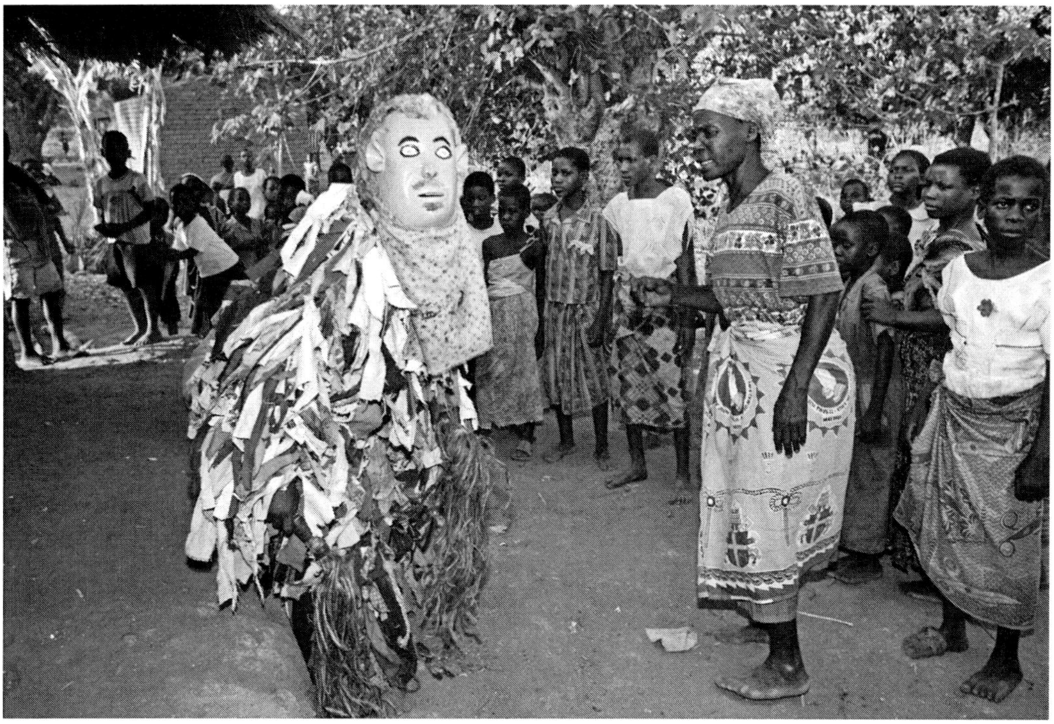

The *nyau* mask of Pombo, a wise and well-respected elder, is danced at *mphalo* (funeral ceremony) at Kanyere village, Kachindamot district, Malawi. Photographer: Douglas Curran.

Creative Protocol and Characteristics of the *Nyau* Mask

Fr. Boucher initially cautioned against positioning a typical *nyau* mask maker as the central creator of the *gule wamkulu* rites and celebrations. "Generally, you do not simply see a carver who creates the mask. A community member or family might commission an individual carver to create a mask that displays the characteristics of someone recently deceased, or a community committee might commission him to create a *nyau* figure, but a new masked personality will undergo significant development via planning and approval by a committee designated to maintain integrity of purpose and quality. Indeed, virtually all serious masks must receive final committee approval before being included in the celebrations."

He describes this group interaction in a way that bears marked resemblance to that of a mask maker on staff at a typical professional theatre company in the United States, where each member contributes creative effort based on group discussions with and approval by the design and technical staff, actors during costume fittings, and directors during technical rehearsals.

Boucher explained that the *gule wamkulu* mask maker describes his process as going hunting (or fishing) and he looks for the footsteps of the mask. He does not think of the mask as being invented out of the blue by himself. The mask maker follows the footprint path of the mask (the character's actions) in order to see the mask revealed. Boucher went on to say, "Whether one carver creates or an entire committee creates, rule out the idea that a single artist inspires the form." He reiterated that mask creation is ultimately a community event requiring participation of many members who set guidelines for each successful mask.

Communities in this part of the world consistently recognize the power of the group over that of the individual. Only recently, he acknowledged, has the Chewa community begun to realize the Western Renaissance concept of the potential for the individual's impact on the group at-large. *Gule wamkulu* assumes a creation process based on the group at-large and this creation process spans preceding millennia way before the formation of Chewa society.[65]

According to Boucher, a successful *nyau* mask must evoke a specific spirit and must clearly indicate its good or evil characteristics. The mask must avoid looking too crude and the opening for the eyes should not be so big that the viewer can see the dancer's face behind it. The costume surrounding the mask typically incorporates everyday clothing and materials to improvise an appropriate effect that no longer resembles the original functions of the wearing apparel. The masquerade itself must follow set rules and proceed in an appropriate order. Two versions of the same spirit can dance together, but each will dance according to a different beat and look slightly different.

Boucher described two categories of *nyau* masks: those created and used at night, primarily for the initiation ceremonies, and those created for use during the day for community funeral rites and coronation celebrations. The initiates improvise the creation of the night masks, supervised by their mentors. They work in the moonlight or within a patch of darkness at the graveyard near a body of water. The masks primarily function to hide the face of the performer and are destroyed immediately after the performance. The initiates are taught how to use local materials such as bamboo grass and palm leaves and how to incorporate them into figures with weaving techniques. Some initiates go on to create exceptionally interesting masks. The costumes are made in the same way, improvised with natural materials. The day masks can include carved masks which can return for repeated performances and sometimes they are specially commissioned by skilled carvers.

Some masks for characters like *Chadzunda* (the archetypal depiction of an old wise Chewa chief) are immediately recognizable even though they vary greatly in terms of facial features and color. Usually *Chadzunda* has a black (or deep red) mask and has middle-aged or elderly features. He projects wisdom and a kind heart as a fatherly figure. A recently deceased Chewa chief might actually inspire the appearance of an upcoming *Chadzunda* mask, making features of the deceased quite recognizable.[66]

Not all *nyau* masks are created in the graveyards, but all masks intended for *gule wamkulu* events are created in a secluded area. The mask maker needs to create the actual physical aspects of the mask privately. Even the materials must be gathered during the night or surreptitiously. Because the *nyau* mask holds such close association with the dead, it also holds potential associations with witchcraft, and a mask maker must be very brave to begin one. One mask maker told Aguilar that it took three days to make a mask, but that was working at top speed. They usually take a week or longer.

From my personal observations, confirmed by Boucher, three basic colors are seen in *nyau* mask work: black (generally considered the most powerful because it signifies aspects of both fertility and death and signals the coloring of the soil for both planting and for burying), red (and versions of pink and brown tones indicating both positive and negative forces of intensity), and white (considered least indicative of power as the color of faded produce, ash, and bones). No set ruling is apparent regarding specific colors for specific masks though some characters tend to maintain certain characteristics or colors such as *Chadzunda*, who is consistently black or deep red.

The *Kasiya Maliro* also utilizes a consistent color; seen as white or the natural light straw color of the grasses or maize husks that form the body of the mask,[67] which ordinarily would imply a lack of power according to the use of color for the masks in general. Yet in this specific case, the light or white coloring of the *Kasiya Maliro* predictably makes a strong statement regarding its dual functions. On one hand, it is made from the dried, light-colored straw grasses thrown away with the trash. Yet it comes to life during the initiation rites; making a gleaming statement in the moonlight that evokes states of new beginnings in birth and regeneration. Aguilar quotes Chewa descriptions of the *Kasiya Maliro* as "rising from the pure, lustral waters, white and bright. The deep pool is on the underside, the depths of the world, the darkness of the womb and grave, the place where the sun hides after setting, the place of the moon during the day. In the season of dryness, it comes from the rains, and performs in the white, pale moonlight of the nocturnal dance, and in the brilliance of the sun in day. The bright white light is said to shine on the white-like maize husks as a vision of life even in the clothes of its own dead husks."[68]

Of the three mask makers that Aguilar interviewed, one is a dancer as well as a carver. Each learned his basic craft techniques from other mask carvers (rather than from formal training) though each has his own distinctive style in carving.[69] Not all *nyau* masks resemble the physical appearance of an ancestor; however, Aguilar states that likenesses to real people compound the metaphorical potential of the mask for the community to witness. I paraphrase her insightful descriptions below because they point to the inherent artistry of these mask makers as well as their technical virtuosity in capturing likenesses:

1. The mask is merely a wooden image of a human face, but at once human and at once wooden.
2. The mask, as an ancestor — especially a recently deceased one — resembles the deceased when he or she lived and yet the mask maker does not always have knowledge of the actual resemblance of the deceased.
3. The mask represents the deceased; at the same time, it is present again as in life.
4. The mask is an ancestor but also a spirit; it is at once dead and at once alive.
5. The masked dancer is at once the ancestor and at once his own being.
6. The mask is at once the ancestor in death and at once the ancestor "alive" as he used to be.[70]

Aguilar presents the concept of the *nyau* ancestor mask as an iconic summation of the deceased that allows for the audience to actually "feel" the presence of the ancestor as the dancer creates former actions of the deceased as he or she lived. "The fiction, the suspended reality [of the deceased], was 'felt,' I believe, as the people stood silently and almost breathlessly as the masked dancer appeared beside the grave."[71] Her observation underscores the necessity for tremendous talent on the part of the masked dancer to create this cathartic event.

Again, we can reflect back on the Chewa chameleon, with its ability to see forward and backward simultaneously. In Chewa cosmology, one recognizes eternity aided by the masks of the ancestors. Curran cautions that *nyau* masks and rituals have a range of meanings for different individuals even within the ranks of the Chewa.[72] And yet *gule wamkulu* masqueraders strive to perpetuate a state of certainty within the fluctuations of existence by relying on the ingenuity of their mask makers.

American Mask Maker and Master Teacher Bruce Marrs

Most serious mask makers — those who spend years developing their craft and reputation — acknowledge that they do not become wealthy based on their efforts. Yet muses of all sorts beckon them to continue in their work, as my recent interview with Bruce Marrs confirms.

Bruce Marrs, a mask maker/performer/teacher for Dell'Arte International School of Physical Theatre for the past two decades, likes to work with his hands. Bruce Marrs' muse insists that he have his hands on form; he must grope and wonder and learn through his hands. He explains that "then there is the hand/eye thing. I see a face, in reality or in my mind, and then I try to transfer that vision through the 'mind' of my creative hand back to what my eye sees (again) which contemplates further what my hand hath wrought. My hands proceed to contemplate by sculpting and editing once again. The love affair between my eye and hand continue."[73] For Marrs, the paradox that masks reveal more than they conceal makes them personal tools to explore the mystery of who we are. Marrs' obsession rests in the ever compelling, ever constant mystery of the essential, distinctive humanity in each individual he tries to portray with his masks.

Bruce Marrs began his theatre career as a dancer, dancing with, and choreographing for, The Oregon Dance Theatre, The Human Dancing Company, and Southern Oregon Light Opera. He studied mime in Paris with Marcel Marceau, Etienne Decroux, and James Keylon. He acted a season with the Oregon Shakespeare Festival, and was a solo talking mime nightclub performer. He appeared with Vincent Price who called him the funniest mime he ever saw. In addition to teaching at Dell'Arte International School of Physical Theatre, he has been a guest teacher and director at various universities across the country.

Marrs understands the power of movement and music when combined with the mask. While living in Ashland, he had a friend whom he admired as a dancer and as a mask maker named Leo DeFlambeau. Leo's masks spoke to Marrs. Marrs says, "They invited character and movement from me. I had kinesthetic responses to his masks, and I wanted to act; to give them life and let them live in me and through me."

> I was also somebody who could "see" and draw, to some extent. Later, in 1985, I took a *commedia* workshop at Dell'Arte International. We did mask making. I was an arrogant student, the kind I don't like to teach. I wanted to be left alone to make masks, and not have the intervention of my teacher. Actually it was more passion than arrogance. My first mask was a demon-priest. I called him the Inquisitor. It was a good mask. I was interested in materials and usage from my first teacher, but not art, as I felt he didn't have much to teach me there.
>
> Later, I learned from a lot of teachers and mask makers. Gina Bastone, the crazy genius clown from Canada, taught me about large eye-holes so the actor could act with the eyes, and about shading the perimeter of the mask to give depth as well as the necessity to really sand spackle to make papier-mâché smooth. Then I taught mask making, and eventually taught students who had more talent, or more of a history of inquiry into art than I did. They went on to become mask makers, took everything they learned from me, and advanced on their own talent. I stole from them, competed with them, learned viscerally, and essentially learned a great deal from these students. They included Joe Dieffenbacher, Xstine Cook, and even students of theirs. I am so grateful for their creative leaps forward.[74]

While Marrs often performs solo using his own masks, he has a history of collaborating with others on theatre, film, television, and dance projects. He adapts well to various situations. He says:

> If I have plaster positives of the actors, or if I have the good fortune of time and resources to make those positives of the actors, then in working with those positives, I am both consciously and unconsciously responding to the relationship between the actors' faces and

> those of the characters they will play. In other words, I do my best, but something better than my best frequently emerges. There are qualities and life essences that come into the mask that I didn't consciously design. Here again is the mystery that makes this work so fascinating. Then, if the production team is smart, they will allow me time with the actors and the masks, to give the actors a few mask-performance/craft notions that will help them to play the mask and to discover the unintended nuances of the mask.
>
> I enjoy directing physical theatre, but I greatly enjoy working under a director, too. I enjoy the relationship with a director, not being responsible for all that a director does, but the way that music directors and choreographers and designers work with directors. I enjoy taking what vision the director can communicate with me, running it through my own vision, and advancing the whole of it. I enjoy the co-discovery with a director and a cast. We are all artists. We are using the known to explore the unknown. Why else would we do this?[75]

Most muses demand some sort of quiet personal preparation that involves focusing or praying or meditating when beginning a project. How does Marrs psychologically and emotionally prepare for a new project in mask work? "This question reminds me of Krisnamurti's considerations about the notion of meditation. One meditates, one finishes meditating, and then is not meditating?" he responds.

> I'm never not an artist, and the bank is never empty. Well, that's probably not true. I'm often stupid and dull. But I think that my own interest is almost always at work. Paddling a kayak against a wind is like the drama that ends up in a mask. The pain for the price of existence doesn't get dissipated between life experience and the process of creating a mask. Beauty, a Goddess herself, thrashes us around and demands our witness. Yes, I acknowledge her demands, but I know her biblically through my own hands. So when I begin a mask, I know that I have begun already, long ago. My hands are ready to discover. There is already a question that I have been asking, about eyes, about corners of the lips, about movement as large as the human scale and as small as the nuance of mannerisms. I'm already prepared to investigate these questions through clay and the movement of my hands. I don't want to purify or clear anything out first. Life does not exist independently of my torture and stupidity and glory and loss and foolish hope. I do not want to disavow all that experience from my new investigation. Rather, I want to learn, to reflect on all that muck, mire, and beauty of the movement that moves me to create.[76]
>
> All this does not diminish the need to consciously prepare. If I am to make a mask of an African Queen, then I will want to look at African masks, I will want to study African faces, and wonder about queenliness, the price of power, aloneness — all that — but that inquiry is wonder about all that, wonder about animals, about the notion of awareness that makes us supposedly different from animals, about the paradox of our animal and divine nature, and about the formlessness that is the design behind all form. This is my meditation. There is no place to rest from it.[77]

Masks have such power in exaggeration that they often relate on some mythic or archetypal level. When asked how extensively he incorporates myth and archetypal images in his mask work, Marrs replies, "Well, I don't know about myth. I guess if it is a true myth, then the images are archetypal. Archetypal means that the images, or memories, or invocations transcend any particular culture, and translate through the limitations and prejudices of any culture. I don't respect anybody's culture. I'm not multi-cultural at all. I hold that your particular culture embarrasses you more than supports you. Get over it. Honor your ancestors, but get over their silly cultural limitations. Be a cultural traveler, a borrower, a wanderer, an artist at the service of evolution."[78]

He concludes with the following idea: "The archetypal image moves forward from the mystery of the past. It takes something truer than culture forward — it advances the human drama and the unfolding of all that through the beliefs, prejudices, and limitations of current or past cultures. It is true that some archetypes die and some are born new from an evolutionary standpoint. Stereotypes don't transcend cultures. They live and flourish in the limitations and prejudices of a particular culture, and die in the light of education, or a greater perspective. But archetypes live, and lurk, deeper than the light of our inquiry can shine, and we, as storytellers, can catch a ride on them as they move forward, beyond us."[79]

When asked how his sense of honesty and criteria for a successful mask factors into his final product, Marrs responds, "I hope I get lucky. I believe in luck. I think luck can be cultivated. I don't know about honesty. I am as honest as I am and I don't worry about it. I don't mind stealing from everyone. Any notion that I steal goes through my own fingers and that is as much purification as I might need. I don't know what honesty means. I guess it begins first with one's self. I'm in search of knowing this self. But I'm also hip to the notion that the search itself can be a distraction from knowing what is probably too close to be noticed. So, I don't know about honesty. It will take care of itself."[80]

Marrs admits that he is not interested in recreating what already exists in his conscious mind. He believes he is here to make mistakes, to take risks, to be affected by forces he doesn't necessarily understand. He wants to discover and be surprised. "If I make a good mask," he says,

> it will have something of what I intended in it, but it will have something in it that I didn't know I intended, and I will be able to see it and say, "Ah-hah!" A good mask must be interesting to look at, and remain interesting. A good mask must inform the actor, enrich, and compel. A good mask must work without the need of the actor to work so hard. A good mask requires the actor to relax and trust that the mask is working; it will require the actor to get out of the way a bit. I need to be reminded of this last notion all the time. All of us actors seem to need this reminder: to not work so hard, to trust that the mask is working, that the magic is there, and to give it the time and space to work.
>
> Those of us who make masks, though, do not perform in them need to remind ourselves of the mask's ultimate purpose. What looks good on a wall or at the crafts table does not necessarily have the power or ability to facilitate the performer's story. The temptation to incorporate extraneous detail, textures or color can too easily distract the audience.[81]

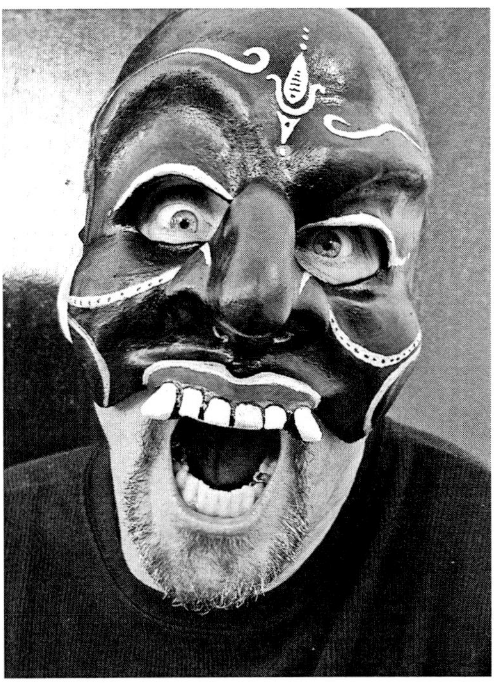

Dell'Arte International School of Physical Theatre mask maker Bruce Marrs wearing "Will's Demon," a neoprene mask.

Marrs insists that the mask either has magic or it does not. It can easily look more like a lampshade on someone's head. While the craft of the performer bears much responsibility for the success of the mask, good acting craft cannot compensate for a dead mask. There is the amazing fact that any mask, plus the actor, combines to create a third thing. With good masked performance, the whole is greater than the sum of the parts, but a great mask will shape the actors more than be shaped by them.

Marrs' techniques in mask making are discussed later in chapter 3. He has taught for over two decades at Dell'Arte International, which has been a primary influence on mask makers worldwide and its significance is examined in greater detail in chapter 5.

Trinidadian Carnival Masks Makers

Communities worldwide have used masks throughout history as a distinctive theatrical art form. Masks offer similar functions to every culture by disguising or hiding the identity of the performer; transforming the performer's personality into another personality, animal, or spirit; and protecting the performer (as well as the audience) against harm. Also, masks possess distinct characteristics and significance within each cultural community's aesthetic experience. The Carnival street masquerades found in numerous countries invariably utilize such masks and typically reflect distinctive cultural style and values in its costumes as well. Barbara Mouldin in *Carnival!* lists eleven European and American communities (several blend Asian and African festival traditions) where Carnival remains an important part of the annual cycle of festivities: Laza, Spain; rural Bulgaria; Venice, Italy; Basel, Switzerland; Basile, USA; Tlaxcala, Mexico; Oruro, Bolivia; Recife and Olinda, Brazil; Port of Spain, Trinidad and Tobago; Haiti; New Orleans, USA.[82]

Historically, Carnival street masquerades took the form of pre–Lenten secular celebrations in preparation for the sacrifices required by Christianity's Catholic concept of Lent. The Latin root word "carnivale" ("farewell to the flesh") actually refers to this break with the rigors of the upcoming Lent sacrifices which fostered atonement with Christ. But also many non–Christian communities have celebrated Carnival-styled festivals or rites of passage as an escape from the winter doldrums and as bacchanal parties acknowledging the advent of spring's fecundity. Frequently, the Christian Catholic traditions of Carnival have blended with these pagan traditions, creating unique celebrations worldwide.

Regardless of the sacred or secular motivations behind Carnival street masquerades, they still encourage ordinary citizens to display personal, cultural and spiritual values (or paradoxical/controversial values) they hold most dear. "Through ritual masquerade, and play, which exaggerate and invert everyday behavior, the celebrations lead people through this time with irony, disguise, laughter, and revelry, helping to ensure a proper renewal and growth for themselves and their communities."[83] The masks and/or costumes invariably take on whimsical, sometimes mysterious, but always exotic, exaggerated qualities. During Carnival, the most reticent citizen on the street has the freedom to masquerade as a powerful protector, an idealized beauty, king, queen, or mythic/heroic figure, a mischievous demon/devil, an esteemed ancestor, or satirical clown. Carnival masquerade need not be confused with Halloween masquerade, which has entirely different traditions and occurs more often for children's events than for entire community celebrations.

Some of the best known Carnivals invariably blend the cultural influences of more than one country, such as the annual Carnival in Trinidad, representing the diaspora movements of Indian and Chinese indentured servants, indigenous tribes, and African slaves with eighteenth-century French and British settlers. Other Carnivals reflect the clash of historical and religious values between dominant and indigenous cultures such as those seen in the Mexican pre–Lenten *Pastorela* festivals or the French Mardi Gras celebrations. Upper-crust seventeenth-century Venetian merchants and aristocrats took time to "play" with the surrounding Italian peasants in the street masquerades of Carnival in Italy and this continues today with the addition of tourists. Still other non–Christian but Carnival-styled spring festivals such as the West African Yoruba *Egungun* and *Gèlèdé* masquerades celebrate the rich ancestral heritage of a community. African celebratory traditions and characters frequently morphed into new Carnival masquerade versions as African slaves were brought over to most of the countries associated with Carnival festivities in North and South America, such as Brazil, Venezuela, the Caribbean, and the United States, but also in Great Britain as well, as seen in the Trinidadian festivities at Notting Hill.

"Masquerade" evokes related meanings and images. Playfully speak the word several times and one will hear its resonance in a number of Latin, Greek, French, and Spanish root words. Contemporary ritual or musical images also come to mind. For instance, the Greek root word *maza* and the Latin equivalent *massa* mean "to knead/to mingle"—perfect images for lively street theatre.[84] Likewise, the connotations of religion and ritual associated with the Catholic mass point to the sacred origins of Carnival. "Mass" also refers to "a large body of persons in a compact group" or "the body of people as contrasted with the elite." The French root word *maschera* refers to "partial covering or disguise" (or even the contemporary word for the type of makeup used to decorate a woman's eyelashes), while the Spanish *mascarada* refers to people at "a social gathering wearing masks and fantastic costumes." And finally, the term *massa* is an old Southern slave term for "master" or "one that conquers the masses."[85] "Masquerade! What a sublime name for such street theatre, where much of the energy is in playing the slave, if you already define yourself as a princess amongst the masses."[86] "Masquerade! How exquisitely appropriate for the sort of street theatre considered vulgar and unacceptable by Trinidad's elite British citizens during much of the nineteenth and early twentieth centuries."[87]

Trinidadian Peter Minshall has probably reached more audiences with his spectacle as a commercial mask maker/designer than any other mask maker in the world. Vividly original, brilliantly visual, Minshall draws on elements of Carnival and *mas* in his work in theatre and contemporary special event spectacles. His work has reached international audiences at stadiums, concert-spectacles, and festival performance events such as those at the Pan American Games, the 2002 Salt Lake City Winter Olympics, a Parisian Bastille Day Spectacle, and a city-wide concert spectacle in Moscow. Theatre companies in the United States, England, Scotland, the Netherlands, and Germany have presented his theatre designs and visual art. He possesses the urban sophistication and experience enjoyed by few traditional mask makers (those relying primarily on their native cultural heritage and values). Until 2004 (some speculate that he has gone into retirement) he worked locally in Trinidad while also producing major international spectacles seen via television by millions of people worldwide. He has taken the art form of the masked performance to new dramatic levels with mass audience appeal. His magnificent "dancing mobiles" and "walking sculptures" point toward a new way to define what we mean by the term "mask" while they demonstrate the mask's power on contemporary popular audiences.

The complex intercultural dimensions of Trinidad's Carnival and *mas* have given Minshall a unique worldview that spans religions, myths, political dogma, and social expectations. Trinidad's hotbed of creative energies serves as a microcosm of current world tensions as cultures collide and clash within the increasingly global economy and internet landscape. According to Victor Reece, a Northwest Coast Indian mask maker, "The Hopi believe that there are great changes during any conflict arising from the merging of two or more cultures. When things change, the people who rise from the ashes of lost traditions are the artists.

Today, with so much change, there is room for many artists, particularly mask makers." Out of the ashes of pre-colonial native Trinidadian custom and ceremony has risen a strikingly diverse cosmopolitan center. Minshall, a twenty-first-century prophet, uses his innovative, newly defined masks to project mythic masked and "mobiled" characters that effectively evoke the new century's expanding worldview.

Minshall credits his childhood memories of *mas*, the largely improvisational street theatre of Trinidad, as having most influenced the spectacular effects he has created over the past thirty years. "I start doing the *mas*, even as the *mas* is undergoing certain social changes," Minshall acknowledged to Richard Schechner and Milla Riggio in a 1997 interview. "It used to be very much a male thing, but at the point of my return it was becoming what you now see, very much a female thing. It was going through all kinds of visual changes. At this point, I really came into it saying, 'This is a theatre of the streets.' Which is obvious to me, but no one here [New York] understands the terminology. 'Oh, you're trying to turn it into theater.' Oh my God, don't you realize it's always been that?"[88]

Why is Minshall so attracted to the elements of Trinidadian *mas*? What is *mas* all about?

Milla Riggio describes "*ole mas*" as "traditional *mas*, basically a satirical form, usually involving skits with much word play and many puns."[89] In Trinidadian Carnival celebrations, "pretty *mas*" or "fancy *mas*" contrasts with "dirty *mas*" as dialectical forms of entertainment. Pretty *mas* displays its rich carnival masquerade characters representing beautiful women, Carnival kings and queens, and luxuriously colored and textured mythic characters and creatures.[90] Pretty *mas* characters strut and glide elegantly in the light of day. (Similarly, we still see vestiges of the elite Italian Renaissance characters during Carnival in Venice — which emphasizes more eye candy and fantasy than substance or historical detail.)

On the other hand, dirty *mas* celebrations, like the Renaissance street *commedia* performances, express the dark underbelly of a community fraught with the tensions brought by low incomes and a sense of powerlessness, though dirty *mas* seems much more participatory and less presentational than *commedia* performances at the Venice Carnival. While some participants in dirty *mas* simply want to loosen up and "get down" more than they want to "get angry," the communal nature of these "night events" allows people to release pent-up frustrations and anxieties by participating alongside "low down" characters, minority figures, misfits, and legendary drunken sailors and devils.[91]

Pretty *mas* is high spectacle featuring elevated characters while dirty *mas* has the gritty, home-spun qualities of low spectacle and lowly characters. Incidentally, a number of Carnivals include versions of both characteristics, but Renaissance Italy offers one of the most vivid examples of rapid development into such dialectical entertainment. Renaissance Italy saw the evolution of high and low spectacle elements within a short century as its economic base rapidly increased with international trade from Venice. Its burgeoning forms of elaborate costumes and masks for the elite's masques, operas, and ballet contrasted dramatically with the scrappy, sweaty *commedia dell'arte* costumes and masks for the common people with performers touring in and on rickety wagons to various cities and towns. Italy's newly wealthy elite, wanting beauty and escape from their everyday realities of complacent boredom, produced grand masques/balls and theatre. The commoners, on the other hand, could afford little material beauty but also wanted escape of a different sort — from the frustrations of poverty and anger with the people in power. Touring *commedia* troupes offered street theatre to the masses — witty, subversive, and vulgar laughter against the elite. The troupes' much less costly gymnastic routines and simple yet bold costumes and masks helped the town's poor ignore their sense of helplessness and inability to change their lives. Both forms of high spectacle and low spectacle still grace the Venice Carnival and attract tourists worldwide.

The high and low spectacle in the Trinidadian *mas* events suggests a dialogue between dualities reflecting civilization and order in pretty *mas* versus chaos and its consequences in dirty *mas*. Minshall sees this dialogue as one dialogue — in the same manner that he sees our world and all living things as one. In his 1997 interview with Richard Schechner, he expressively describes a crystallization of this concept that occurred to him while still a teenager witnessing the pre-dawn *jouvay* celebrations of ole/dirty *mas*: "And another thing about the *jouvay* then was the mud. Sometimes when I think of people putting mud on their bodies in the predawn, when I try on my own to figure out what the carnival's about, I say: The ritual of putting mud onto the body for *jouvay* is about the myth of man being made from that mud. It is returning to the source, it is being one with the universe. That mud is of the earth, but it is also of the Milky Way. That river of people is a river of stars, it is not your everyday."[92] This concept surely has much to do with how he uses each nuance of color, sequin, tassel, and suspended mobile unit. The seemingly irrelevant artifices weave and undulate through the magnificent membranes of the dynamic, mythic, larger-than-life creatures and characters.

Today, Trinidadian Carnival excludes no one from celebrating, as long as the spectators can afford the price of airfare. It depends on the money derived from tourists who are eager for their own escapes from boredom and frustration. The global economy, while volatile, encourages Trinidadian tourism on an unprecedented scale. The democratic combination of participation by the elite with the common people ensures that a larger number of citizens can delight in both the high and low spectacle found in versions of pretty *mas* and dirty *mas* Carnival celebrations.

ARTISTIC ACCOMPLISHMENTS OF CONTEMPORARY TRINIDADIAN CARNIVAL MASK MAKERS

Mask makers in Trinidadian society are known as masmen — and they often perform in the masks they create for the annual Carnival celebrations in February. When Minshall decided not to design and produce for 2004 Carnival, masman Brian MacFarlane, who has designed for several *mas* bands, specializing in Carnival king characters, acknowledged the increasing dominance of bikinis, feathers, and sequins at *mas* without the more substantial theatrical Minshall-esque conceptualizations. He decided to design and produce *The Washing by Fire by Water* in 2005, partly in homage to Minshall and partly in response to Khalil Gibran's *The Prophet*, which had inspired him to call for a community-wide spiritual cleansing in the midst of rising crime rates in Trinidad.[93] After seeing MacFarlane's 2005 *mas* extravaganza, *The Guardian*'s Anne Marie Henry declared that "Peter Minshall's style of Carnival will not die if Brian MacFarlane has anything to say about it. On Carnival Tuesday he did not bring *mas*, he made theatre. The headpieces, which looked like mops, draped from the heads of the revelers, bounced up and down as they moved across the stage."[94]

The press has also paid attention to other innovative mask makers besides MacFarlane. "Minshall has lamented that no young designers have emerged to challenge [late twentieth-century masmen]," writes Kerrigan and Laughlin in *Caribbean Beat*. "Bikini *mas* reigns. Yet there are still flashes of brilliance, perhaps in the form of a headpiece or the combinations of colors in a section. Promising young designers like Brian MacFarlane and Marlon Griffith familiar with the achievements of the [Minshall] golden-age masquerades are deserving of praise and publicity."[95]

I interviewed Marlon Griffith at his studio seven months after he had lost most of his sketches, paintings, art supplies, and personal possessions in a flood. Fortunately he still had remnants of work from his recent designs for his 2005 children's *mas* event and a few surviving masks, lithographs, and paintings. He also had carefully documented much of his work on disc. Curator-in-residence Claire Tancons at Caribbean Contemporary Arts quoted the reaction of an unimpressed older Trinidadian's fatalistic response to Griffith's catastrophic loss: "If he is a real masman he will start over." Tancons continued, "Nothing can characterize Griffith and the spirit of *mas* better than a tested endurance to renewals. But Griffith never really has to start from scratch. At its most experimental, his work is always in progress and he is always ready to improvise it into new configurations."[96]

Tancons asserts that Griffith learned a great deal from working with Minshall's Callaloo *mas* camp for several bands, most recently the 2002 Ship of Fools band. ("Band" here refers to the group of performers during *mas* who purchase the costumes for the event from the designer/band leader.) Griffith, like other artisans working at Callaloo, learned a "wide range of skills and techniques, such as wire-bending, papier-mâché molding, cane work, wood carving, and metal repousse, passed along in typical fashion from Minshall or Minshall's supervisors" (Tancons, 2004, online). She reminds us that *mas* celebration bands for children often give emerging masmen their start, such as Minshall's and Griffith's early designs for children.[97]

Griffith's work, like Minshall's later work, tends to keep his *mas* mask imagery ultra-simple and features low-cost materials and bold decoration. He remembers the magic he experienced as an eight-year-old in 1986 while watching Minshall's *Ratrace*. "Everyone had rat heads with giant rat tails out of tubing, many of them wearing pin-striped business suits. The stage image was so powerful."[98]

Griffith, like Minshall, frequently focuses on mythical characters, zoomorphic animals, and energy forces. Various examples can be found in his *mas* mask designs for children. He has created *burroquite* masks (similar to hobby horses) for some of his performers to ride, making them elegantly abstract with white wire. Griffith's child queen character, called Little Princess, and the child king, called Run Jack Run, represent the innocent and mischievous aspects of childhood. Elaborate wire and macramé headdresses combined with abstract costumes dominate other children's faces and become large walking sculpture masks that evoke parading "dream catchers."

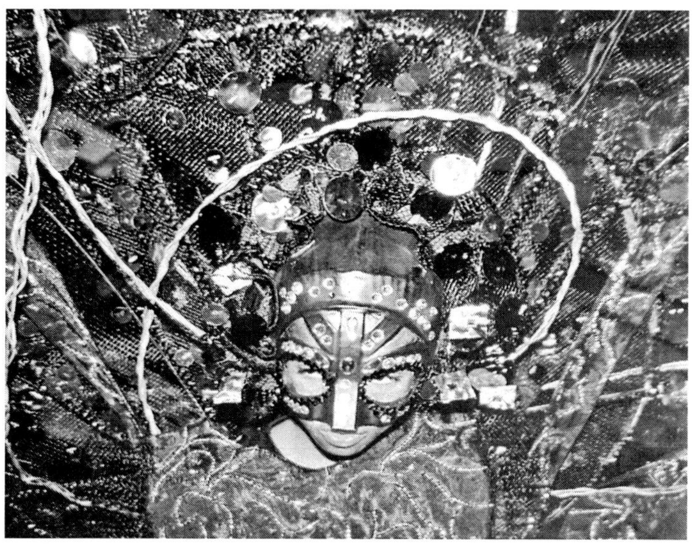

Trinidadian mask maker Marlon Griffith's "Run Jack Run" mask for the Children's Carnival celebrations.

Griffith has created a bird mask accompanied by rigged leg harnesses for huge feathers for his lead character in an American Indian myth version of Icarus, but in this case the bird is a sister to the Thunderbird. The anxious bird tries to challenge her brother to fly closer to the sun and burns the tips of her wings. *Arrow to the Sun,* a Pueblo Indian folk tale, resembles *The Magic Flute* with its own self-validating trials including encounters with lions, bees, serpents, and lightning. The tale involves a son who seeks his father, the sun, as an arrow and becomes a spark of light. (Child band members masqueraded as sparks of light.) Griffith created an herbal energy mask called "the bush doctor" as the cumulative representation of valuable medicinal herbs found in Trinidadian backyards. Various children in the band became herbs that surrounded the masked bush doctor.

"I do not like static costumes. Basically I design by trial and error. I believe the children not only develop a sense of *mas* while participating in these bands, but they also learn about myths, folktales, and even medicinal remedies for herbs. *Mas* has become so commercialized that you rarely see the sort of spontaneity that used to be its primary characteristic. Only with children's *mas* do we truly carry on our Carnival traditions while also allowing the stories to evolve with the new perspectives of child-like wonder."[99]

Like Minshall, Griffith ventured out internationally at a young age. He found inspiration while serving as an artist-in-residence for Johannesburg, South Africa's Fordsburg Artist Studios. For several months, Griffith worked with leading African artists and two Indians also working as artists-in-residence. A Dutch company financed his travel for this highly competitive position after seeing examples of Griffith's work. Just as Minshall created a number of *mas* works for the British version of Carnival at Notting Hill, Griffith created a *mas* experience for these international artists by giving each of them the same prototype of a mask. He then asked them to "decorate" their mask in a way that reflected the current style of their paintings, jewelry, and sculpture. The masks reflected a wide range of considerations and fantasies. Near the end of Griffith's residency, the artist group surprised him one evening by organizing a *mas* ball. His colleagues and members of the community all came wearing their own South African versions of fancy sailors, blue devils, and Carnival Kings and Queens. He says he felt at home in South Africa that night. (Griffith recently returned from another international artist-in-residency in Japan in 2005, and the Victoria and Albert Museum invited him to display his costumes and masks in an exhibition on Carnival.)

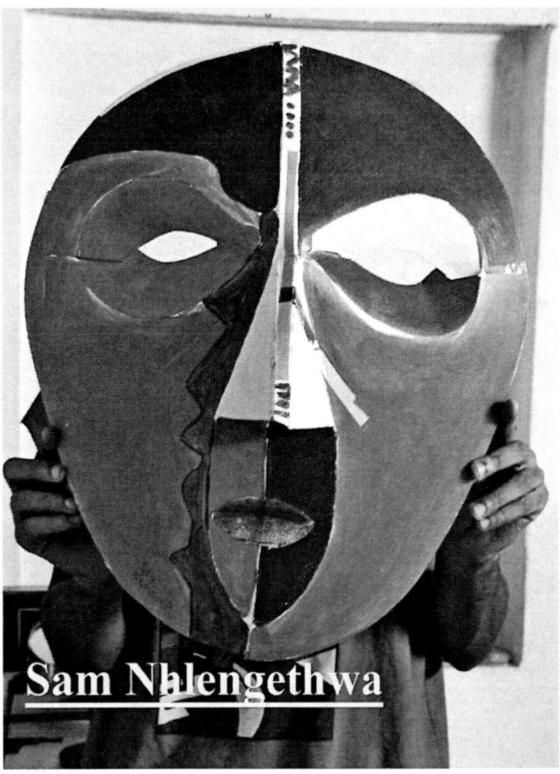

A contemporary papier-mâché mask created by Sam Nhlengethwa at Griffith's mask-making workshop in South Africa. Photographer: Marlon Griffith.

The son of Portuguese immigrants to Trinidad, septuagenarian Geraldo

Vieira supports his passion for Carnival costume and masks by molding industrial plastics. His designs have won in the King of Carnival category at least seven times since 1971, and he frequently wins other competition categories as well. He fell in love with Carnival at the age of fourteen and has been obsessed with the art form ever since. He has worked for other *mas* band designers, including Berkeley (whom he most admires) and Minshall (for whom he made Minshall's sister's harness for her Queen costume in *Splash*).[100] He smiles as he fondly quotes his late wife, "Geraldo, we could have purchased a fine house with all the money you've spent on your Carnival creations!" But he feels that he has maintained his autonomy and full creative range by not accepting backing from a demanding patron in the typical manner of Carnival financing.[101]

Annan Boodram has called Peter Minshall the "wizard of the dancing mobile."[102] Yet Minshall's brilliant conceptualizations have met their match in the masterful engineering skills of Vieira, who continues to search for the quintessential *mas* experience in his rambling and rolling larger-than-life creations. The sparkle in Vieira's high-energy sorcerer-like countenance makes him at least as enthralling as his *mas* characters, who harness rain on stage, or command the coming of dawn and sunset, or evoke the effect of riding into hell with the gyrations and pyrotechnics of their costumes and masks. He oddly insists, however, that he is no artist: "I'm not moody or temperamental enough to be an artist — I am an engineer, an artisan. I want to see my creations come alive. I start with a small idea and

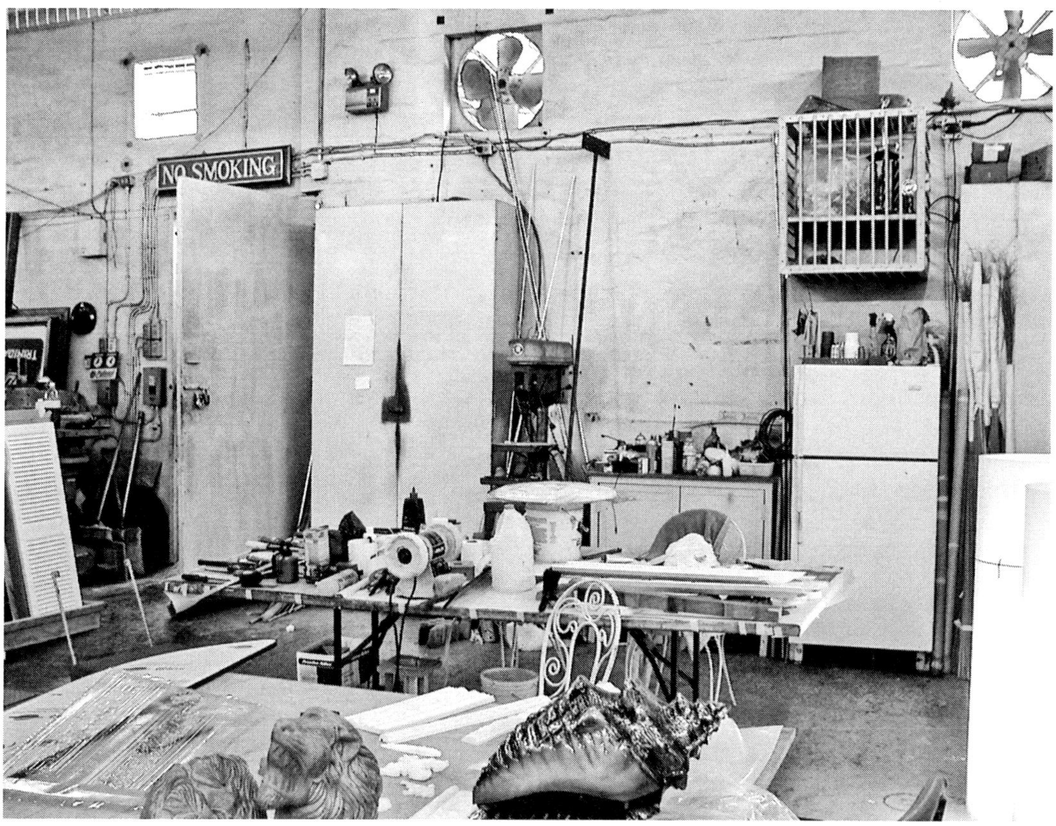

Trinidadian mask maker Geraldo Vieira's plastics studio. Vieira specializes in vacuform masks for Carnival.

then I think of the geometrics and the logistics of the idea. Hardly anyone can beat me in structure. I often use pneumatics and even radio waves and robotics for remote controlling the movement of my characters. I am a pattern maker by trade, and I can produce the machine that makes the molds. Technology is the greatest thing in the world. I can design, construct, decorate, sculpt, mold, paint it — and sometimes I even masquerade it. Next year I will be the oldest masquerader in the history of Carnival to win the King Costume. I'm sure of this!"[103] Vieira did indeed win the King Costume in 2006.

Two of Vieira's recent mobile spectacles, *Aladdin's Last Ride* (2003) and *Trouble in de Bamboo* (2004), both designed by his son, Geraldo Vieira Jr. (who won the Carnival King title in 1996 performing in the *Rainfest* mobile), possess humor and pathos. Aladdin, a figure of death, rides into hell as a king on a huge griffin controlled by robotics. Aladdin (performed by Vieira Jr.) seems to be having a grand time. A closer look at the blue devil in "de bamboo patch" reveals that he is eternally pestered by ants who are the real devils. The ants move seemingly at will, controlled by "radio waves." Both moving mobiles have several "masks" that interact with one another. Earlier versions of spectacle produced in the mid-nineties, *Splendoria* (homage to the dawn and sunset) and *Rainfest* (homage to the rain) easily compete visually with the environmental themes found in Minshall's characters in *River* and *Song of the Earth*. For over seven years, the junior Vieira has designed or crafted work for Trini-Revellers, a major *mas* camp, and also for Carnival events in Barbados.[104]

Sheldon Clemdore credits Geraldo Vieira with mentoring him as he developed into a first-rate masman. Clemdore started making costumes and masks at age eleven and describes himself as "a total *mas* camp because I'm so multi-task-oriented." He has a wide range of skills, such as fabric painting, wire-bending, and sculpting (for which he has a particular talent). He says that Vieira taught him how to make molds for plastic and foam products. Now he makes molds for commercial uses such as lamps, furniture, and three-dimensional sculptures for storefronts, movie houses, and the island's international airport. Like Minshall and Griffith, Clemdore first started by making King and Queen costumes and masks for children's *mas* events. He also believes that children's *mas* events encourage more creativity than the more commercialized Carnival competitions — though he's worked extensively for those events as well.

Clemdore not only made the King's costume and mask for MacFarlane's *The Washers,* he also performed and danced with MacFarlane's band. He believes the mask traditionally inspires the dance. "I see the whole costume and mask and then I begin to feel the personality or spirit of them. My performance and mold mask-making work is very intuitive. I edit ideas quickly and evolve the character's essence to the point where it can live through me." He assisted Vieira Jr. and Vieira with the mask molds for their 2004 *Aladdin's Last Ride* and their 2003 *Trouble in de Bamboo* (both won in several competition categories). His mask for *Trouble in de Bamboo* required twenty-seven molds for the eyes, teeth, jowls, and ears. Several parts of both Carnival masked mobiles moved with hydraulics, presenting Clemdore with a more complex challenge.

Like Peter Minshall, Clemdore talks about the need for more community awareness in his country. He wants to establish a community center where he can inspire underprivileged children and uphold and continue the best aspects of *mas* tradition for them the way Vieira has done for him.

Minshall's legacy has always embraced Carnival's traditional and ever-present Saturnalia motifs of bare-skinned, muddied youth at dawn or highly decorative, bikini-clad women that acknowledge and even celebrate our internal devils. But we will probably remember

Minshall more for his inclination to uphold Carnival's other traditional emphases that often engage with the broader and frequently controversial social issues of Trinidad. A cosmopolitan man of his time, he has dramatized and magnified Trinidadian issues to reflect the even more complex tensions of our current global society at large, using Carnival to search for a more profound sense of community and a quest for better appreciation and care for the earth.

MacFarlane, Griffith, the Vieiras, and Clemdore continue to champion these issues with humor and panache as well as with spirited, beautifully vivid imagery found in the Carnival *mas* celebrations and street theatre. Unsolicited and in separate interviews, the masmen all remarked at one point or another that, "It takes a village." Sheldon Clemdore added, "Each child needs my grandmother ready to beat him after searching for him if he stays out too late. She once beat me and then took on each of my friends. Their parents thanked her when she returned them to their homes. We never were out late again. We knew someone on the street cared."[105]

Each masman declares his hope for rejuvenating and reinventing our global community and planet. They firmly believe that rejuvenating and reinventing Carnival lies with the lessons to be learned from Trinidad's children — particularly in "making *mas* and playing *mas.*" *Mas* allows adults to be imaginative, innovative children again. In Carnival, the children and their spirit create new insight for the world. Peter Minshall's career grows out of this fundamental truth and current masmen continue on with this fundamental approach.

Universal themes magnificently come full circle in Trinidad's street *mas* celebrations and at the Queen's Park Savannah grandstand competitions, crystallized most effectively with the children's *mas* celebrations and the walking mobiles — the gigantic masks that no other international Carnival artists can create with more zeal or artistry than a select group of Trinidadian masmen.

Contemporary Masks Used in Healing

Comparisons Between Mask Maker, Art Therapist, and Shaman

The term "therapy" refers to remedial treatment for people suffering from either physical or mental disorders. But one does not need a major physical or mental disorder in order to experience a sense of imbalance and disharmony. Imbalance, disharmony, and a general state of tension constitute a larger part of the human experience.

Whether conducted by the amateur artist facing mental or physical disorders or the professionally recognized artist facing disturbing personal, social, or political issues, the actual process of the creation of a mask challenges was to both identify and confront disturbances. Successful effort assists with establishing new ways in which to define or express, and ultimately confront the tensions at hand. The expanded perception gained in the act of creation becomes entirely personal and thus original (at some level). This expanded perception offers the potential to encourage profound positive change for the creator.

Susan Makin, in her book *A Consumer's Guide to Art Therapy*, reminds us, "shamans from many other cultures have used art for centuries in their healing rituals."[106] We see similar healing rituals today in masked performance. The presentations encourage the mask makers, masked performers, and audiences to enter another state of reality, a more intense state of reality that promises better harmony and understanding. Shamans no doubt promoted similar intense states of awareness during their healing rituals and performance presentations. Descriptions of their rituals involve a great deal of theatricality, often using masked characters or spirits with special ceremonial costumes that "framed" the mask and headdress. Their drums or rattles established ritualistic beats to conjure the life force.

Consequently, the use of mask making for therapeutic purposes should not necessarily be construed an inferior process of creating art. Did Picasso see African masks as great artistic efforts or as therapeutic efforts by Africans to confront and understand their inner demons and ancestral spirits? Does it really matter? One could argue that it depends on the artist's and viewer's interpretations. In *Art Therapy and Dramatherapy*, art therapist Sue Jennings underscores this point, "Dreams, masks, and images come to life in art therapy and dramatherapy and assist in our soul-journeys."[107] The amateur mask maker grappling with serious illness or issues of alienation can create a mask with the same degree of intensity as a professional artist. Similar intensity might occur for the mentally disturbed amateur mask maker who makes a protective mask in response to perceived feelings of imbalance and disharmony. A skilled shaman might likewise portray and confront demons.

The creative process for the amateur or professional mask maker/masked performer and the ancient shaman ultimately enables each to identify, more clearly understand, states of disorder. Yet Jennings makes some distinguishing comments between the professional world of art (in this case, theatre and masked performance) and the world of art therapy (or specifically, dramatherapy):

> Are we, therefore, encouraging our clients to be actors? No more than art therapists are encouraging their clients to be painters in the sense of a career or profession. However, we are engaging with our clients through the processes of theatre art as actor, director and technician, i.e. the art and the craft of the theatre, with the aim that they will experience new insights, new experiences, and new perspectives about the world as a whole, and their relationship with it.... The theatrical distancing enables this to happen in a contained way; as in the theatre, no one is totally involved. There is always a part of ourselves watching ourselves and others; therefore we are not overwhelmed.[108]

Jennings proceeds to more clearly describe drama's vital place in our lives: "Drama, as an art form in which we are participant as actor, technician, director and audience, is crucial for survival. If we do not have the opportunity to participate in 'the drama that is larger than life,' then maybe we will create [life] dramas that are larger than life in more destructive ways."[109]

Masks in Mental and Physical Therapy

Living near each other in the Arcata/Eureka area of northern California, distinguished mask makers Joyce Radtke, Donvieve (no last name), Lauren Raine (currently living on the East Coast after living for over a decade in California), and Bruce Marrs are familiar with each other's work though they rarely work together on projects. In addition to their artistic pursuits, they all serve as mentors for mask making, though each offers a different approach. They introduce the provocative power of masks as they work with people facing critical illness, at-risk children, juveniles in rehabilitation centers, or children simply experiencing the complex pains and pleasures of growing up.

Radtke, Donvieve, Raine, and Marrs acknowledge that they are not art therapists, and indeed they have no formal training in art therapy. But they frequently function like art therapists by serving as mentors, counselors, and educators while they teach mask making.

Although they do not professionally diagnose and treat seriously disturbed individuals, these skilled artisans assist their clients, students, and community groups in understanding daunting life challenges. They guide their clients toward valuable self-discovery, while helping them find voices for their frustrations as well as their celebrations, using masks as highly expressive devices.

Obviously they are not shamans, but their therapeutic approaches can occasionally seem "shamanistic" since each of these mask makers focus on the mask's potential to access one's spirit within to an alternative reality where one can harness unconscious knowledge and healing benefits.

Artistic Accomplishments of Mentors

Joyce Radtke has particular fascination in exploring "passage rituals" for theatrical productions and religious ceremonies. In addition to her work as a mask maker, she is also a painter and writer. Her paintings have been displayed nationwide, including a gallery in New York, and are most popular in Alaska, California, and New Mexico. Many of her paintings are about the mask (representing a transformational journey). She has published her paintings in a Chronicle book called *Art. Rage. Us*, and has included pieces in its traveling exhibition which has toured throughout the United States and Hong Kong. Her paintings were a part of an invitational group show that went to Kumasi, Ghana. Published in several magazines including *MAMM*, *Access*, *Cure*, and *Northcoast Journal*, she has also had her work printed in calendars by the Breast Cancer Action and *WeMoon*.

Donvieve, a weaver/textile artist as well as a costume designer and mask maker, won the American Conservatory Theatre Festival's Meritorious Achievement Award for her Uber Puppets and an award from the Kennedy Center for the Performing Arts for her theatre prop designs. Donvieve creates masks, puppets, and scenography for theatre and has received numerous awards for her performance masks, which can be seen in galleries from San Francisco to Portland. The Annesbrook Nelson Museum in New Zealand accepted her masked pageant costume entry as part of its World of Wearable Art Exhibit. She has worked in Japan while on a fellowship with the JUCEE NPOP in Osaka and was project coordinator with at-risk youth for a consortium grant between the National Endowment for the Arts, Humboldt Arts Council, and the Ink People Center for the Arts, creating collaborative projects in the community by teaming up local business and youth in alternative high schools. She has studied Balinese mask making techniques with I. Katut Molog in Ubud, Bali. She designs courses on teaching mask making as a tool for art therapists and teaches elementary, secondary, and university students regularly at guest workshops and special seminars.

Lauren Raine spent her teenage years in Afghanistan during the 1960s where she experienced the conservative (pre–Taliban) policies of that culture's discriminatory practices against women. Consequently, influenced in part by those years in Afghanistan, she has developed an ongoing masked performance project in which she champions the "divine feminine" and showcases her multi-cultural masks of ancient goddesses.

Raine received an MFA degree in cross-disciplinary arts at the University of Arizona in 1987. Early in her career, she attended the New England Institute for Art Therapy and was introduced to shamanic influences in mask work at the 1989 New York Renaissance Festival. A choreographer as well as a visual and performance artist for over three decades, she developed her mask making techniques after studying with Balinese master I. Bodus Anom. She has also helped plan several annual Spiral Dance annual rituals in San Francisco and created thirty-five goddess masks for it in 1999 which were used again in 2006. She eventually sold them in 2007 and has published a book showcasing them entitled *The Masks of the Goddess, Sacred Masks and Dance*. This book describes her work with producers, ritualists, and choreographers over a seven-year period, touring and directing productions using the masks in several cities in New York, California, and Arizona. Also, in 2007 she received the Alden B. Dow Creativity Center Fellowship to develop her "Hands of the Spider Woman" project. She received an additional grant for this project from the Puffin Foundation and in 2009 served as resident artist at the Henry Luce Center at Wesley Theological Seminary in Washington, D.C. Her mask and doll work, as well as that of her students, focuses on archetypal masks that incorporate myth and women's spirituality.

Bruce Marrs (introduced earlier in this chapter) has extensive professional performance experience in mask making and masked performance, and local audiences have often seen him perform as a tango dancer and as a mime. His mask making and masked performance summer workshops at Dell'Arte International School of Physical Theatre attract students worldwide and he has studied mask-making techniques with Balinese mask maker I. Katut Molog. He sells versions of his neoprene *commedia* and carnival masks to institutions and theatre companies across the country.

These mask makers have taught classes in mask making and mask performance or have served as mentors/guides for student and community groups. As with many art therapists in the process of demonstrating mask-related techniques, they create a "safe place" to initiate a personal dialogue between the mask maker and the mask, whereby the mask maker can more effectively confront the issues and conflicts dominating his/her life. Students frequently feel so confident and positive about the personal artistic dialogue they establish for themselves that they look forward to extending that private dialogue to public group theatrical presentations as well. This allows the audience to share in the revelations of the masks and lends a supportive atmosphere for the group at large. Likewise shamans encouraged their communities to witness masked performances, as ritual (to make the group feel more secure), and also to introduce alternative worlds and realities more powerfully.

JOYCE RADTKE'S MASKS AS INNER GUIDES

Joyce Radtke has direct, large luminous eyes and walks with the assurance and centered demeanor of a person who takes time for daily meditation and contemplation. She has a calm, thoughtful disposition and looks younger than her fifty-something years. Masks, body maps, body sculpture, and paintings grace her walls and tables. She obviously holds high esteem for the artistic effort represented in the room.

Radtke utilizes the medium of mask making to create representations of inner guides for clients participating in her workshops. Her clients often describe this inner guide as a warrior mask who protects the individual from harm, but Radtke prefers the more gentle term "guide." She adds that another type of mask can help cleanse the darker forces within us by projecting and contrasting these darker forces in full view, thus diminishing their internal, invisible negative power.[110]

Radtke knows a great deal about internal negative power because of her harrowing experience with breast cancer. She explains that while she was struggling with the disease, her paintings and poetry reflected her fear of two daunting challenges. The first challenge required an extensive search for a cure for her survival. The second, perhaps even more daunting, was her need to create some sort of transformation within her psyche to reclaim personal empowerment. "Serious illness strips us of our power. External influences such as doctors, insurance companies, and family pressures impact our decision-making ability. I initially felt alone and relatively helpless," she says. "But we can all reclaim our power by reclaiming how we perceive our dilemma."

"We are spiritual beings practicing in a physical world," she continues. "We yearn to connect both to the earth and to our bodies. Consequently, during times of extreme stress, we often want to work in the garden or go to the beach or take long walks. Connecting to the physical world as spiritual beings brings us a level of simplicity and contentment. Art is another way to connect our physical world with our spiritual world. When I experienced this overwhelming sense of powerlessness during my battle with cancer, I decided to direct my artistic expression toward issues that enhanced my self-esteem. I explored various projects that utilized my abilities as a ritual maker, painter, and writer, and these projects offered me hope, balance, and a sense of integrity. I decided to share this process with others experiencing similar serious illnesses and initiated the Persephone Healing through Arts Program."

Radtke's Persephone Program has had remarkable success. Megan Fulmer writes: "Radtke sees herself as holding a light at the entrance of a sacred space as the founder and coordinator of Persephone: Healing through Art Program. Ink People Center for the Arts in Humboldt County initially helped fund this program and eventually California Arts Council and NEA funded it as well. For over seven years, Persephone has offered free workshops for people going through life-threatening or catastrophic illnesses. Participants in Radtke's program engage in diverse forms of artistic expression, such as poetry and doll making as well as painting and mask making, boosting their self-esteem, confidence, and joy."[111]

The workshops in this program have evolved into four or five classes per week with four to six people in each class. Each group meets for several hours each week and commits to a twelve-week cycle. Some of the initial Persephone group members continue to participate. One of Radtke's current groups has essentially been together for several years except for those who have died from the illnesses that first brought them to Persephone. All of the group members serve as a powerful support system for one another, though Radtke does not allow them to kvetch for the sake of kvetching. She and the group challenge each other to decide how to live life one day at a time. Insisting that she is not a therapist, Radtke wants to work with the spirit. She tries to find ways to acknowledge, reclaim, and make visible that spirit in the physical and emotional world of art.

"Before my breast cancer in 1994, I had been involved with passage rituals and theatre design as well as mask making. I had earned a graduate degree in costume design and was active in theatre," she said. "But this illness knocked me flat. I finally acknowledged that I could use my art exploration to reflect my spiritual journey. Though I was terribly depressed, I found a surprisingly rich, fertile area for growth, while going into that shadow world of retreat."

Each member of Persephone begins by making a mask as the first project. Each person contemplates the image of an inner guide and voice of wisdom. Each member's mask begins as white clay formed into a unique inner guide vision. The clay model of the inner guide or inner healer image will always support its maker when confronting the fear of pain and death. This "shaman" guide puts the "critic" voice aside and serves as a nurturer and advisor for the spirit. Unique to each person, this personal guide makes visible its creator's quest and yearnings. Each mask serves as a memory of its creator's inner landscape, including buried grievances and yearnings. The guide knows and understands all. The guide from within will help when the going gets rough.

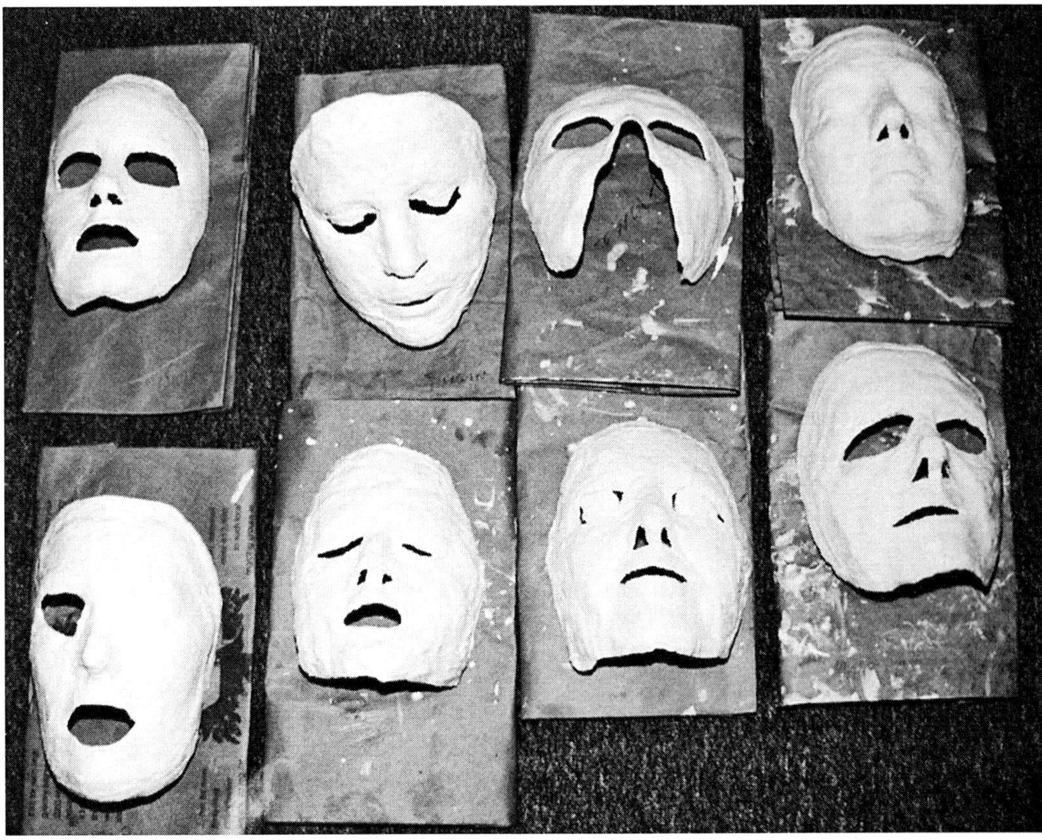

Plaster strip masks created by the Persephone members working with Joyce Radtke at her studio in Arcata, California. The Persephone members are in various stages of critical illnesses. Radtke assists in empowering them to cope with their illnesses by creating inner guide masks.

After completing the white clay masks, the members of the group take them to a pit fire in an outside location. They observe the purity of their masks before the trauma of the pit fire burns, breaks, cracks, and colors them in distinctive, individual ways. Yet the masks are not totally destroyed. They become stronger, more resilient, and even more beautiful in their unique disfigurements. The shattered but resilient masks reflect brilliant beauty in the harsh reality of trauma that perpetuates the human condition. Like Persephone embarking into the underworld, each person accepts and embraces one's personal and unique trauma, striving to appreciate the tensions of living and thus dying. The group members take their scarred masks and embellish and embrace the pieces their masks have become and the compounded power they now hold. What is the voice of each mask now? How has the reality of its journey changed, and how will the creator listen to and accept the mask's vision for the wearer?

Radtke acknowledges our society's intense fear of aging and death, particularly dying with pain. But we each have an inner core and depth of self-understanding and acceptance that can grow when we are faced with serious life-threatening situations. The inner guide mask mirrors and enhances the strength of this inner spiritual core. Each mask challenges, indeed beckons its creator to continue to live and thrive in what remains of life on earth.

Other masks can become monsters, reflecting darker aspects of the soul. Radtke encourages workshop participants to bring their demons "to light" in the form of this other mask, the foil to the inner guide. "We are incredibly rich, powerful, complicated human beings," she says. "This type of mask allows group members to visually identify and acknowledge the monster mask. They can then reflect on the negative aspects within all of us, and the mask maker is no longer forced to manage the terrible secret alone."

Radtke says that leading her workshop participants as they explore their spiritual realms rarely evolve into tangible, predictable outcomes. Even so, this effort usually impacts the whole community by becoming a bridge and dispelling alienation. In Radtke's world, however, the mask maker doesn't necessarily need to "perform" with the mask in view of other group members. (Often members are too ill to physically perform.) The healing journey rests within. The process of creating the mask allows individual release and contemplation for its creator, affirms life, and re-energizes the spirit. By openly acknowledging the heart and inner spirit through the mask, its creator can achieve a peaceful awareness with less internal conflict.

Ed Duddleston, one of Joyce Radtke's workshop participants for the past five years, has lived with AIDS for over fifteen years. He acknowledges that her magic as an artistic mentor lies in her strength of spirit. "She has a genuine and honest spiritual core in spite of her debilitating illness," he adds. "If I'd never met Joyce, I'd still be fighting with myself and my disease. Joyce helped me see my illness as a special journey and that this journey is exactly what it should to be. I now realize how pointless it is to try to control the events that come our way. We forget that we are all mortal. If I hadn't acquired AIDS I'd probably still be working fifteen hours a day, waiting to retire so I could figure out who I am. I'd waste a lot of time. In the process of making my inner guide mask, Joyce helped me vividly understand that regardless of the path I was waiting to take, I couldn't avoid the path life inevitably presents to me but I could choose my response to that path."[112]

Donvieve's Masks as Self-portraits

Donvieve shares a studio with Joyce Radtke in Arcata, California. Each acknowledges the other's influence, though Donvieve specializes more in mask making for performance. Radtke works mostly with adults, while Donvieve works more often with elementary and secondary school children.

I first met Donvieve in Bali, where we studied Balinese mask woodcarving and Balinese *Topeng* dance together. An energetic dancer, Donvieve has a ready laugh and enough self-confidence to try almost anything once. Well-traveled and well-educated, she does not take herself too seriously, though she has sold many masks and has exhibited her work with the support of several northern California grants.

Perhaps most importantly, Donvieve is a teacher and comes from a family of teachers. Numerous family members have long been active in the arts, particularly in painting and playing musical instruments. Donvieve entered the world of mask making through her love of dance and international music, including African, Balinese, Japanese, and South American. "I've always made a living through my art and through my teaching. The dual roles seemed natural when one considers my family background," she explains. "My interest in masks also comes from my work with fiber arts and metal and clay sculpture, as well as leather crafts created for furniture shows. My former husband and I created fiber and wood furniture chairs, screens, and crafts which we showed in San Francisco galleries for several years."[113]

After assisting her mentor, Professor Lynn Pauley, a costume designer and mask maker at Humboldt State University, in making a video of Pauley's mask making process, Donvieve felt she had learned traditional techniques of mask making with plaster casts and leather. Before that Donvieve had simply (and rather successfully) experimented by herself. Pauley especially liked one of Donvieve's unique creations that had come from abandoned leather hides she found thrown over a sawhorse at a dump. Donvieve had quickly "seen" faces in the leather that she then struggled to "free" by using leather craft techniques she had developed while working in her furniture crafts business. Pauley encouraged Donvieve to do more work with leather masks. But Donvieve, essentially a northern California spirit, has considered it more important to use leather from only dead animals not killed for commercial profit. "I've always liked the idea of somehow bringing the animal back to life by using the leather in a mask that lives for its creator and an audience."

The late Italian Carlo Mazzone-Clementi, who lived and worked in northern California for much of his life, was a well-known clown, mime performer, director, and co-founder of what is now Dell'Arte International School of Physical Theatre. (Mazzone-Clementi's work is discussed in chapter 5.) He encouraged Donvieve to create more masks, especially ones that incorporated Donvieve's preferences for fur and feather additions. Seeing Mazzone-Clementi's masked performance work caused Donvieve to appreciate the power that masks can have when combined with the appropriate movement created to complement the mask. She saw Mazzone-Clementi incorporate masks as a way of generating and influencing movement rather than movement influencing the masks, and she started to understand how masks could live more profoundly in this type of presentation.

Donvieve realized that the process of mask making had several applications for class projects, ranging from geometry calculations to geography. She enjoys creating masks as inspirational educational tools and encourages her students to use masks to project self-portraits. The self-portrait masks allow pre-adolescents and adolescents to achieve more self-awareness and confidence in themselves at a time in their lives when a positive self-image is critical.

She approaches the process of creating self-portrait masks in several ways, depending on the ultimate goal for the class as well as its skills level and its designated time allotment. But the process generally starts first with some sort of visualization technique. She has found several visualizing techniques successful. They all encourage a sort of initial exploratory meditation before beginning to create the mask.

Donvieve particularly favors a visualization technique in which each student creates a mandala to represent a personal inner core. The term "mandala," meaning "circle" in Sanskrit, is a universal art form involving a balanced, central design within a circle parameter using abstract line, color, and texture. This abstract design can profoundly affect the mandala's creator when that person has an open mind and is ready to experience the mandala's power. The mandala, associated historically with the sacred, emerges from within the individual and can help transport its creator into a more focused and heightened state. The mandala allows its creator to contemplate a problem or personal issue in a more concentrated way by aiding in the release of unconscious solutions. One experiences a sort of meditation while creating the mandala.

Mackey-Kallis takes great interest in identifying mandalas found in film in her book, *The Hero and the Perennial Journey Home in American Film*, and points out a number of masked characters that underscore mandala images such as E.T. as well as the aliens in *Close Encounters of the Third Kind*. I discuss this insight in greater detail in chapter 6 but here it is useful to mention Mackey-Kallis' reasoning regarding the value and implications of mandalas within a creative process as we look at Donvieve's work with mandalas in her classroom. Mackey-Kallis cites Carl Jung's statement that "Mandalas are birthplaces, vessels of birth in the most literal sense, lotus-flowers in which the Buddha comes to life. Sitting in the lotus seat, the yogi sees himself transfigured into an immortal world." She goes on to remind us of "significant mandalas appearing in the natural world and humanity's experience of that world including the sun and moon, the planets and the solar system, the mother's womb, the birth canal, the circularity of passage of time, of the seasons, and of the ages of consciousness." Finally, she summarizes the use of various mandalas incorporated in a number of modern films which attempt to "reconcile the tensions between scientific/rational ways of knowing and spiritual/nonrational ways of knowing."[114] (I will discuss the ramifications of this argument in chapter 6 when I introduce transcendent masked characters for contemporary stage and screen.)

To begin creation of a mandala, Donvieve suggests that her students start by making a circle and filling it with a color if they can't think of anything else to do. Start by thinking about something as simple as the activities of the day, and let the thought of these activities radiate outward from within the circle, visualizing the activities as an overall rhythm-of-life routine for the day. Some students find it helpful to write and doodle about the day's routine while they create their mandalas. Each mandala becomes a map or guide for its creator. Sometimes the mandala creator ponders an animal totem or elements of the earth (earth, air, fire, and water) and how they relate to any given day. Whatever comes to mind should be "recorded" somehow in the drawing in an abstract way. Mandalas should never be edited.

Donvieve also uses paintings/drawings of abstract form and color that juxtapose various rhythms as another way to help visualize and focus on the upcoming mask.

If the process of drawing intimidates students, she suggests that they try other visualizing techniques as simple as taking long walks and observing birds and nature images. They can jot down notes about their observations and how they might be applied to their thoughts about their own self-image. For her own personal work, she likes to focus on a mask project by using Tarot cards or collecting crystals, though she admits that students can't take advantage of these techniques unless they understand the significance of such interpretations. They can, however, explore the idea of keeping a daily journal that records their dreams and immediate daily concerns.

Whatever the visualizing technique, Donvieve then has her students experiment with clay sculpture, concentrating on proportion. "Once we achieve the visualization ideas of character, the mask will come. I tell them to put away their drawings and journals. Let the clay speak to them, and

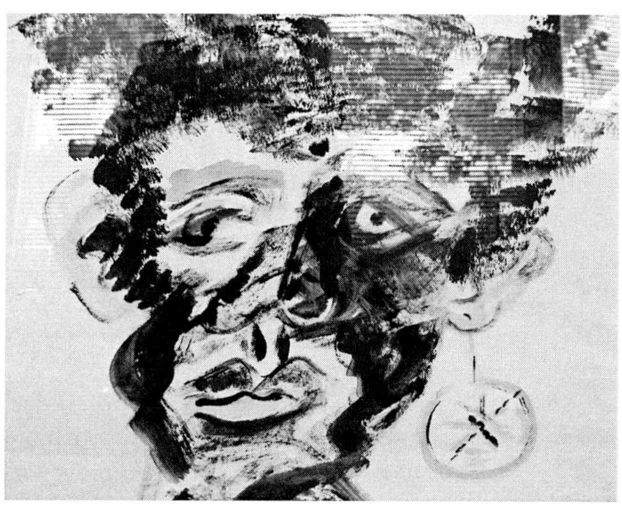

A self-portrait drawn by one of Donvieve's students in Arcata, California.

their mask will develop." Sometimes she has them create plaster gauze masks on their faces at this point, and then they paint the gauze and frame the mask with major lines (responding to their visual imagery ideas).

"Next I usually have them perform skits or improvised scenarios. Sometimes I have them write *haiku* and the *haiku* frequently inspire spontaneous movement, as they wear their masks. Or I might ask them to write their own personal story inspired by their *haiku*. After that point," she continues, "Each student might attempt to write a rough script. They begin to perfect their masks with an emerging personality evolving from the ideas gathered for the script. Presenting themselves in the beginning stages of their masks before a group can also generate ideas for improving the power of their masks, helping them to understand how each mask communicates and specifically what each person's mask should communicate."

Eventually a sense of their own self-portraits (presented in part by the masks) begins to solidify for each participant as well as for the group, especially as each student's masked character copes with conflict within the class skits. Each self-portrait in the form of a masked character can "play" at creating various responses to conflict, realizing that some responses are more acceptable to the performer (and the group members). Because it all takes place in an atmosphere of experimentation and play, each student can perform safely without fear of external admonishment. "If the student can identify a preference for an ideal self-portrait and its ideal internal characteristics, the student can more easily apply appropriate behavioral patterns (or reject patterns they do not want) to their own life struggles."

Donvieve considers the mask a success (that is, a successful healing event) when the student actually acknowledges a positive change in behavior resulting from the mask experience. "This is kinesthetic learning rather than verbal learning," she says. "Class skits almost always end up identifying family dynamics." In fact, she suggests that the students try wearing their masks at dinner and "see what comes up. The mask doesn't hide in this situation if presented seriously," she explains. "The mask always reveals."[115]

"I had my first son when I was eighteen and perhaps because I was such a young mother, I especially relate to teenagers. I'm very honest, committed, and connected to kids in my community. I try to listen to them carefully and I don't use a lot of extraneous philosophy when working with them." Her students create not only self-portrait masks, but warrior/inner guide masks, inspirational heroic masks, and personal totem masks as well. Like Radke, Donvieve believes mask making that acknowledges the self-reflections and personal spiritual dimensions of her students ultimately affects her entire community in positive ways. Indeed, shamans would agree.

One of Donvieve's students, Sandy Phillips, said that while taking one of Donvieve's mask workshops, Donvieve could laugh at herself and be who she wanted to be as a masked character, allowing the students permission to trust the spirits of their own alter egos in their masks.[116]

LAUREN RAINE'S GODDESS MASKS

Lauren Raine focuses primarily on masks of goddesses throughout history, spanning many cultures. She has worked with numerous community arts projects across the United States that involve participants who develop masks and performances based on goddesses who inspire them. Her extensive web site displays examples of her own masks and photos of goddess performances that have evolved during the workshops she has led.

In the spring of 1999, during a camping trip as she looked out on the valley under a full moon in Ojai, California, Raine recalled that the native word for Ojai means "valley of the moon." She stated that "It seemed an auspicious place." That night she had a vivid dream that a long line of women in a rainbow of colors stood before her. Soon afterwards, she attended a planning meeting for the Spiral Dance, which takes place annually in San Francisco to pay homage to *Samhain*, the Celtic Day of the Dead. The group wanted to emphasize cultural diversity themes and decided to celebrate the divine feminine cultures worldwide. Raine was commissioned to create twenty masks of ancient mythic goddesses, and researched corresponding myths for each one. She kept a journal of her dreams during this project and began to recognize the power of myths. She became particularly drawn to the Hindu Kali (a dark goddess) and the Tibetan White Tara (a white goddess). An on-line video shows a glimpse of this event: http://www.reclaiming.org/rituals/samhain.html.

When the Spiral Dance was presented, she indeed saw the procession of twenty colorful goddesses in masks and knew her dream had come true. In later years, she witnessed the masks used by ritualists, producers, priestesses, and dancers. She saw her masks evolve with proceeding presentations, filled with energy.

Raine believes that the goddess is returning to collective consciousness. "Whether we call her Mary, or Quan Yin, or Corn Mother, or Mother Earth, her return gives hope that the goddess can redeem the equilibrium of life. The balance can be restored," she says. "Myths are the templates of art and religion. These templates define the sacred and the profane." Raine believes that we are at a critical time when we need to revise the mythic assumptions we currently hold. "When I was a child my first paintings were of the bull dancers of ancient Crete along with their bare breasted, snake-entwined Goddess. I don't know why I wanted to paint her, but I do know my fifth grade teacher was embarrassed by my obsession with the imagery. Forty years later, I still believe that the goddess with a thousand faces has been driven underground, but has never left us. She lives in our archetypal memories, and is reborn in our contemporary mythic imaginations."

"In the '80s, as a graduate student, I joined a group of women artists. Initially we came together to have 'channeling sessions,' but what we really sought was mutual support as we confronted a competitive arts aesthetic that seemed incomplete. The underlying modern myth that viewed great artists as alienated genius seemed to us to present creativity as an awfully lonely process. Although I was a visual artist, I wanted my work to be a shared participatory art form between our group as we meditated and made moon rituals. I began to create community ritual dramas, not realizing I was naively re-discovering the origins of theatre." Raine added:

> All arts have sacred roots. Ritual enactment, with masks and dance, is one of the primal ways people have petitioned the gods, enacted rites of passage, and achieved heightened states of consciousness since ancient times. And people, everywhere, make masks. Art historians may view tribal masks as art objects, but their original use was as power objects. They were meant to be threshold tools that literally brought the gods to earth. Sacred masks were never made lightly. They required important procedures in order to function effectively, including choosing the right materials from the right place at the right time, asking ancestral spirits which masks were needed for specific ceremonies, and consecrating the finished work. A great deal of psychic preparation was necessary, and the masks were activated and de-activated with great respect. In Bali, I saw dancers carefully anoint them with holy water before and after each performance.
>
> Masks and all artistic effort appear ultimately as tools. The creative process is seamless, intimately personal, and equally transpersonal, involving our lives and many other lives at the same moment. I believe when we are in "flow," we find ourselves within a network of

> invisible collaborators. Some people call it synchronicity. Others call it synergy. For me, it's a grand conversation any creative person is privileged to join.[117]

Raine goes on to describe ritual dance as a way of embodying what is personally sacred, petitioning the spirit. "We open a temple within ourselves, bringing that temple to the theatre. Remembering is a gestalt experience."[118]

Lauren Raine has great interest in creating circle rituals with groups because "Theatre of the Goddess," as she calls it, "appears as circular motifs. We speak of becoming 'powerful,' but another way of viewing power within a group might be 'power-flowing,' by creating a stage upon which a complimentary exchange flows throughout the group. As the group generates synthesis, it generates energy, energy that can flow to the audience and beyond."

Raine explains that circularity is the essence of the ancient religions of the Great Mother. In Ireland, Malta, and Crete, prehistoric sites are covered with spirals and serpentines. The Great Mother moved in concentric and interwoven circles; the wheel of the year and the moon's passages are within a circle. Water and wind move across the landscape like a sinuous snake.

For Raine, masks are also about circles, the circle of personae that encircle our souls. The Greek word for mask is persona. She believes that we're all multiple personalities with varying degrees of conscious recognition of our multiplicity, and during the course of our lives we engage in many personae, which collectively become a council of the self, engaged in noisy and conflicting discourse. When the interior conversation is harmonious, we experience aspects of love and creativity. And at circle's center, beyond the last mask, there is the mystery of the spirit. Raine asserts that we become beings who are more compassionate when we can witness, embrace, and celebrate our "circle of self," from the mundane to the divine, the angelic, and the demonic. She concludes that the "so-called shadow self, the denied personae within," has an enormous reservoir of energy when brought to conscious expression within the appropriate arena of theatre.

She suggests that women (and men) expecting the goddess may decide to work with an archetype for many reasons, both personal and devotional. She mentioned one woman in her workshop who discovered a joyful opportunity to reconnect with "the wild woman within" when she decided to dance as Artemis for a community event. The adventurous, ecstatic relationship with nature she had as a young girl flooded back into her life. The mask of Artemis gave her the freedom to remember and renew those energies.

Raine recalled another one of her workshop participants who found new meaning for an ancient myth when she decided to dance as Sedna, the Inuit sea goddess (known for balanced restoration) during a community ritual at the Muse Theatre in Tucson. She enacted Sedna's traditional story, but also offered a conscious ritual of benediction which restored forgiveness and reconciliation to the forces of ignorance that had brought injustice to the performer herself.[119]

Raine writes, "In 2004, a few weeks before our first performance of *Restoring the Balance*, we learned that a new planet, in the cold depths of space beyond Pluto, was discovered by NASA researchers. The little planet was named Sedna, who was also the primary character in our production. For our cast, this striking synchronicity affirmed that we were, somehow, part of a larger telling."[120]

BRUCE MARRS' MASKS AS FAMILY-PORTRAITS

In addition to teaching at Dell'Arte International and other universities abroad, Bruce Marrs works with underprivileged teenagers across the country by using masks to help identify their conflicts at home and as burgeoning adults. Marrs admits that his best students are the ones who have had the most traumas in their lives. "They invariably lead the rest of the class, taking the masks and their dramatic power most seriously."[121] After all, both "trauma" and "drama" come from the same Greek root word meaning conflict. Both words can refer to physical or emotional conflict. Conflict, a basic component of drama and storytelling, most effectively expresses the universality of the human condition.

And Marrs has had his share of conflict. A colorful, energetic, vitally creative, and charismatic personality, he grew up in a single parent household with limited means. He struggled to adequately fit into the typical high school environment too structured and inflexible to accommodate his robust zest for life along with his deep teenage yearnings for recognition and appreciation. In hindsight Marrs did not have a complete perspective on the issues he faced in his youth, often feeling rather alienated. He now understands that many young people face similar challenges, especially those who feel vulnerable and unappreciated in rigid educational environments where class sizes remain too large. Over the years he has developed a special propensity for identifying these more frustrated students and enjoys working with them in his workshops and classes. He believes that his work as a mask maker and performer, in addition to his own experiences in school, helps him to better understand and assess these at-risk individuals while he assists them in blending, as well as standing out, in improvised family-portrait skits.

For over three decades Marrs has successfully managed to merge his professional work as a performer, mask maker, and instructor for Dell'Arte International while developing an international reputation as a commercial mask maker and as a director/teacher/performance coach for secondary and university-level students. His mask workshops for adults and young adults at Dell'Arte are especially popular every summer, where he regularly demonstrates his improvisational performance skills.

For several years Marrs has worked once a week with the at-risk elementary and preadolescent students at a ranch called Burt Ranch School near Blue Lake, California. Many of the students in this program have first-hand encounters with poverty. Some have parents who are in prison or addicted to drugs or struggling with long bouts of unemployment. Frequently these students find themselves as caretakers in their relationships with their parents.

Marrs has these students improvise family-portrait settings, often wearing masks (or conjuring a masked exaggerated state) while presenting their parents. He says he learns everything he needs to know about their individual situations through these workshop presentations. He has these students present their ideal parents in the form of similar presentations. Invariably these disenfranchised students show themselves baking brownies with their parents, or doing some other one-on-one activity where they share skills and conversation. He points out that these students realize that they do not have standard living situations. These group presentations allow them to see that they are not alone as they "reveal" their self-portraits in relationship to the group of masked self-portraits surrounding each other. The group of masked self-portraits becomes a family-portrait, encouraging trust and appreciation for the family at large.

Often these workshops offer the single opportunity for these troubled students to act out their frustrations. Marrs provides a safe place where his students can be heard. He offers encouragement with advice that many have not heard before: "So what if you've had a crappy childhood — you are surviving it. When you grow older, you will have survival skills and gifts to offer others. Don't quit school. Continue to change and ultimately take charge of improving yourselves and your situations." Marrs believes his students should understand that constructive awareness and empowerment can come from such difficult life situations. Some of them gain at least a glimpse of how they might improve their lives.

Donvieve, who has worked with teenagers in lock-down prison facilities, agrees. "Students universally like working in the masks. Ironically, the masks allow them to be themselves, and they are often terrified of being themselves. They want very much for these self-portraits to fit into a larger cultural group/family-portrait. Instead of presenting a devil character, the kid accused of the most serious crime invariably presents some sort of spiritual character, one that has the potential to be accepted and respected by the participating group members."[122]

Kate Hamm, a teacher for a magnet performing arts program for secondary schools in Iowa City, brought Marrs to guest direct one of her productions, *Wiley and the Hairy Man*. Hamm produces very physical theatre with aerial acrobatic work often incorporating a masked *commedia/Cirque du Soleil* style. "Marrs reaffirms their work and pushes them to next level," she says. "He is a brilliant collaborative artist. He loves all aspects of theatre—the mask, movement and design work, directing, and coaching. He recognizes magic all around him. He accepts his mistakes with humor, making it safe for those around him to make mistakes. He can give and take ideas and he is always respectful. The academic programs are intense here and he allows the students to escape the rigors of their classes with the very physical, spontaneous ensemble world of performance. He's a big kid and gives people permission to be kids as well." Each rehearsal begins with Marrs greeting the group and he announces, "Now we will simply play."[123] With that playful spirit, they improvise and work together toward performance solutions, building their confidence levels and trust in each other.

Radtke, Donvieve, Raine, and Marrs all serve as mentors with this premise of play in mind. Accordingly, drama and masked performance can serve as valuable therapeutic experiences and encourage vital powers of perception, healing, intensity, self-awareness, and a stronger sense of community. These are ultimate aims of any successful artistic experience as well.

In summarizing the therapeutic benefits of mask making, note that shamans sought these benefits millennia before as vital processes for artistic and spiritual development. Early on, shamans understood the mask's exceptional power. Each of the four contemporary Californian mask makers introduced in this section serve as guides, much like the Pacific Northwest shamans who preceded them by carrying out contemporary healing versions of creating masks in response to or to confront adversity. These mask makers understand the significance of personally committing to the act of creating a mask, knowing that in this process, even the amateur mask maker can become stronger, wiser, and more sensitive in accessing psychological worlds not fully recognized before.

International Mask Conferences

Professors Loyce Arthur and Ralph Hall of the University of Iowa Theatre Department organized the first International Mask Conference in 2001. This inspiring and provocative event attracted over two hundred mask makers, mask performers, educators in the art of masked performance. They gathered an impressive international group representing United States, Canada, England, Sweden, Indonesia, and Italy to share their skills, insights, and artistry. A substantial number of the mask makers I have interviewed for this book either attended this initial conference or were mentioned by participants during their presentations.

Both Arthur and Hall have extensive backgrounds in mask work. Arthur has held a West African Research Association Fellowship and has trained with Italian mask maker Donato Sartori. She has designed several productions which used masks based on African, Asian, and Native American styles, most notably Langston Hughes's *Black Nativity* at Saint Paul Community Baptist Church in Brooklyn, New York. This show received a Village Voice OBIE Award. Hall, who graduated from *L'École Internationale de Théâtre Jacques Lecoq* (Jacques Lecoq's International School of Theatre) in 1981, worked as a teacher, school director, and company actor with Dell'Arte International from 1982 to 1998.

The organizers attracted some of the best-known mask artists of our time. Outstanding mask makers and performers such as Rob Faust (Faustwork Mask Theatre), Ralph Lee (Mettawee River Theatre Company, NBC-TV's *Saturday Night Live*), I. Made Suryasa (Indonesian mask carver and performer), Joan Schirle (Founding Artistic Director of Dell'Arte Company and School Director), and Torbjörn Alström (sculptor, mask maker, and performer based in Sweden at the National School for Theatre and Opera at the University of Gothenburg) were all at the conference. Never before had so many distinguished artists been together. Their presence and contributions, along with the participation of authors Judy Slattum (*Masks of Bali*) and Sears Eldredge (*Mask Improvisation*), made the conference a landmark event.

The conference participants also had the opportunity to learn and observe from a number of other dynamic and knowledgeable artists. These artists offered a full range of work representing a number of diverse cultural communities ranging from Tsimshian tribal performance in British Columbia (Victor Reece and the Karen Jamieson Dance Company), Japanese Kyogen Theatre (Marsha Paludan and Laura Ramberg), West Coast festival and street theatre masks (Newman and Xstine Cook), African-influenced Shakespearean drama (Loyce Arthur and Nefertiti Burton), Celtic drama (Gateway Performance Productions), Greek drama (Betty Monroe), and Italian *commedia dell'arte* masked performance works (Newman, Bruce Marrs, Ralph Hall, Don Jordan, and Xstine Cook.) Bob Croghan demonstrated new techniques and approaches for making non-toxic wonders such as thermoplastic mesh and neoprene masks work effectively, easily, and beautifully. Charlie Oates, Bruce Marrs, Leslie O'Dell, Rick Kemp, and Robin David all offered insightful training tips for the novice mask maker and performer and demonstrated several typical mask-training exercises.

Other conference coordinators could learn from Arthur and Hall, who organized the conference presentations so that no session overlapped, giving everyone the opportunity to hear and observe all of them. The conference participants appreciated the community spirit that easily developed within the four-day period. Mask performers and mask makers (many of whom are both performers and mask makers) could approach content and form issues at the same time, focusing on perspectives of performance, style, and audience perception effortlessly along with technical perspectives on mask making and training. Consequently the conference had a strong sense of integrity.

Audiences delight most in recognizing the concept of "less is more" when watching a top performer combining great visual stylization and implications of the mask with technical virtuosity, evoking clear characterization with carefully controlled rhythmic movement and action patterns. Joan Schirle (with Dell'Arte Company) achieved all this and more when she performed *Second Skin: Stories of the Mask* during the first evening of the conference.

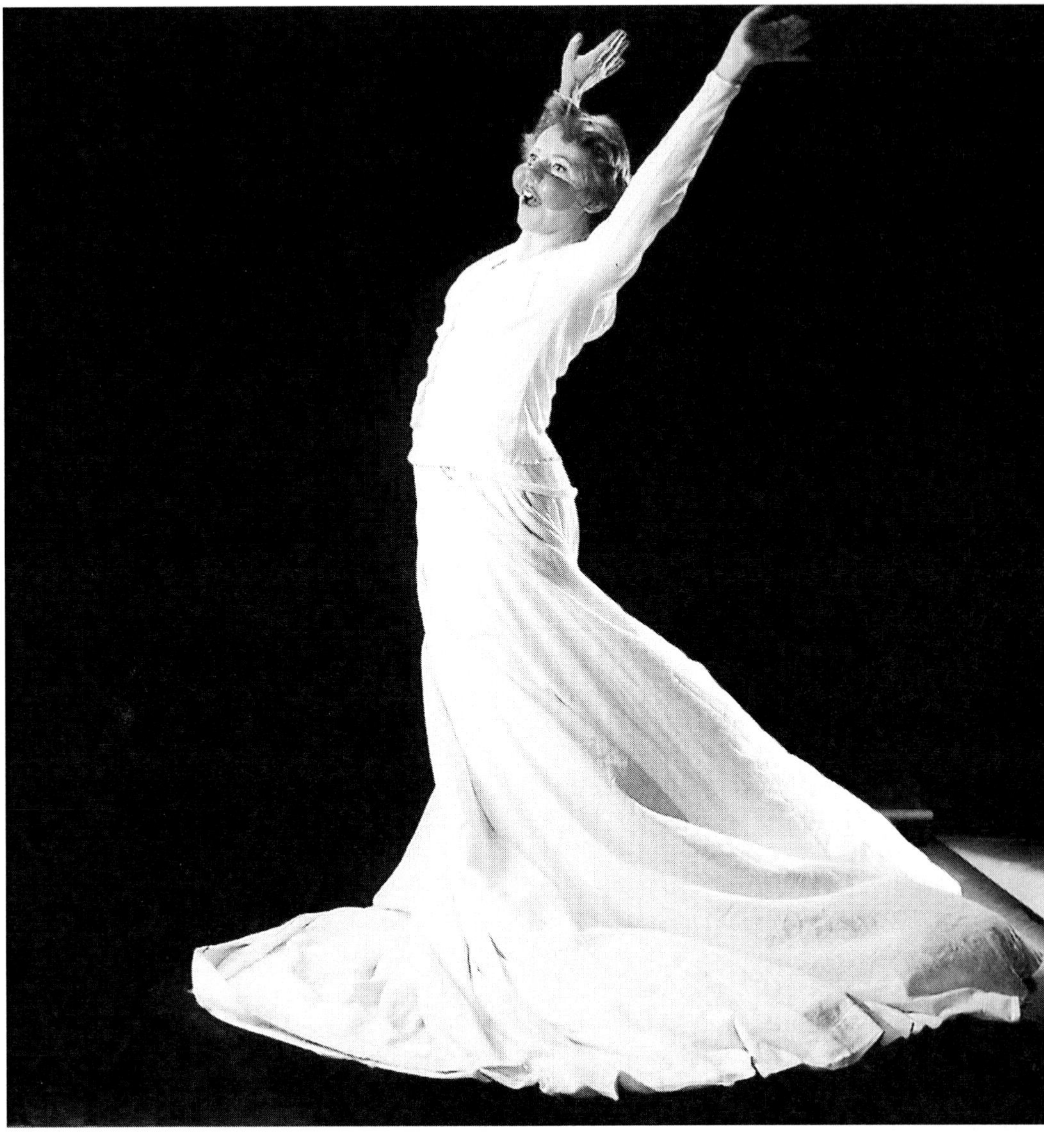

Joan Schirle in her one-woman tour of *Second Skin: Stories of the Mask*. Photographer: Robin Robin. Courtesy of Joan Schirle.

Schirle's program note described her as having created a "vivid series of masked characters (and wildly disparate characters at that) who coalesce around the threshold of the afterlife, as Schirle weaves multiple character portraits into an all-souls journey." Schirle then stated during her performance that "the image of a second skin is evoked by masks themselves, as well as from the very human desire to be someone other than who we are. Many of us long to have a life other than the one we find ourselves living. I'm fascinated by how self-image becomes obsession. It's funny and scary at the same time."[124]

Schirle's masked characters, like the remarkably specific characterizations of mask maker/performer Rob Faust of Faustwork Mask Theatre (in his *Mask Messenger* performance the following night), were so detailed that the characters moved into the realm of universality.

I recognized personalities and characters that the artists portrayed as unique personalities that surprisingly resembled my own friends and acquaintances in my personal surroundings, far from Schirle's and Faust's life experiences. Their stylized characters went beyond exaggerated cartoon (though somehow they fit that description in mask and movement), and became "more real than real" in a stunning, magical, theatrical way.

Numerous presentations during this conference in Iowa centered on *commedia dell'arte* themes. These themes particularly emphasized related movement issues and achieving rich characterizations. Other presentations included descriptive traditional processes of making commedia leather masks as well as contemporary techniques using papier-mâché and thermoplastic. Ralph Hall's *The Troubles of Love* played to a full audience on the Iowa City Festival Stage. After having set up the basic scenario via email, the performers (seemingly) effortlessly improvised a roughly sketched-out dialogue, much as sixteenth-century *commedia* performers did. Bruce Marrs shared insights into how *commedia* characters move and respond while always aware of balancing intuition with craft. His demonstrations, as well as Don Jordan's demonstrations of *commedia* characters in action, displayed the sort of technical virtuosity, flexibility, and spontaneity that develops only after years of work. Marrs insisted that almost all the *commedia* characters (except the lovers) start with movement that evolves from the knees at a slightly bent position. His Capitano and Jordan's Harlequino expertly romped across stage with wit and flare, using beautifully constructed traditional costumes. Newman discussed some of the techniques he uses to create leather *commedia* masks more easily, using frozen oil-based Plasticine clay (or Pastilina clay) rather than a wooden matrix and slits placed under the nose. Another talented mask maker, Teodoro Dragonieri, who has lived with *commedia* and Venetian masks since his childhood in Italy, shared humorous anecdotes on various devils, gamblers, lovers, and fools he has helped bring to life on stage. Sara Romersberger demonstrated ways of unlocking the physicality of Shakespeare's comedies with the masks of *commedia*. Some of the exercises that harkened back to those she had learned from Lecoq still serve her students well.

With a series of pictures and demonstrations, Charlie Oates vividly described successful characters created by his students, choosing plastic bags in all shapes, sizes, and contortions, imaginatively worn around the body. Oates showed how creating narrative through messy, accidental means could break through the doldrums of predictable, boring, and lifeless characterizations. The students had a sense of play while intuitively creating invigorating characters that seemed to evolve from the plastic sculptures they put together in less than an hour.

Indonesian mask carver/performer I. Made Suryasa and his wife, scholar Judy Slattum, presented an authentic *Topeng* or Balinese Mask Dance, demonstrating the traditional characterization of the Minister character and the Old Man from a *Topeng* Mask Drama, complete with an elaborately draped, colorful Indonesian costume. Slattum pointed out various characteristics of successful Balinese dance, such as short staccato movements occurring at odds with the overall directional flow. This dance particularly emphasized the head, hands, and feet — rich with ancient East Indian and Chinese-influenced iconic references, though altogether distinctly Balinese. Balinese convention insists that the performer must raise his/her toes at all times, walking on the balls of the front feet. The rhythms of the music are at odds with the dancer's movements of head, hands, and feet. Still a regular feature of everyday Balinese life, masked performance takes on greater significance for Balinese audiences, allowing for satirical comments on topical political situations.

Mask carver/performer Laura Ramberg performed the marvelous masked crab in *The*

Crab and the Yamabushi with performer and director Marsha Paludan. Paludan, who has an extensive background in Japanese *Kyogen* theatre, has worked with the eminent Japanese artist, Andrew Tsubaki. Together they have toured in the United States as well as Japan with their performances. Ramberg explained at one point, "My performance is simply a memory of making the mask." Together, Ramberg and Paludan provided a wealth of information on how *Kyogen* theatre developed, pointing out that *Kyogen* began in rural Japan, much the same way as *commedia dell'arte* did in rural Italy. *Kyogen* and *commedia dell'arte* use similar archetypal characters and carefully orchestrated movements unique to each character. *Commedia* works with spontaneous story lines and improvisational dialogue. However, *Kyogen* theatre has highly structured movement, dialogue, and vocal intonations. Only men traditionally wore the *Kyogen* masks, while women frequently performed female characters (with or without masks) in commedia performances.

The crab character in their *Kyogen* performance reminds us how important animal personalities and totems are to masked performances worldwide. The performances of many Native American, African, European, and Asian cultures incorporate animal masks. *Commedia* characters have certain animal and bird traits as well. Harlequino, for instance, has agile, cat-like traits, and Columbina means "Little Dove."

This concept tied in nicely with Rick Kemp's presentation, when he led conference participants in several demonstrations incorporating intuitive techniques when evoking animal totems for the creation of contemporary masks. With rhythmic drum sounds, he had conference participants imagine meeting or encountering their own individual animal totems in a far-off "field" residing deep in their subconscious. These animal totems have tremendous spiritual energy and potential to protect, empower, and disguise the performer as animal totems have done since primitive times. We still see this force at work in such contemporary productions as Julie Taymor's *The Lion King*.

The most profoundly moving presenter, Native American Victor Reece, paid tribute to his ancestors with his exquisitely detailed masks. He described how the masks contained their spirits and their love for him and their Tsimshian tribal community. This community currently confronts extinction. Dominated by Christianity for the past two centuries, its new generation has lost much knowledge of its language, religion and traditions. While he spoke and performed in Tsimshian for conference participants, Reece observed that he is one of the few remaining fluent Tsimshians. He can only hope that his masks, representing the last remnants of his culture, will live on after he is gone. His masks project a sense of his grandparents smiling at him and encouraging him. He wants the rest of the world to experience their spirit and warmth and power as well.

New York mask maker Ralph Lee presented photos of his remarkably grand, gigantic, and impressive puppet and mask figures that towered over audience members in outdoor settings. His masks depict the theatricality and dramatic tension inherent in diverse traditional and contemporary cultures. His themes and styles ranged from those found in *Arabian Nights* and Winnebago trickster stories to Welsh legends and Irish sagas to Mayan, Greek, and Iroquois creation myths.

The 2005 International Mask Conference, bearing the all-inclusive theme *Masks of Transformation* and rivaling the first International Mask Conference in 2001, brought together mask makers, masked performers, mask vendors, masqueraders, and scholars of the mask to Southern Illinois University Carbondale from such far-flung countries as Nigeria, Sweden, Israel, Mexico, Canada, Iceland, Hungary, Greece, Bali, the United Kingdom, and Brazil. This four-day conference became the mask Mecca of the world, with opportunity to explore masks from many vantage points, ranging from detailed descriptions of mask-making techniques to the healing potential of masks used in art therapy and performance to retrospectives on mask makers such as Stanley Allan Sherman and early-twentieth-century mask maker Benda as well as those in Iceland, Trinidad, and Greek folk festivals found in Sardinia. The conference included a comprehensive historical and international exhibit of masks; native masked performances representing Nigerian ancestral masquerade, Northwest Native-American archetypal matriarchal spirits; performances by master masked performers Rob Faust (United States/Canada), Larry Hunt (United States), Torbjörn Alström (Sweden), and much more.

Ron Naversen, Hilary Chandler, and Segun Ojewuyi organized this comprehensive, action-packed conference that embraced both the sacred and the profane worlds of the mask. For four days, mischievous clowns, aspiring angels, ancestral and matriarchal spirits, demons, and tragic heroes all lived under the proscenium arch of Southern Illinois University Carbondale's McLeod Theatre, its University Museum, Carbondale Convention Center, and onto the city's streets for a Saturday mask celebration festival.

The coordinators seemed undaunted by the intricate up-front planning; quests for corporate and institutional funding; large public turnout; and execution of twenty-two scholarly presentations as well as the logistical challenges of publicizing the event and mounting six fully produced masked performances. The coordinators assembled (or co-hosted) a Mask Cabaret at a local nightclub, twenty-one mask-making or masked performance workshops, eleven mask poster exhibits, a mask bazaar and vendor exhibits involving the artistry of over thirty-four mask makers.

Conference participants undoubtedly displayed their greatest enthusiasm for the masked performances presented by performers held in particularly high regard by aficionados of the world of masks. One of the most provocative pieces, entitled *Margie*, created and performed by Rob Faust, looked at memories of his childhood nanny, Margie, while growing up in a privileged environment in New Orleans. The conference took place only a few weeks after Hurricane Katrina, so the audience found itself with double reflections on the losses of the city as well as Rob's loss of childhood innocence.

> After more than thirty years of having no contact with my childhood nanny Margie, I called her on the phone. We'd talked for a mere three or four minutes when she told me she still loved me, and was still proud of all her four white children. The stage piece in which I relive that phone call, both as myself and as Margie, was originally entitled *For True*, which is what she exclaimed when I said into the phone, "Hello, Margie, this is Robbie." The performance story is my attempt to get at a deep truth. Growing up white, with a conscience, in uptown New Orleans in the '50s and '60s, you couldn't help feeling the contradictions of face-to-face vs. race-to-race. In spite of the legacy of slavery, the many power imbalances, and the tilted playing field (recently shown so clearly by Hurricane Katrina) white and black people in the deep South get along and even love each other. Imagine that.

On stage Faust transforms himself into the flamboyant, large-bosomed African American Margie by seemingly effortlessly donning a fat suit on stage and then wrapping himself in a large rectangular white and black print dress topped with a red bolero jacket and beaming, rosy-cheeked mask — all set to New Orleans' jazz. "Performing *Margie* and actually becoming Margie onstage was a way for me to acknowledge and to explore, with both humor and utter seriousness, the relationship I had with a black woman — a surrogate mother — without having to dwell on, figure out, the gargantuan issues, past and present,

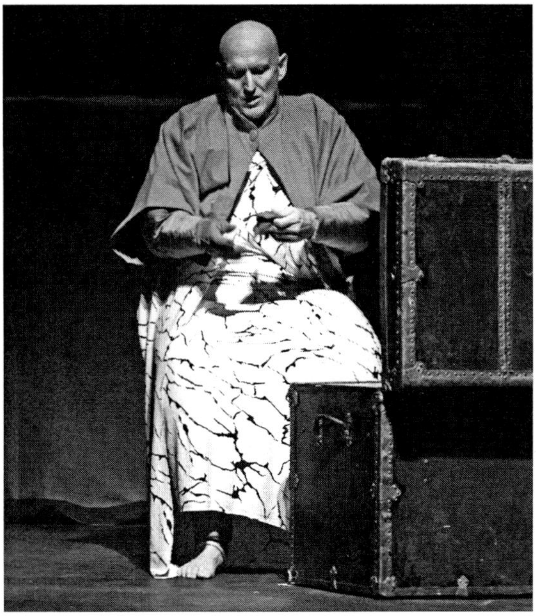

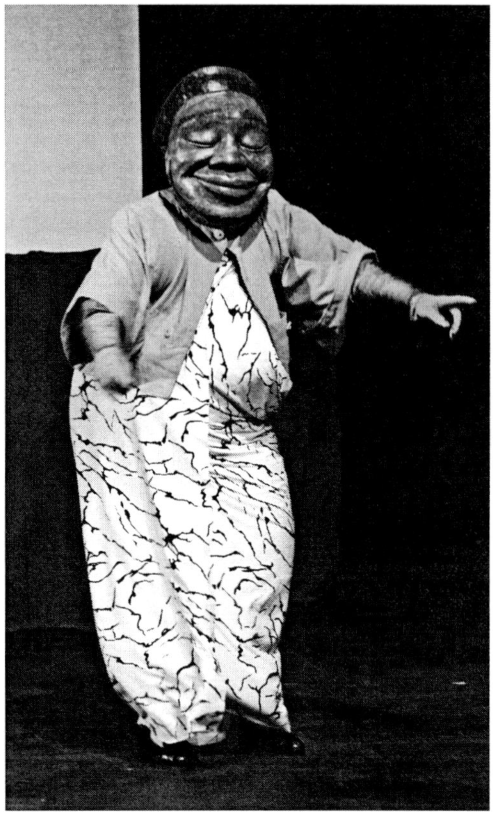

Above: **Rob Faust transforming himself into his childhood nanny during his performance of** ***Margie*** **at the 2005 International Mask Conference at Southern Illinois University Carbondale.** ***Right:*** **Faust fully transformed on stage as Margie. Photographer: Ron Naversen.**

of racial inequality. Of all the work I perform, *Margie* is the deepest felt, the most personal, and perhaps the most satisfying. Ironically, it disturbs the political sensibilities of some audience members, while causing others to both laugh and cry. As a writer and performer, what more could you ask for?"

Larry Hunt, of Masque Theatre, combined masks, mime, music, and dance to explore the essential mysteries of the human condition; the magic of hope re-kindled, the soul's flight in the guise of a great bird, and the cycles of human life reflected in the phases of the moon. This range of exploration was all done with lively humor, panache, and an ability to depict specific "street characters" in universally recognized ways.

Torbjörn Alström displayed his genius in mixing informal lectures on mask work (offering a broad range of its historical and cultural comparisons) with staged presentations of some of his best loved characters, such as his Pulcinella (who always manages to transcend Italian *commedia*), and several versions of his grotesque Everyman masks, projecting ultimate pathos, despair, entrapment, and hope. He also performed in some of the wooden masks he's developed that use stringed inside sections placed carefully in juxtaposition to varying levels of carved space which allow for the masks to emit human and animal sounds that carry out easily into the audience. He has developed this technique through significant, extensive experimentation spanning several years. The resulting innovative masks evoked audience delight and wonder.

The native performance of a typical Nigerian ancestral (*Egungun*) masquerade held the audience spellbound with rhythmic drumming, music, and dance as the *Egungun* paraded on to the stage to prophesize, pontificate, admonish, and inspire the surrounding village people. (Some were members of the audience who came on stage to participate.) Ojetunji Ojeyemi conversed and consequently revealed the masked *Egungun* ancestral figure, offering expertise that only he as the son of a Nigerian chief, born into the lineage of the Oje (Yoruba traditional cult of Masquerades) could possess. As a boy of six he was initiated into the guild of mask dancers and acrobatic performers. He has since been a pivotal presence in the annual Nigerian *Egungun* Festival.

Northwest Tsimshian master mask maker and performer Victor Reece along with his prolific wife, Sharon Jinkerson-Brass (film-director and writer), and dancers Mariko Ohara and Melina Laboucan-Massimo presented a highly ambitious, distinctly original combination of film imagery and text with masked performance and dance that explored the Native American matriarchal spirits of Copper Woman and Spider Woman (keepers of women's ritual, dances and songs) as a way of maintaining the most important life-affirming values of the village community.

Morgyn Owens-Celli, curator of the American

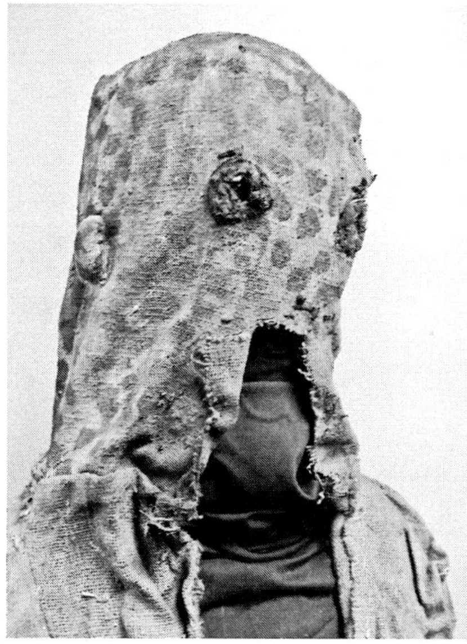

One of the authentic Nigerian *Egungun* masks exhibited at the 2005 International Mask Conference at Southern Illinois University Carbondale.

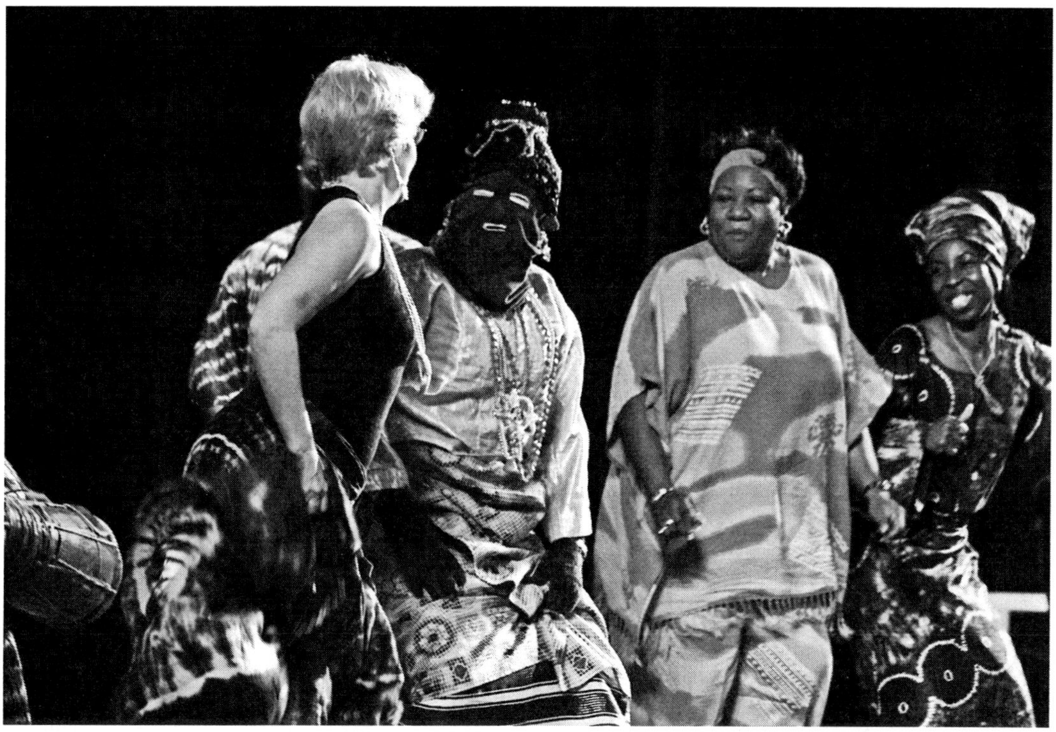

Audience members performing with Nigerian *Egungun* character played by Ojetunji Ojeyemi. Photographer: Ron Naversen.

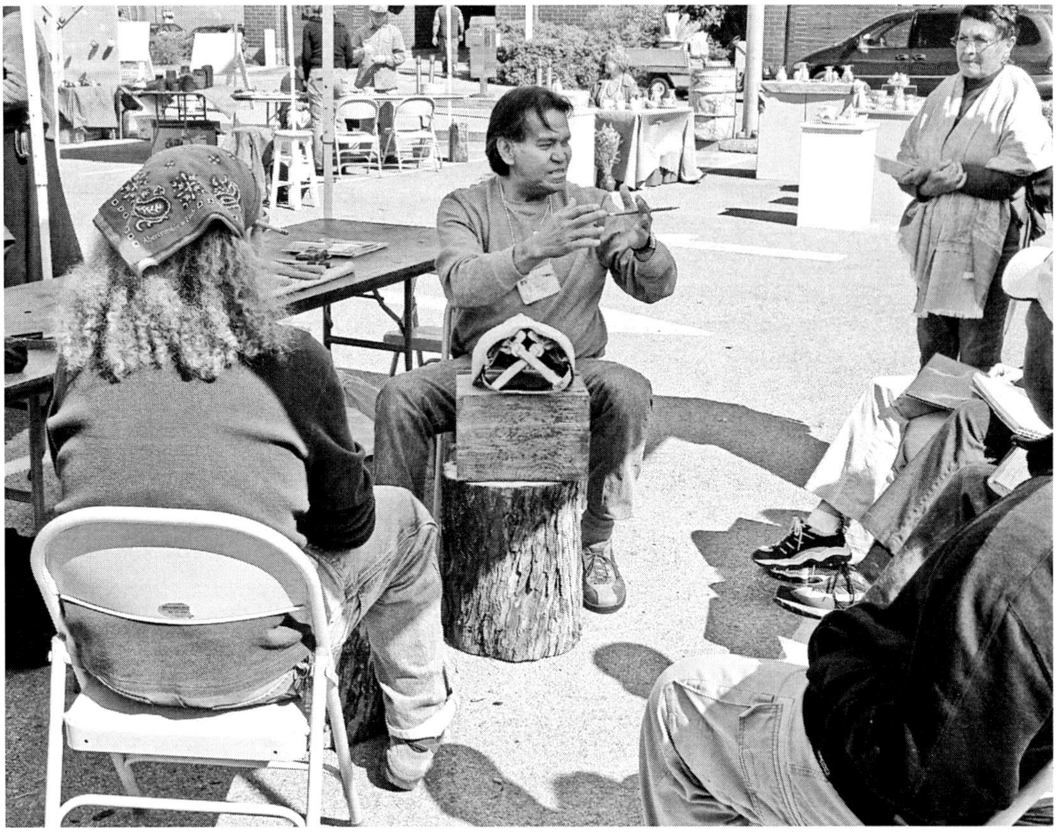

Tsimshian mask maker Victor Reece demonstrating how to carve one of his masks at the 2005 International Mask Conference at Southern Illinois University Carbondale.

Museum of Straw Art surveyed a photographic history of straw masks from many cultures, identifying some of the customs in straw-mask masquerades. He demonstrated how straw masks were often seen in the ceremonies of agrarian societies. He also described various types of straw, how they can be colored, as well as their potential for various ways of braiding. He presented some of these braiding techniques for a smaller, more informal audience after his conference session.

The first decade of this century saw two universities in Iowa and Illinois that have sponsored the first two international mask conferences. These events have offered camaraderie and inspiration for mask makers. The mask conferences showcased the remarkable variety of masks and underscored their relevance in contemporary as well as traditional settings.

These two conferences also exemplified the sense of community found in live masked performances. Recall earlier in this chapter Trinidadian mask maker Sheldon Clemdore who remarked that sooner or later, "it takes a village."[125] He expressed the sentiments of masmen, but also the sentiments of mask makers worldwide who understand the potential of masked performance to build strong bonds of community within a range of diverse cultural values. Masked performance especially works as a type of intimate performance within small audience groups, allowing both performers and audience members to share complex truths imaginatively. Of course, we enjoy masked performance in film as well. But the smaller community circles of live masked performance events, when conducted successfully,

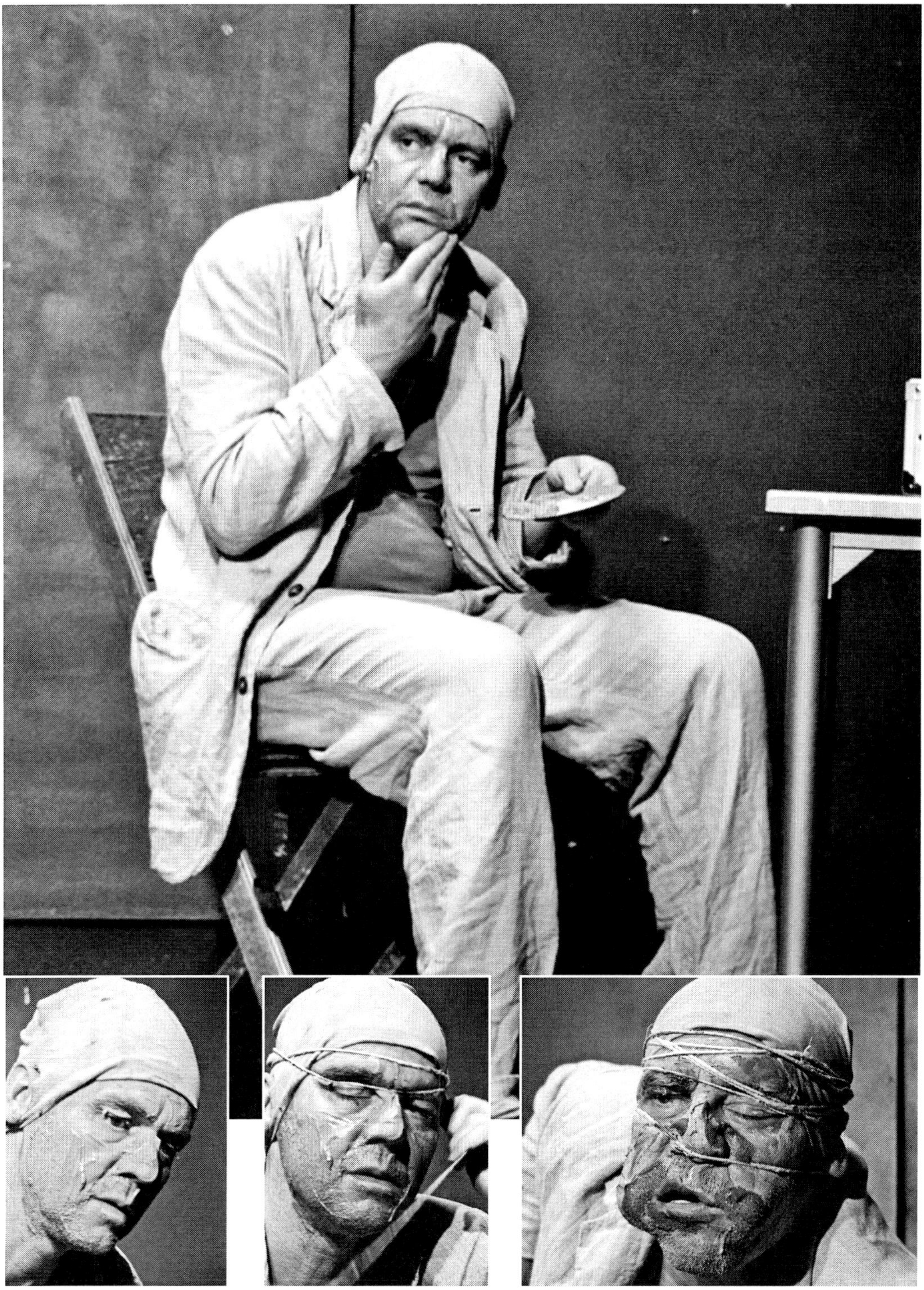

Swedish mask maker Torbjörn Alström becoming his version of Everyman on stage in his performance ***Tales from the Mask*** at the 2005 International Mask Conference. His haunting performance of the grotesque Everyman evolves on stage, taking almost five minutes to achieve this final effect while Arvo Pärt's ***Spiegel im Spiegel*** plays in the background. This mask is inspired by Greenlandic masks which are thought to be at least three thousand years old.

have substantially more potential to present the vital, ancient experiences of ritual and community. These intimate community performances can "create a village" of audience members even when amidst strangers.

Displaying the Mask

Amleto and Donato Sartori International Museum of the Mask (Museo Internationale della Maschera Amleto e Donato Sartori)

On December 30, 2004, the International Museum of the Mask opened in Abano Terme (near Venice), Italy, featuring the work of Amleto Sartori and his son, Donato, sculptors, painters, poets, performers, and world famous mask makers, along with masks from their extensive international collection. This opening was officially celebrated five months later by the Nobel Prize Laureate Dario Fo and his wife Franca Rame with a play Fo created and presented entitled *Masks, Puppets, and Painted Men,* which focused on the history of the mask and of the Sartoris. In this way Fo offered homage to the Sartoris as superb mask sculptors. In his welcoming speech, he singled out Donato's wife, Paola Piizzi, curator of the museum, declaring that she was "the true soul of this museum."[126] Dario Fo reminded the audience that the mask has its roots in performance ritual; consequently, contemporary performers must always remember its ties to realms of the sacred.[127] He also paid personal homage to Amleto and Donato Sartori:

> The Sartoris are straight out of the Renaissance, like the Carraccis, the Venezianos, the Pisanos. Usually the father passes the baton on to his son, who seems to be the father's reincarnation. But when it comes to Amleto and Donato, the two form a single, unique pair.
>
> We are talking about the craft of the mask sculptors. I myself have worn hundreds of their masks, in performances, during exhibitions and lessons, in conferences and in universities, from Copenhagen to Paris, from New York to Beijing. With my eyes closed I can distinguish Biancolelli's Arlecchino mask from the one that is presumed to have belonged to Tristano Martinelli, the first Arlecchino.
>
> But it is easier for me to discover whether a mask has been carved and beaten in leather by the Sartoris or whether it is an imitation. I don't want to be hysterical, but I assure you that more than once, in an emergency, I have had to wear a mask made by imitators: after only a few minutes I couldn't go on with the performance. It stuck to my face, rubbed my cheeks, scratched my nose. Above all the voice that came out of the leather lip was distorted, hissing, even opaque. Few people know that a mask made by a master is above all an extraordinary acoustic tool, a musical instrument that amplifies and catalyzes the balance of tones, of high and low pitched sounds.[128]

This three-day celebration of the opening of the International Museum of the Mask included several performances and attracted over 4000 audience members. These events would not have taken place without the dogged perseverance of Donato Sartori and Paola Piizzi, as well as public funding and support by international performers and scholars. For more than two decades Donato and Paola had dreamed of establishing a mask museum and, after various political hindrances, they discovered that Villa Savioli Trevisan, an eighteenth-century Veneto villa, was an excellent location to house part of the enormous Sartori collection. The collection includes masks, other works of art, and documents from all over the world. The Museum represents the fruit of the artistic activity of Amleto and Donato, tracing an arc of time from 1928 to the present day, documenting a varied and complex series of experimentation and research.[129]

Donato Sartori could see the potential of this site to serve as a unique, substantial setting to house his permanent, cyclical, and temporary mask exhibits. He had always wanted his masks displayed in a setting which was not only a place of conservation and memory, but also a modern, dynamic, and experimental museum, unique in the world, with lots of material to see. He wanted a site accessible to young people who could learn about the art and functions of the mask, as well as to scholars who could investigate the subject. He envisioned a "non-museum" setting where the masks could become alive as "sculptures in movement" rather than simply being hung on walls. At this site, performers could actually wear his masks in staged events while scholars could also come to study his extensive collection of documentation relating to mask work. Sartori's ultimate concept involved establishing a creative environment that could house a studio, theatre, and perhaps even a film studies lab. Students could learn how to make traditional *commedia* masks and could also examine the masks as well as his impressive mask collection. Thus, they could have a rich understanding of how traditional masks function in conjunction with movement and gesture work. Ultimately, the Museum would give his students inspiration to create and perform in their own masks.[130]

Donato considered the formation of the International Museum of the Mask as the capstone to the Centro *Maschera e Strutture Gestuali*, which has conceived and planned all his cultural and artistic activities since 1979, including his annual summer international workshops entitled The Art of the Mask in *Commedia dell'Arte* for the last two decades. Sartori's museum also expresses the historic Italian propensity for masked spectacle, and Padua offered a setting long known for its patronage of sculptural arts.

Not surprisingly, the museum project enjoyed strong support of the Town Council of Abano Terme, which granted use of the Villa to *Centro Maschere*, which conceived the project for the Museum as an integrated center for the promotion, enhancement, and experimentation of culture, art, and performance. Even so, it took over five years to plan and prepare the Museum. Unfortunately, the Museum as it now exists already lacks adequate square footage. "We have thousands of masks and artifacts but very little room to actually experiment in a theatrical setting. Even though there are two full floors of historical exhibits, hundreds of masks still remain stored in boxes in various warehouses," Donato Sartori acknowledges. Maintenance costs have proven daunting. In addition to standard cleaning and upkeep after public performances and exhibit viewings, there are regular expenses for museum personnel and marketing. To help meet these expenses, Sartori is forced to make space available for outside conferences and offices, reducing the Museum's exhibition space even more.[131]

"I sometimes consider selling the collection and disbanding the museum because I'm uncertain how long I can afford to maintain it," says Donato.[132] Artists have visited the museum, but also many tourists, schools, actors, and scholars. After Goldoni, and with the exception of Carnival celebrations, the use of the mask has declined and it is remarkable how, in the second half of the twentieth century, artists like Dario Fo, Jacques Lecoq, and Donato's father Amleto were able to create a resurgence of interest in this ancient art form by striving to re-create the magic of the Italian *commedia dell'arte* masked performances. Many theatres like the *Théâtre du Soleil* in Paris (where another great mask maker, Erhard Steifel, created many masks) were influenced by Amleto Sartori's abilities and his research into authentic Renaissance leather masks. Amleto created masks for plays produced by Giorgio Strehler, Jean-Louis Barrault, and Gian Franco De Bosio as well as for famous actors such as Marcello Moretti and Eduardo De Filippo.[133] Donato believes that such work is classic and should remain archived, documented, and exhibited for future generations of artists.[134]

Perhaps no one has been more influenced by this work than Donato Sartori himself. He admits that when he was a teenager, his father would punish him for doing poorly in school by making him work in the studio as his apprentice-son, cleaning up projects and preparing various materials and supplies for eventual use in sculpting. In this way, he inadvertently became familiar with the processes his father used in creating his masks.[135]

Donato had always held great esteem for his father, who had fought in the Resistance during World War II and had even suffered torture by the Fascists. His mother was Jewish; consequently his entire family was hidden in the Veneto countryside from 1939 to 1945. Donato believes that his father's dramatic experiences between the two wars influenced his artistic themes and expressions. In fact, the theme of the mask as a sculpture appears in his first grotesques in wood and terracotta in 1928, and was to be developed after the end of World War II. Donato says, "The extraordinary thing about the success of my father's masks is that they were created by a sculptor who in his lifetime had already made an enormous number of works such as monuments, altar pieces, and portals in various materials such as

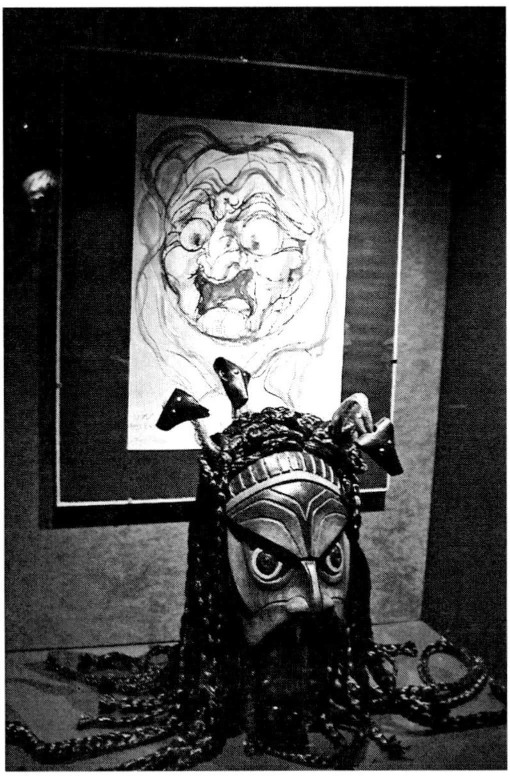

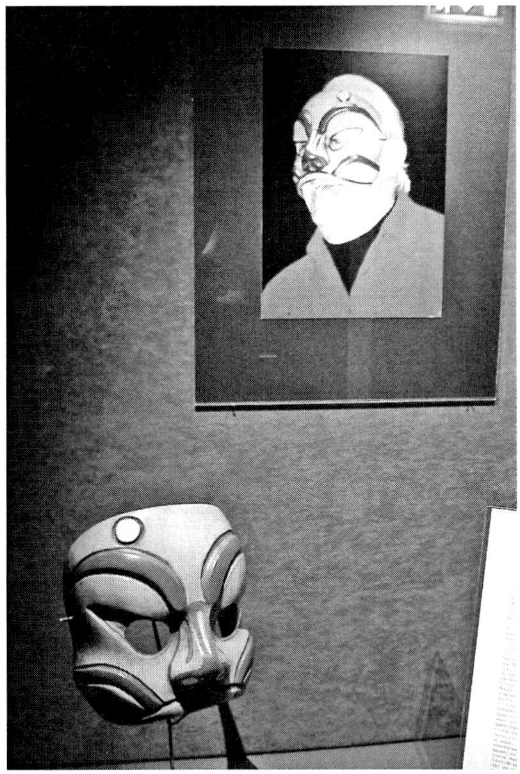

Details of the interior of the Amleto and Donato Sartori International Museum of the Mask at Villa Savioli Trevisan, Abano Terme (Padua, Italy). Photograph on the left presents a study for a bronze Latin mask created by Amleto Sartori in 1948. Photograph on the right presents the painted, dubbed leather Cat Arlecchino mask, one of the Sartori masks of 1980 created for Dario Fo, the 1997 Nobel Laureate in Literature.

bronze, marble, stone, and especially carved wood. The theme of the theatrical mask only appears in the latter stage of his life, that is, as from 1947 when he began collaborating with the theatre at the University of Padua, directed by Gian Franco De Bosio. The dramatic tensions of Amleto's life did not allow him much opportunity to express himself artistically in his younger years." But he made up for lost time when he took strong interest in anatomy and sculpture after the war and quickly became well-known for his masks. "People generally assume that mask makers are simply artisans," Donato said. "My father was not just a fine artisan, he approached his masks with the eye of an artist as the best mask makers do. Interestingly both he and Dario Fo had similar drawing styles."[136]

Amleto Sartori studied sculpture after World War I at the Venice Academy, which specialized in sculptural arts and human anatomy. These studies provided the foundation for his mask making. Later, he taught sculpture at the Art Institute in Padua where Donato eventually took over as one of its teachers.[137] Certainly the son has become the father in terms of artistic success. Donato has exhibited his masks and sculptures in various art museums ranging from Venice to New York, from Tokyo to Mexico City, from Beijing to Moscow, and Singapore. He has regularly worked with theatre companies in Italy and in many European countries, as well as the United States, Canada, Japan, and South America. He has held an enormous number of international workshops on the history, creation, and interpretation of the mask, assisted by the team of *Centro Maschere e Strutture Gestuali* which also manages the affairs of the International Mask Museum.[138] One could argue that Donato has far exceeded his father's expectations.

Donato points out that one can readily see the influence of his father's style on his own early masks exhibited at the mask museum. But his father died, in 1962, when Donato was only twenty years old. And Donato, like his father before him, found his early years full of its own dramatic tensions, culminating in the late 1960s at the height of various student revolutions and avant-garde art movements defined by such bold companies as Bread and Puppet and The Living Theatre. The ethnically diverse music styles ushered in by the hippie generation emphasized communal lifestyles and a return to cross-cultural tribal motifs. The visual arts of this period generated new multidisciplinary and multimedia activity. Donato spent the period of the great student revolutions of 1968 in Paris between *L'École Internationale de Théâtre Jacques Lecoq* and lessons at *École des Beaux-Arts*, which had such an influence on him that he changed and evolved the concept of the mask in art.[139]

Donato Sartori's masks that began to cover the entire body are called "Gestural Structures." These led to the "Urban Masks," huge artistic installations that often cover entire buildings and are art events akin to body art and land art. Major cities like Copenhagen, Venice, and Rio de Janeiro have hosted his masked performance art which leads "tribal" celebrants to spontaneously dance, play, and roam around the giant fabricated masks covering a city hall, an important square in the town center, or a city park, accompanied by lighting effects and the pulsating beats of music generated by elaborate sound systems. He describes a particularly dramatic effect in Lisbon where 40,000 people gathered to experience the Urban Mask and then proceeded to destroy the huge fabric swaths. As Pierre Restany explains, "Today, audiences must participate in these communal events even as they essentially create their own unique art which results from such an experience. This sort of event harkens back to that of primitive tribes, dancing and participating in ritual with masked forces around the light of a bonfire to the accompanying rhythms of drum beats. And like such primitive celebrations, the contemporary urban audience releases pent up energies until the collapse of the giant mask produces a climax of euphoria."[140]

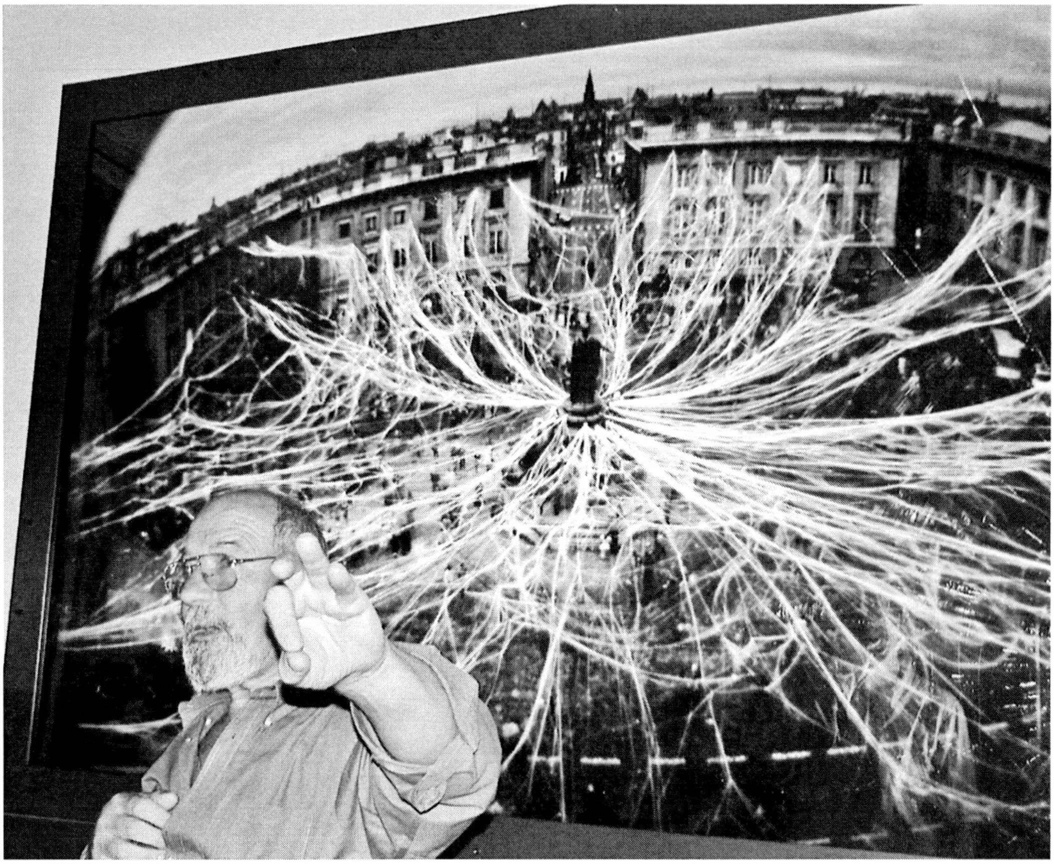

Donato Sartori explaining Urban Masking. Photograph courtesy of *Centro Maschere e Strutture Gestuale.*

Such events of course require a great deal of advanced organization. Donato and the team of *Centro Maschere e Strutture Gestuali* meet with various city groups that work in different artistic fields, such as the visual arts, dance, music, and theatre, to determine a suitable center and to plan how various groups will perform initial responses to the overall activity; much like a jazz musician might cajole an audience into participating in various dance forms. Interestingly, while these giant masked performance art events need an abundance of advanced city support and planning, the aim is to orchestrate an ultimate and inevitable "spontaneous" public response.

One suspects that Amleto Sartori would smile at this ultimate outcome since any consummate *commedia dell'arte* performer could encourage similar "improvised" audience responses in the typical town square amidst the wagons set up to become stages. Masked *commedia* performers understood the dynamic value of interacting directly with street audiences. Likewise, similar spontaneous communal responses between masked performers and audience members in the most successful Carnival street performances are carefully calculated for optimum impact. Donato's grand urban masks covering huge buildings have evolved dramatically from his father's evocations of the original *commedia* masks, but the agendas for both styles (as well as most other masked performances interacting in public celebrations from Paleolithic times onward) remain substantially the same.

Mask makers in Malawi and Nigeria

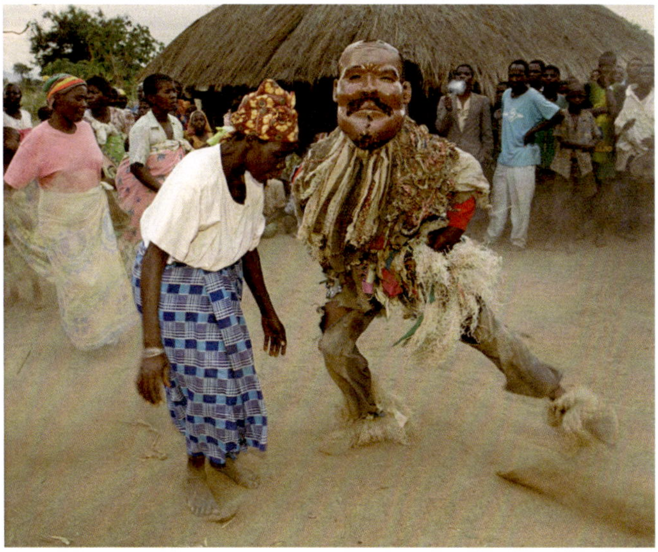

Namkungwi (Mistress of Initiations) dancing with Atsale Adzamange (May the Survivors Prevail) at *mmeto* (funeral commemoration) for a young man who died far from home. This *nyau* character in Malawian (Chewa) cosmology reveals the growing awareness of the depth and virulence of the AIDS pandemic in southern Africa. Unusual for *nyau* masks, this mask borrows its style from the Makonde masks of northeastern Mozambique. The "helmet mask" completely covers the dancer's head. The women's chorus warns, "Run away, run away, the big-headed man is coming." Photographer: Douglas Curran.

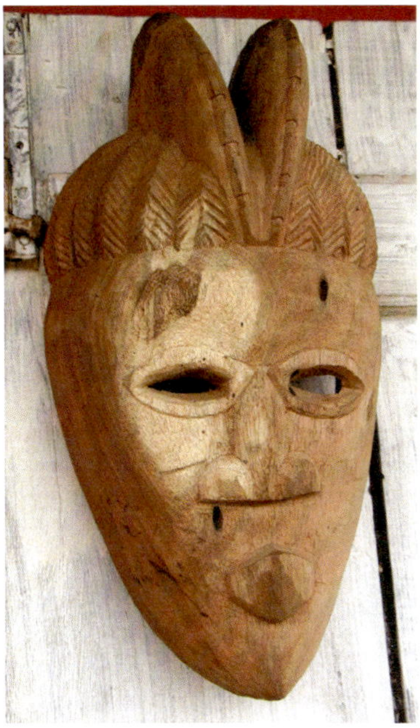

Epa wood mask carved by Nigerian mask makers Olowolafe Rufus and Olurotimi Taiwo.

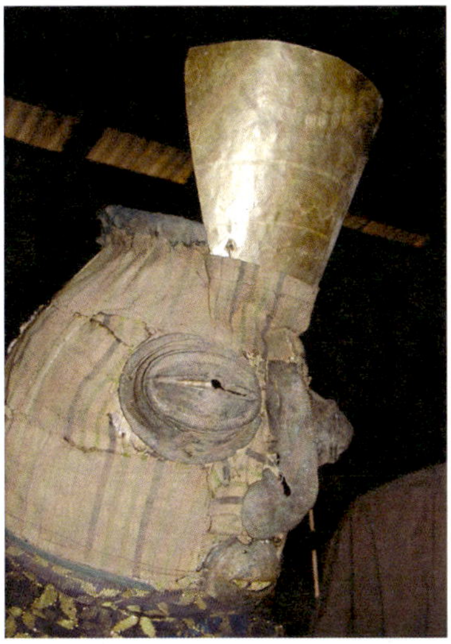

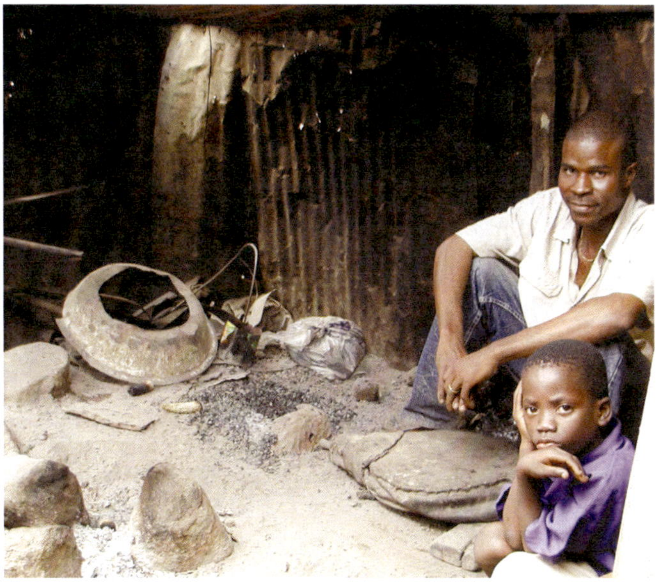

Left—Agbede Adebisi's Nigerian *Egungun* mask. Adebisi's masks are particularly well known in the Osogbo area. This mask features brass sculpture accents created with the traditional "lost wax" process. *Right*—Nigerian mask maker Adebisi and his son at his studio. Note the nineteenth-century bellows.

Mask makers in Northwest Canada

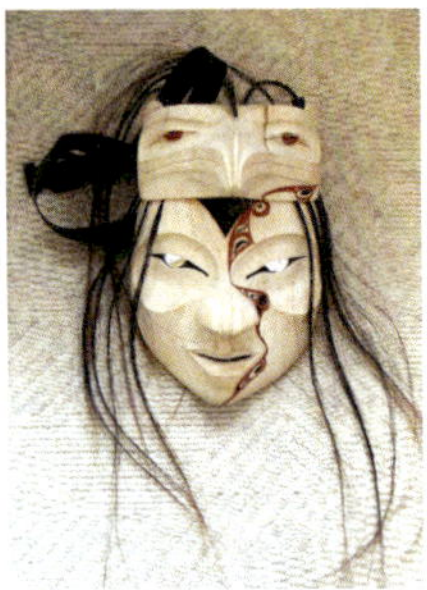
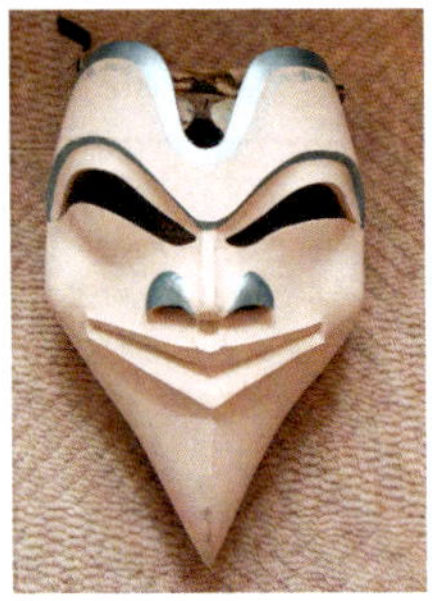
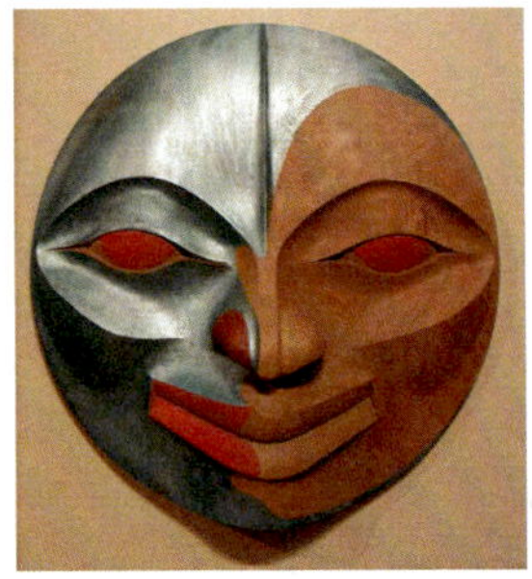
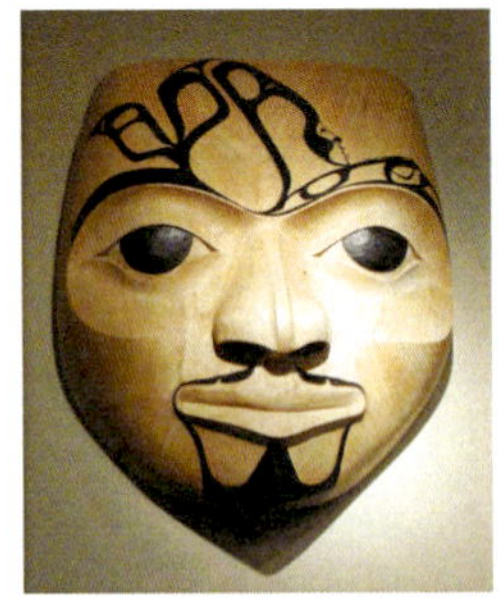

These top four photographs feature carved wood masks byTsimshian Victor Reece on Pender Island. *Above, left to right*—Raven Chief mask (He Who Brings Light). Pacific Northwest Coast Haida, Tlingit, and Tsimshian peoples have all considered the Raven a significant character in their cosmologies; Adolescent Raven mask evokes a mischievous version; Grandmother Moon mask (She Illuminates Our Darkness; Killer Whale Chief (the Chief represents the Killer Whale Clan). Painted lines on the mask refer abstractly to whale imagery. *Left*—*Musqua* (Bear) mask created by Canadian mask maker Xstine Cook and her mentor, Victor Reece, in Calgary. Photographer: Victor Reece.

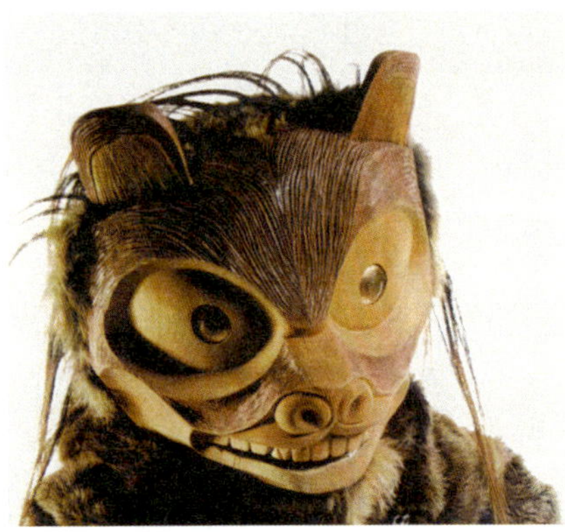

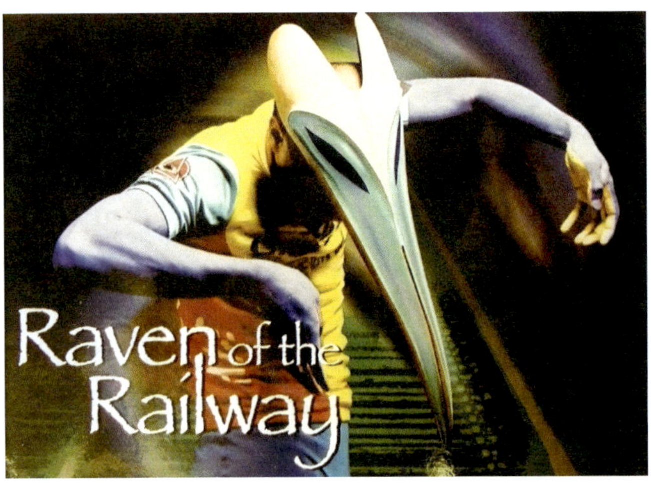

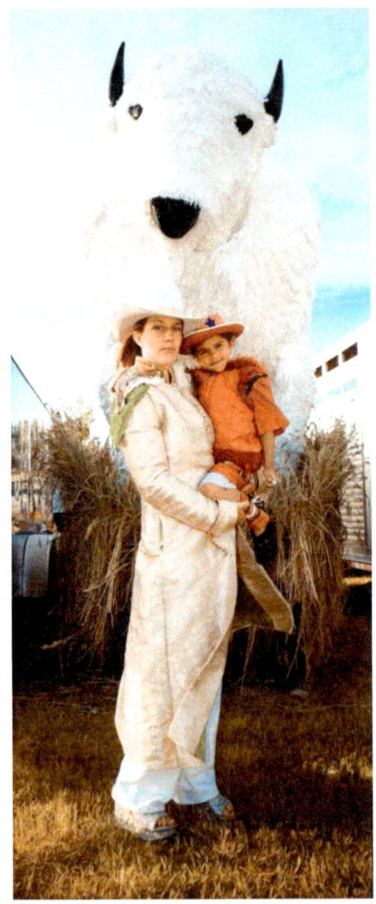

Above—Karen Jamieson Dance, *Raven of the Railway,* 2002. Mask: Victor Reece, Dancer: Alvin Erasga Tolentino, Photographer: Gordon Cooper. *Right*—Xstine Cook and daughter Maezy Dennie in front of "Spirit of White Buffalo" (2007) at the Bricks and Earth Circus in Lethbridge, Canada. Photographer: Sean Dennie.

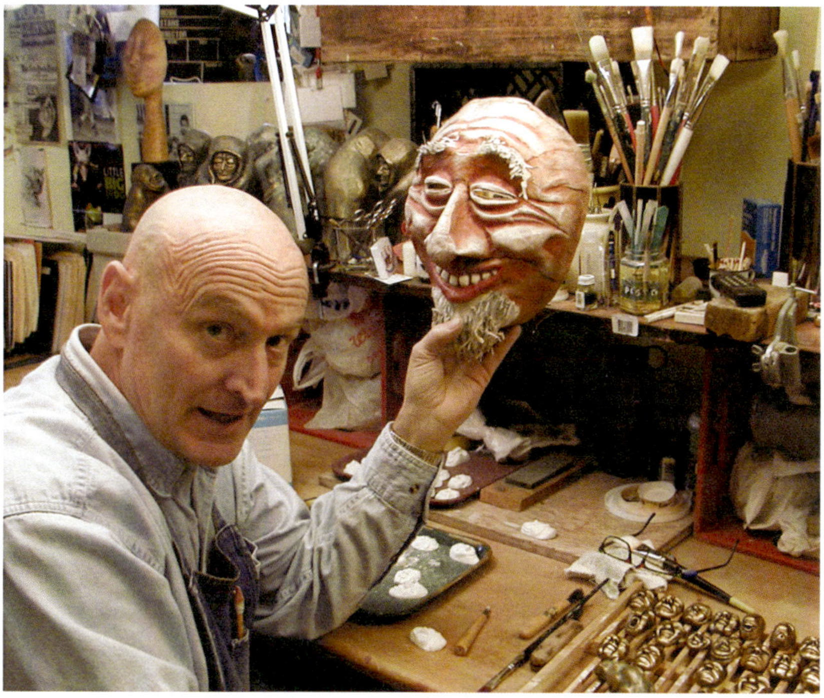

Urban mask makers Rob Faust in Canada and Orangeena in the United States

Above—Rob Faust holds "Smiley Grandpa" in his Toronto mask studio. He has performed and toured in this resin mask (and many others) since 1983.

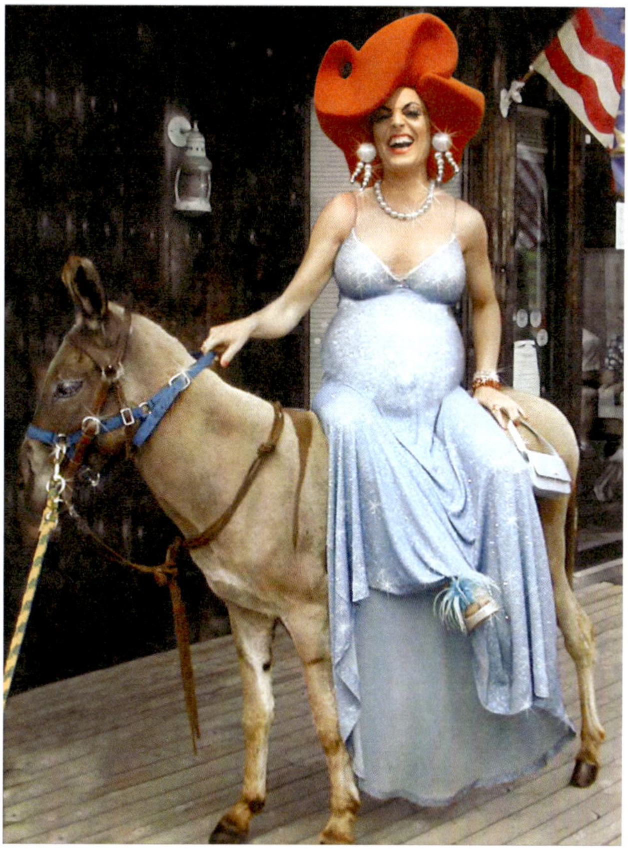

Right—Orangeena has been an award-winning professional puppet maker in New York City for twenty years. She also enjoys masquerading in her own masks and costumes for New York audiences.

Balinese mask makers and performers

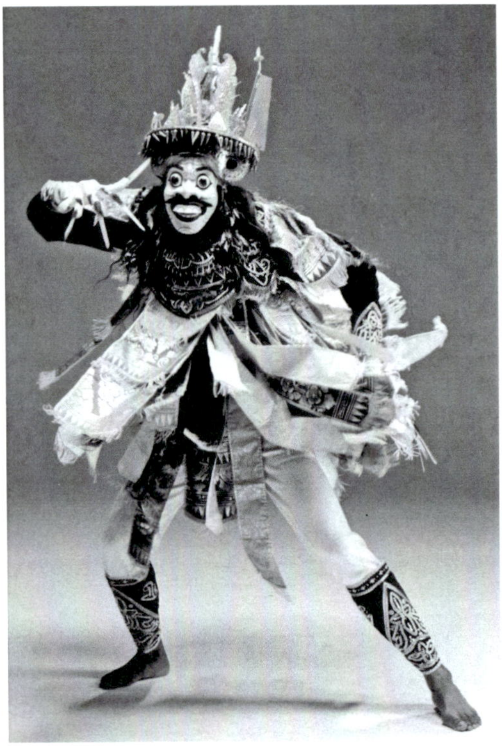

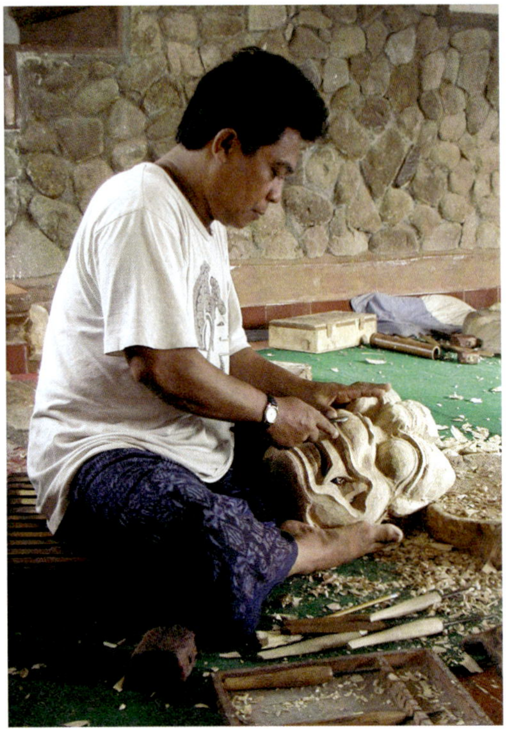

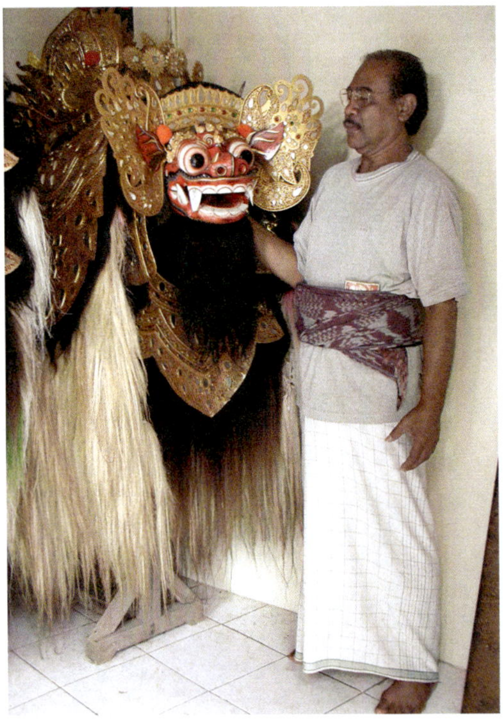

Top left—Suryasa wearing one of his own masks in a *Topeng* dance performance. Judy Slattum, Suryasa's wife and author of ***Masks of Bali,*** points out various characteristics of Balinese dance, such as short staccato movements occurring against the overall directional flow. *Topeng* dance particularly emphasizes the head, hands, and feet. It is rich with ancient East Indian and Chinese-influenced iconic references, though distinctly Balinese. Photographer: Paul Schraub. *Above right*—I. Bodus Anom at work in his studio. "Music and dancing are always with me—along with Balinese stories as I create my masks." *Left*—I. Wayan Dawig with one of his Barong masks commissioned for a festival in Borneo. This mask features leather sections as well as the carved wood facial elements.

South Korean mask maker Kim Dong-Pyo at his studio

Top—Kim Dong-Pyo created, built, and curates the ***Hahoe*** World Mask Museum (the only national mask museum in Korea). Self-taught, Kim creates and performs in the ***Hahoe*** masks. The South Korean government has designated the originals (which he meticulously copies) as national treasures. ***Bottom left***—One of Kim's ***Hahoe*** masks representing the aristocratic character Yangban. ***Right***—Kim's Yangban character was exhibited at the ***Hahoe*** World Mask Museum in Andong, South Korea.

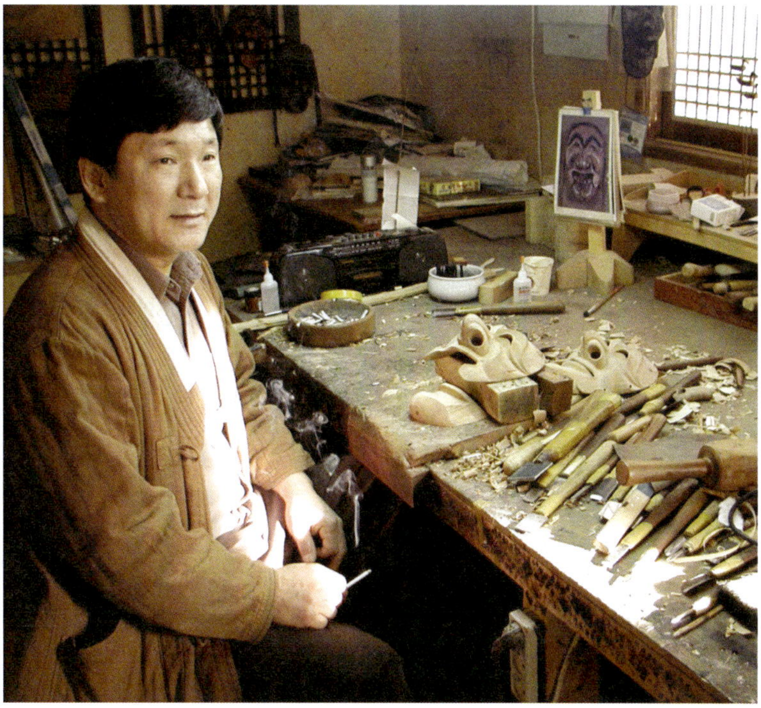

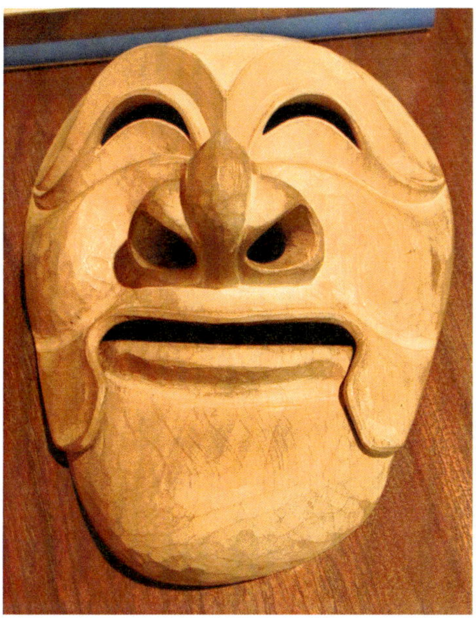

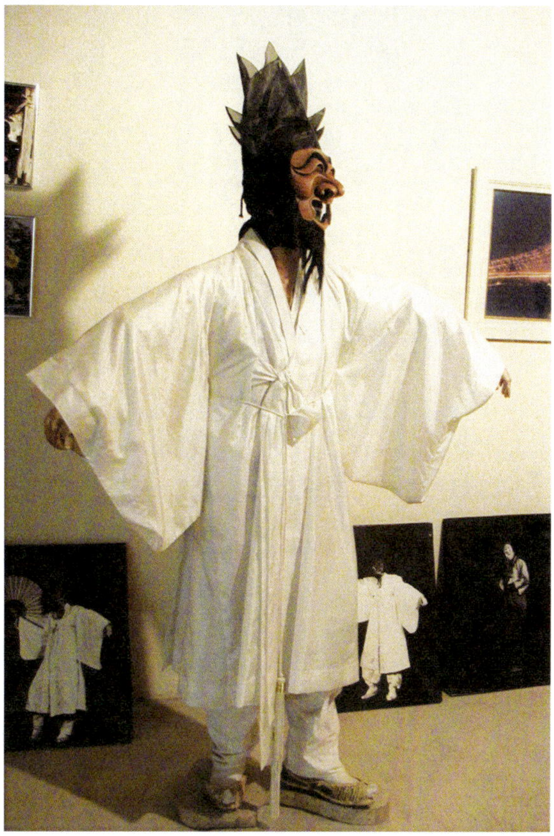

Trinidadian Carnival mask makers Geraldo Vieira, Geraldo Vieira, Jr, Marlon Griffith and Sheldon Clemdore

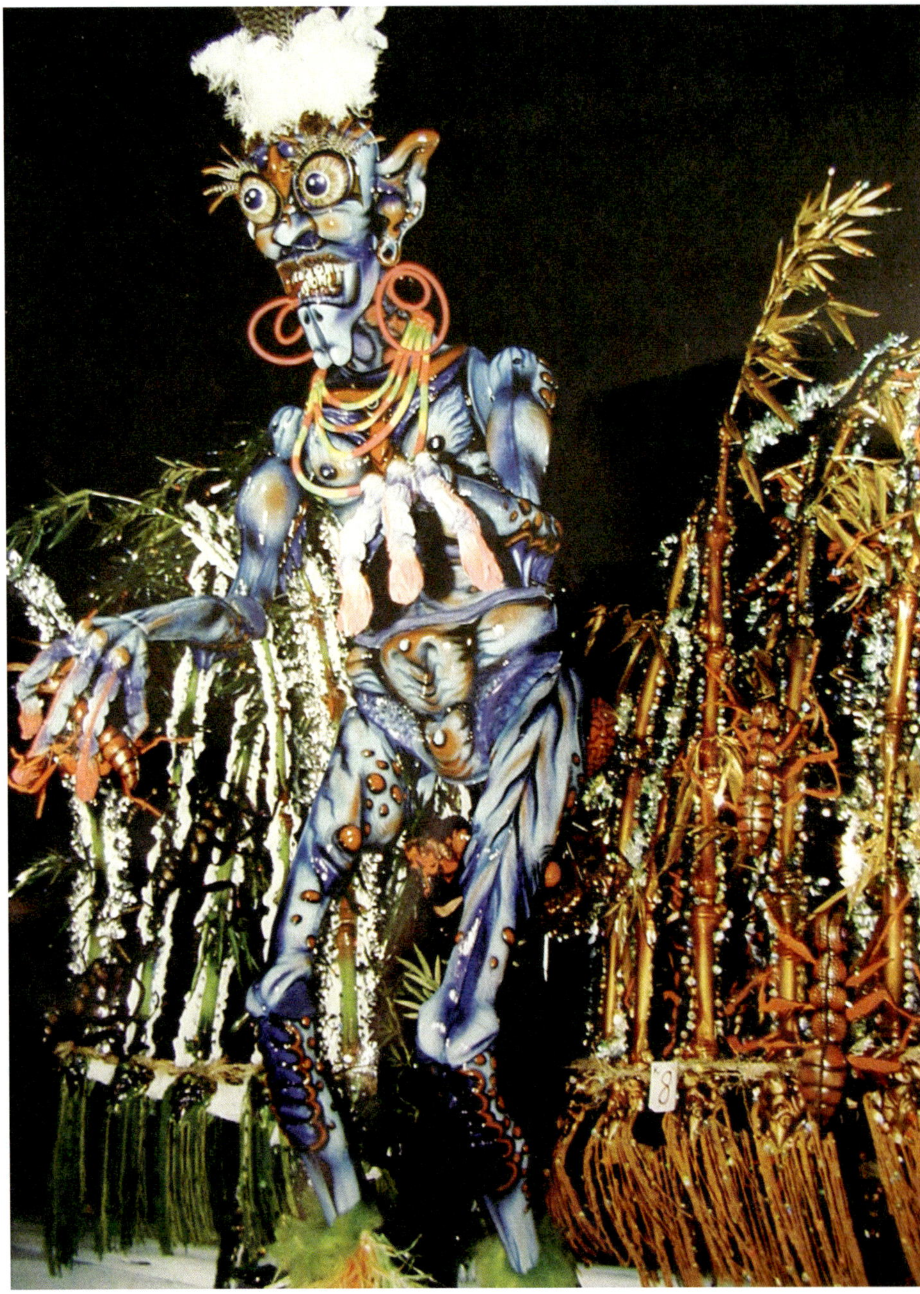

Geraldo Vieira, Geraldo Vieira, Jr., and Sheldon Clemdore annually strut their stuff in Port of Spain with such creations as *Trouble in de Bamboo* (shown in this photograph) and *Aladdin's Last Ride* as seen on opposite page top right.

Top—Sketch by Geraldo Vieira, Jr. for ***Aladdin's Last Ride***. Aladdin, a figure of death (designed to be manipulated and performed by Vieira, Jr.), seems to be having a grand time riding into hell on a huge griffin. *Middle*—Trinidadian mask maker Marlon Griffith has exhibited masks and conducted mask-making workshops in England, Japan, and South Africa. He created his paper mask (top right) in Japan out of ***washi***, a type of Japanese paper made from the bark of the mulberry or ***gampi*** tree. *Bottom left*—Vieira specializes in these mammoth "walking mobiles" controlled by a performer who braces himself with two wheels behind him as he walks. Note the performer's mask, somewhat camouflaged underneath the huge king mask—twice the size of a human head. This gigantic walking mobile mask entitled ***Rainfest***, pays homage to nature, our diminishing rain forests, and the need for sustainability. *Bottom right*—Vieira is shown next to ***Rainfest***'s huge vacuformed plastic mask.

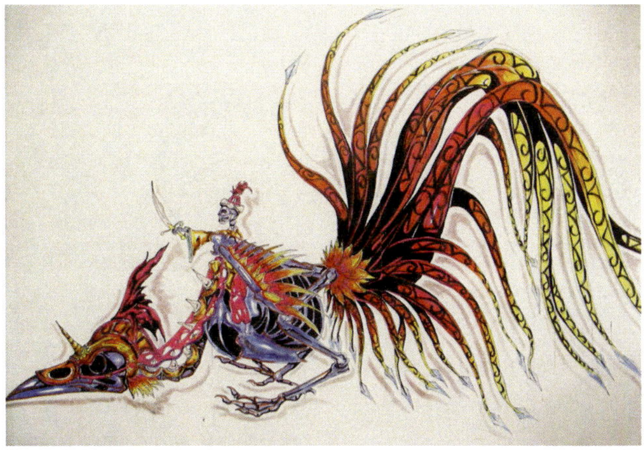

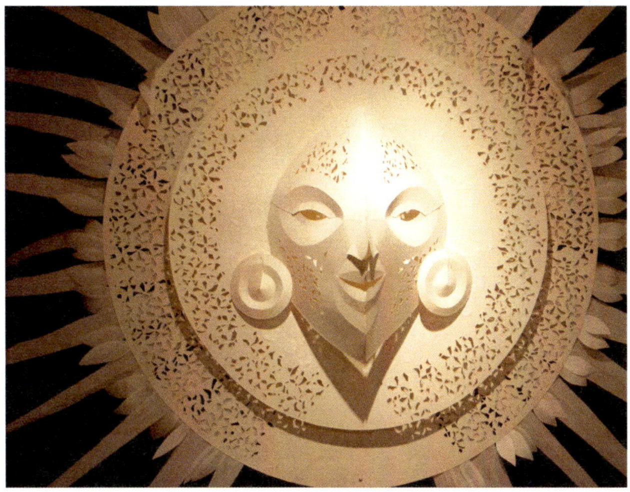

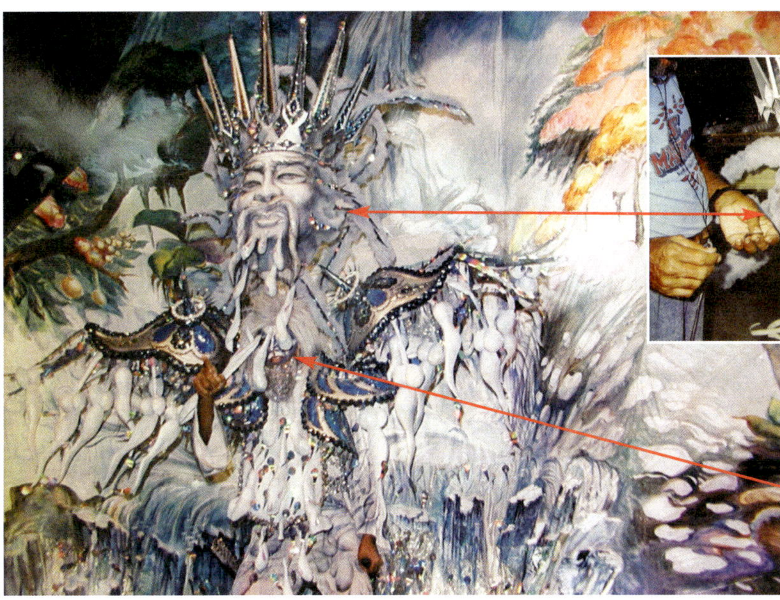

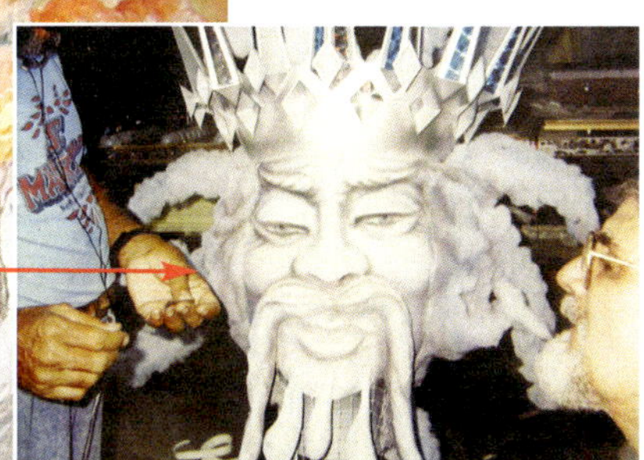

This line points to the performer under the mask.

Bruce Marrs in his studio

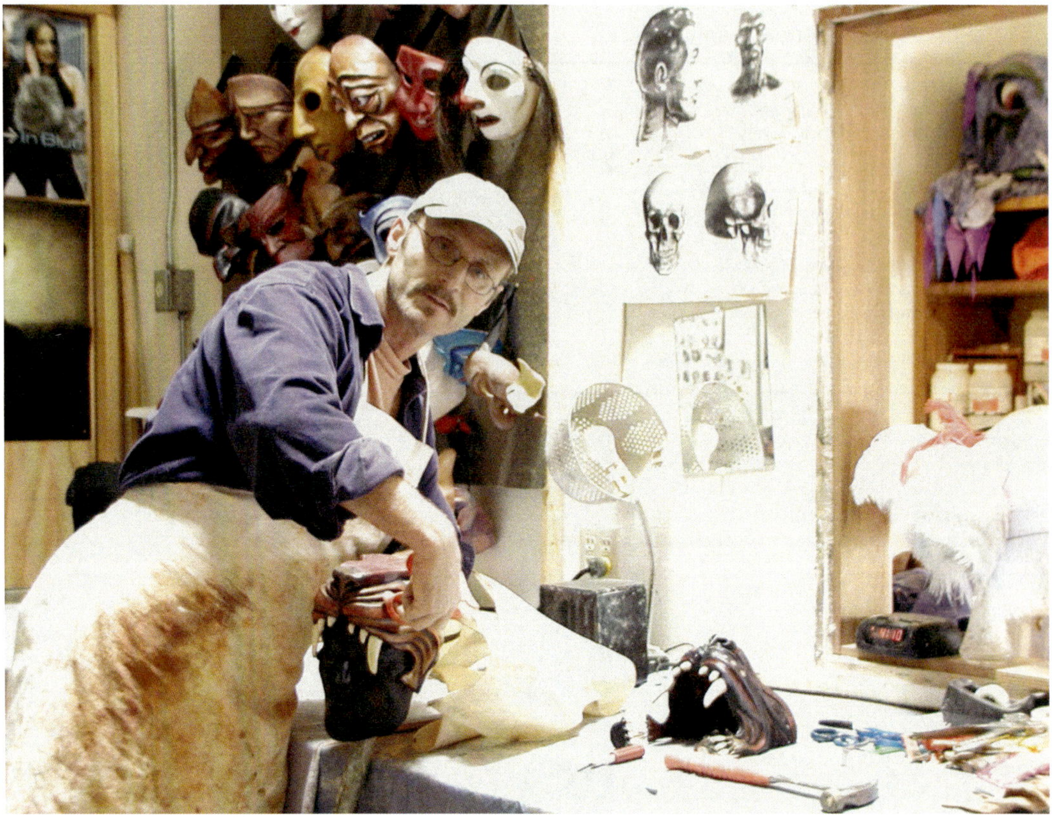

Above—Bruce Marrs in his studio at Dell'Arte International School of Physical Theatre, Blue Lake, California. ***Bottom left***—Marrs' neoprene dragon mask for ***Jack and the Beanstalk in Mime, Mask, and Latina Barbie*** (1997). The mask was inspired by Godzilla and has two distinct angles. One angle presents the mask as the dragon while the other angle presents the mask as the dragon master. ***Right***—One of Bruce Marrs' contemporary ***commedia*** neoprene mask characters. Marrs sells masks like this to universities and theatre companies across the country and internationally.

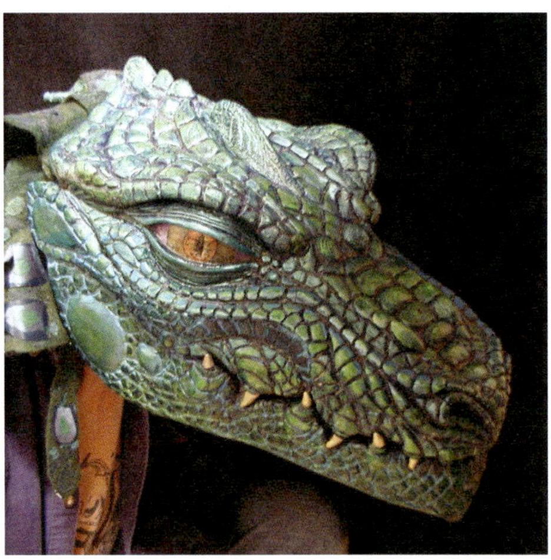

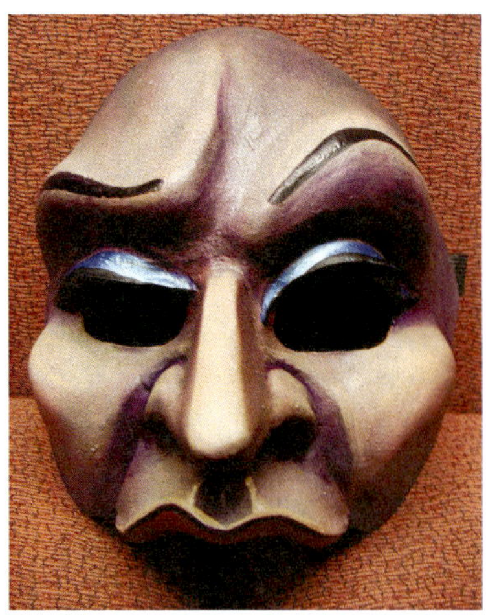

Yet no mask museum can fully capture the visceral, spontaneous qualities of live performance, whatever form it takes. The *Centro Maschere e Strutture Gestuali* can only present a glimpse of such experiences through videos, photos, and projections of the performances. Sartori's International Museum of the Mask becomes a keyhole view into this ultimately temporal world. Still, it does so with integrity and elegance and, while underscoring Amleto's world of sixteenth-century *commedia*, it proceeds to beautifully articulate ancient and contemporary trends in mask work as well. Consequently it serves as an important center for international exchange opportunities.

The first floor displays the modern part of the Italian *commedia* and the contemporary theater, which includes the expressive and neutral masks created for drama schools around the world. One section of the museum is dedicated to the Gestural Structures, life-sized leather structures also called total masks (anatomic busts, human torsos). Finally, there is a room with large slides illustrating the Urban Masks of the last forty years.

The neutral mask shown here remains the high point of Sartori creativity and is also an example of the similarity and diversity of the two Sartoris: Amleto created the neutral mask for Lecoq's School in Paris in 1948 and Donato, continuing and extending his collaboration with Lecoq even after his father's death; the neutral masks still used by Lecoq's School; and another neutral mask for American theater schools. The same may be said about the expressive masks which Amleto created in *papier mâché* and Donato in leather.

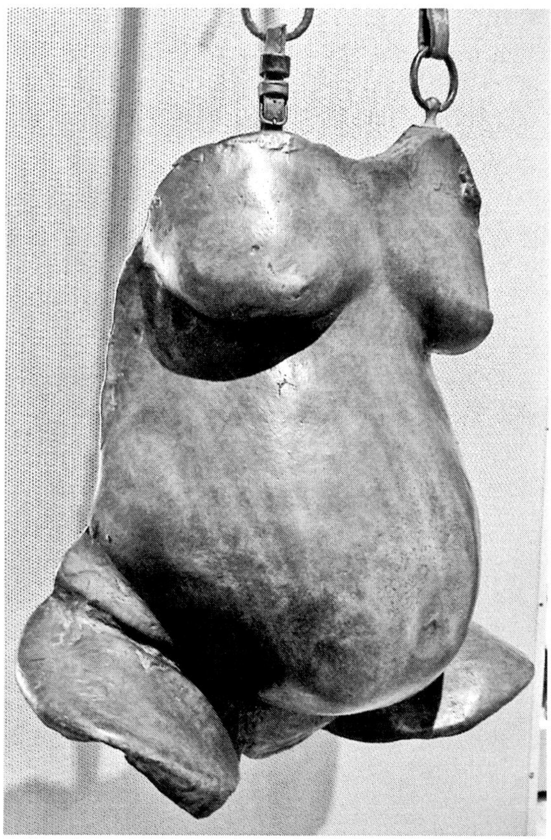

Motherhood, a gestural structure ("total mask") in dubbed leather, created by Donato Sartori at *Centro Maschere e Strutture Gestuale*, Abano Terme, 1984.

Donato, who was a student at *École des Beaux-Art,* but also the son and pupil of a great teacher, continued to collaborate with Strehler and the Piccolo Teatro, creating masks for Brecht's play *Galileo*, an Arlecchino mask for Ferruccio Soleri, the heir of Moretti, and a Pulcinella mask for Eduardo De Filippo. He created masks for theatre productions of Italian director Franco Enriquez and for Lecoq's School. He also collaborated intensely with Dario Fo, and with the Swede Peter Oskarson who directed the *Oresteia* at the Folkteatern in Gothenburg with 140 new masks, designed and created by Donato for the occasion.[141]

The ground floor of the museum displays temporary exhibits from the Sartori Collection, such as the one in 2007 entitled "The Oriental Mask" with examples of Peking Opera make-up (as masks) and headgear, Kathakali and Kutiyattam masks and puppets from India, and *Noh* and *Kyogen* masks from Japan. Scholars and artists added related work to this

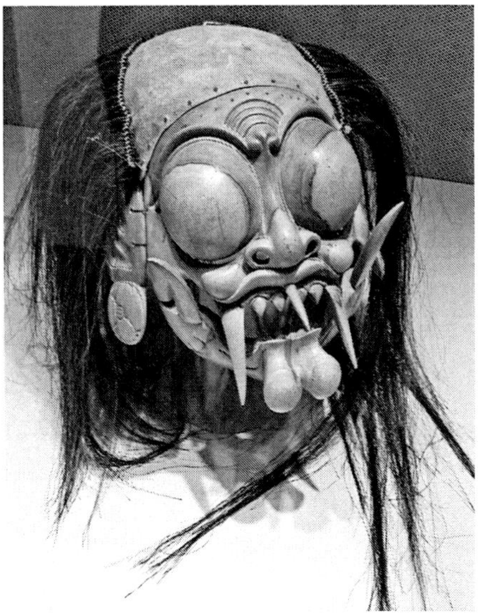

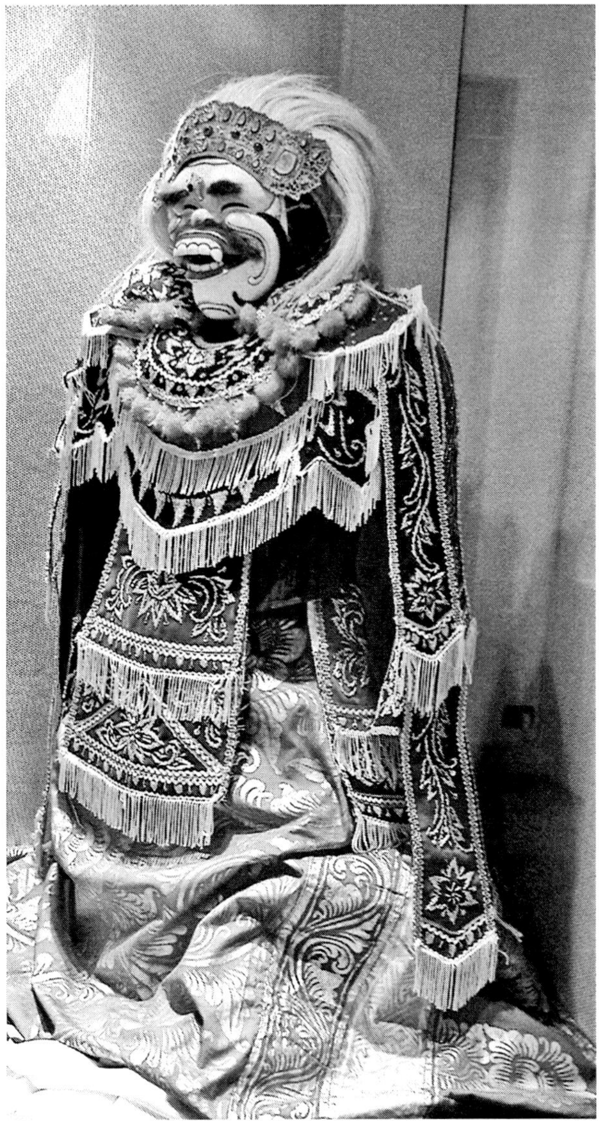

Examples of temporary mask exhibits from the Sartori Collection. Photograph left shows *Buta-Buti*, the wicked servant and counselor of the witch *Rangda* in the Balinese dance of the *Barong*. This unfinished wooden mask features ornaments in horsehair. Photograph right shows the *Tua*, a Balinese mask in treated and painted wood with horsehair finishing for the *Topeng* dance. It represents the wise man who tells the stories and myths of the past.

exhibit. Donato is especially attracted to Japanese mask makers. "Collectively they are some of the world's finest," he says. "With just a few gestures, a Japanese mask sculptor is able to evoke nuanced differences between the mask of a tragic woman and one depicting a young woman. A typical outcome of such deliberation might result in simply projecting just the right shape of the eyelids. For example, a Japanese artist might suggest the wisdom of an older woman lowering or raising the actor's face."[142]

During the guided visit to the rooms of the Museum, Donato pointed out a double array of masks which, though differing in their appearance, materials, and method of production, have the same captions, for they are all characters from the Greek tragedy of the *Oresteia* by Aeschylus. The first set was made in leather by Amleto in the fifties for Jean-Louis Barrault, the great French actor and director, who both acted in and directed the performance; the second set was designed for the same tragedy fifty years later and made by Donato for the Folkteatern under the Swedish director Peter Oskarson. Here we can compare, for example, the Erinyes, one of the furies of the Greek underworld, which Amleto sees as a terrible Medusa, with eyes of fire and hair like serpents; instead Donato presents it almost like a goddess of death, veiled like a chthonic figure, emerging from the water. (In fact, Oskarson wanted the actress wearing this mask to arise out of a pool of water which represented the River Styx, the infernal realm of the creatures of evil.) To enable the actors to work in water, Donato developed (in two years of work) a special water-resistant resinous material.[143]

In Christian iconography, the pre–Christian infernal creatures have been represented like horned devils. The head of the demons, Hellequin, had a name sounding quite similar to what was later to become the most representative mask of the *commedia dell'arte*, Arlecchino. Of course the Church could not allow popular plays with horned devil masks, so the use of these masks was prohibited during the late Middle Ages. Sartori asserts that the actors avoided being condemned by the Church by cutting off the horns, but they left

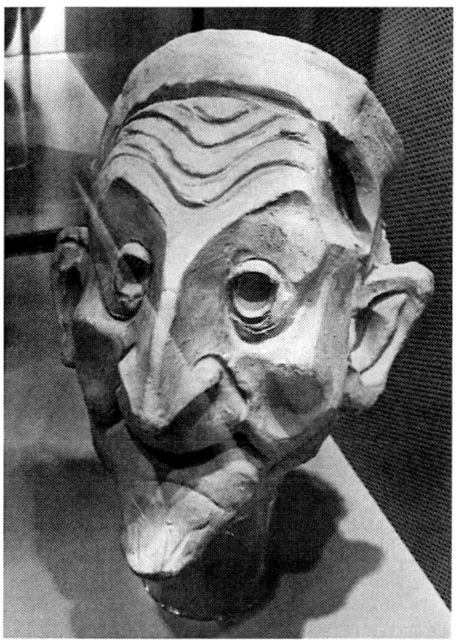

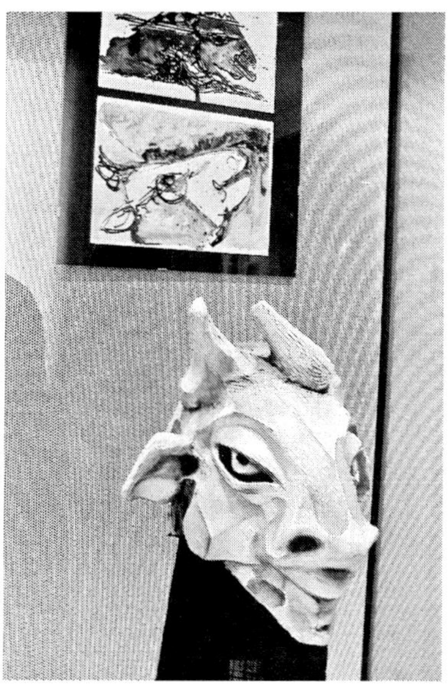

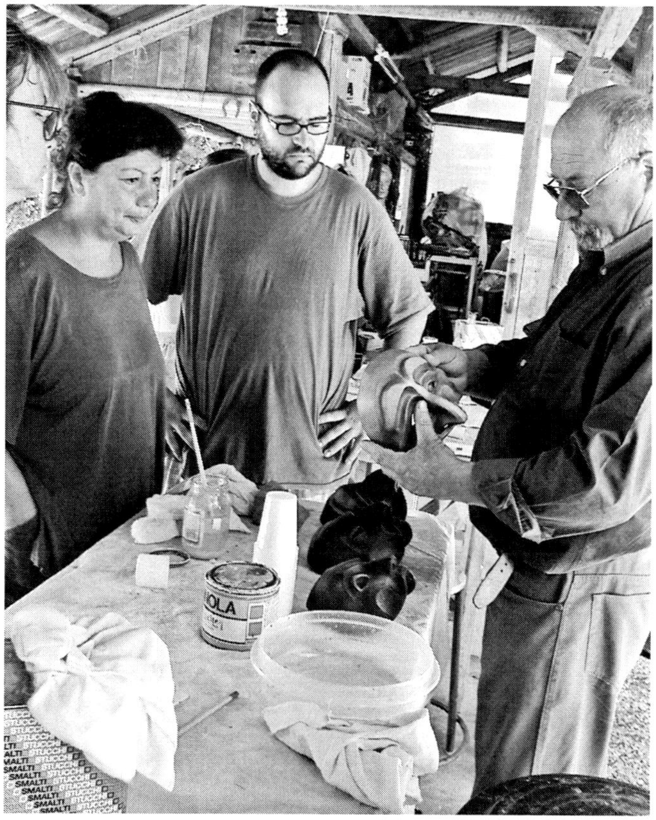

Left top: **Terracotta study for Pantalone by Amleto Sartori, 1951; *bottom:* mask of a zoomorphic cow character, inspired by Chagall's animals for a production of *Fiddler on the Roof,* directed and interpreted by Moni Ovadia at *Arena del Sole* in Bologna in 2002. Donato Sartori created the mask at *Centro Maschere e Strutture Gestuali. Right:* Donato Sartori and Paola Piizzi with a student at the International Workshop, "Art of the Mask in Commedia dell' Arte," a summer course for professionals at Abano Terme, Italy.**

a trace in the form of a small red bump or scar, a characteristic feature that has accompanied *commedia* masks from the Renaissance to the present day.[144] Seattle director Arne Zaslove, Dell'Arte International guest artist and director, considers Sartori's speculation as most credible, but he also remembers Jacques Lecoq or Carlo Mazzone-Clementi saying that the head bump (traditionally found only on Arlecchino — not other *commedia* characters) symbolized the servant's frequent beatings, or implied a cuckold's former horn.[145]

Yet even in acknowledging these universal elements found in *commedia* masks, Donato smiles and concludes that despite such global references, he takes pride in the fact that he, like the great Ruzante who introduced *commedia* to the world, comes from Padua.

Use of Tree Imagery to Display Nyau Masks

Gule wamkulu performances take place at a site near the village called the *bwalo*, always near a large tree. Sometimes the tree becomes the central scenic element of the performance. This communal area is an important site for performances as well as for town meetings. In some ways it can be compared to a European town square and it functions like a church or temple.

Aguilar offers a vivid image of the *Kasiya Maliro* dramatically catching the moonlight as it twirls and circles the tree. She then describes how the tree aids in capturing a grand sense of mystery for other masks, "The light interplays with the shadows from the large tree ... creating its own special effects on the moving masks. These constructions are performed in groups; at times with three, ten, or even twenty large mask forms...."[146] One can easily imagine the theatricality of these as suspended figures, floating as spirits in the air, especially accompanied by drums and the right evening light, or even juxtaposed against the flickering flames of a community bonfire.

Ott states that "trees are regarded as the dwelling places of the ancestral spirits who are the main protagonists during the rain sacrifices and at each *Gule wamkulu* performance." He understands this as the rationale for masks suspended in trees or from stylized tree crowns. He believes that this concept fittingly shows up in Chewa community churches so that the African ancestors are present for the rituals along with the communion of [Catholic] church saints.[147]

How appropriate then, for the *Chamare* Museum's magnificent exhibition of *nyau* masks to hang suspended from branches on a huge thirty-foot replica of a tree in the middle of the central circle of three such rounded spaces. Each space depicts Chewa, Yao, and Ngoni cultural traditions. However, the central space dominates; showing well over 150 masks, suspended from surrounding branches of the tree and capturing the essence of their spirits overlooking creation. The range of positive and negative forces around the space offers only a glimpse into the power that these creations hold and one can easily imagine the compounded effects of these spirits embodying actual dancing masqueraders.

Boucher told me that due to the sacredness of these authentic *nyau* masks the local chiefs had insisted that he promise to forbid photos. (I have photos of selected masks from his private collection shown later.) As with the Grand Canyon, however, one photo or series of photos could never capture the spellbinding effect of this presentation. Even if one were allowed to photograph the space, it is too extensive and finely detailed.

The tree metaphor is, of course, a common African theme. Like the stalk of the maize, the image of the tree succinctly summarizes the contrasting states of life, death and rebirth as do other Chewa mythological figures previously mentioned.

Hahoe World Mask Museum

Korean master Kim Dong-Pyo has an exceptional reputation as a mask maker of authentically based, hand-carved *Hahoe* masks for which people worldwide pay dearly and wait many months to acquire. The *Hahoe* masks evoke humorous servant/master archetypal characters, similar in spirit to the Italian *commedia dell'arte* characters. His masks (along with those of several other mask makers I interviewed) are found in a number of museums. Queen Elizabeth requested a viewing of Kim's *Hahoe* masked performance of Pune (the flirtatious widow) during her 1999 tour of South Korea.[148]

Kim's experienced such demand for his miniature "tourist" *Hahoe* masks that he built a factory to manufacture large quantities for tourists visiting Hahoe Village in the Andong region. He found this endeavor so profitable that he proceeded to purchase a notable collection of Korean masks. In 1995 he created, built, and began curating the *Hahoe-Dong* Mask Museum (the only national mask museum in Korea) in Hahoe Village. Self-taught, Kim creates as well as performs in the *Hahoe* masks. The originals are designated as a national treasure. A member of the organizing committee for the Andong World Mask Dance Festival, which produces work annually during ten days in late September to early October, Kim Dong-Pyo is considered to be a significant leader of the arts in his region. His mask museum received support from the city of Andong and the Korea National Lottery to build an additional wing to house his impressive international mask collection, with masks he's acquired during his world travels. Accordingly, by the end of 2009 he changed the museum's name to the *Hahoe* World Mask Museum.[149]

The most impressive masks are the nine remaining (out of twelve originally) *Hahoe* masks which are held by the National Central Museum in Seoul. But Kim displays his own beautifully crafted copies of the originals at the *Hahoe* World Mask Museum and they are the centerpiece of his collection. These masks project a rich combination of realistic though caricatured facial features and are quite humorous. Several of the masks have moving mouths that project varying attitudes. They (or versions of them) are thought to have been used as early as the twelfth century. In 1964 the South Korean government designated this mask collection and dance as Important Intangible Cultural Property #69 and National Treasure

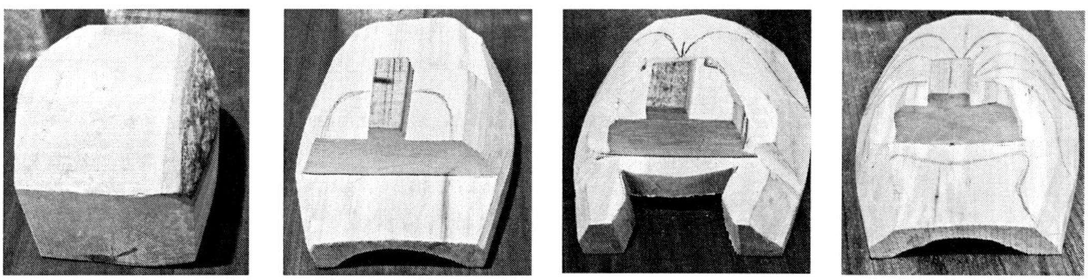

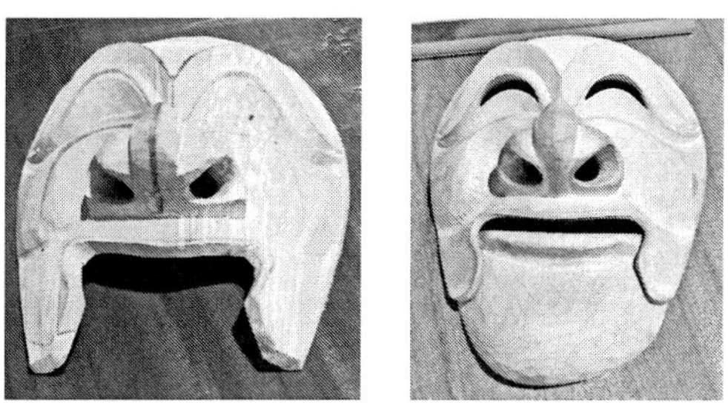

Kim Dong-Pyo's wood carving process for his *Hahoe* masks. This particular mask renders Yangban, the Aristocrat, one of the major characters in the *Pyeolsandae* stories

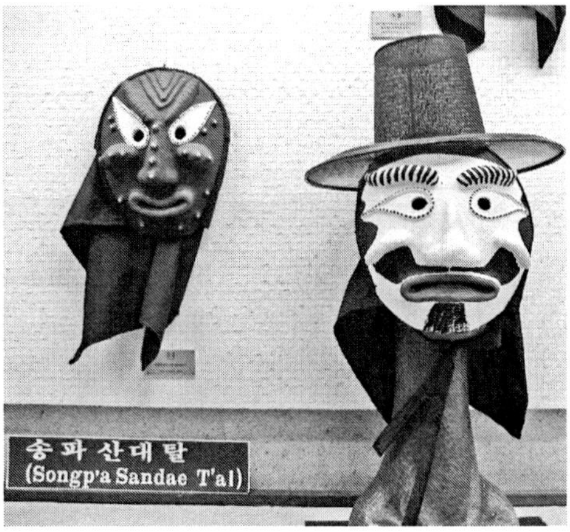

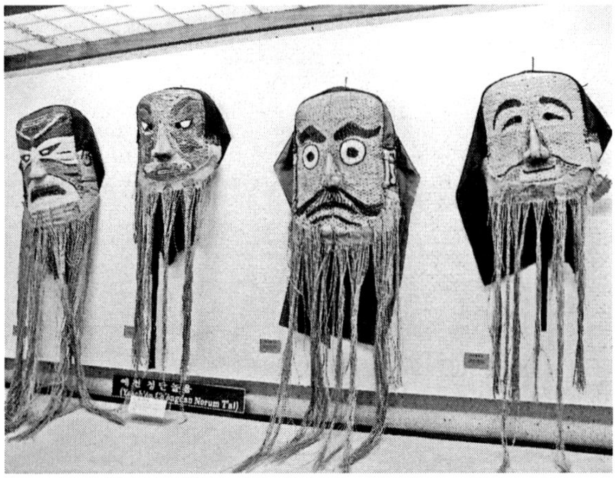

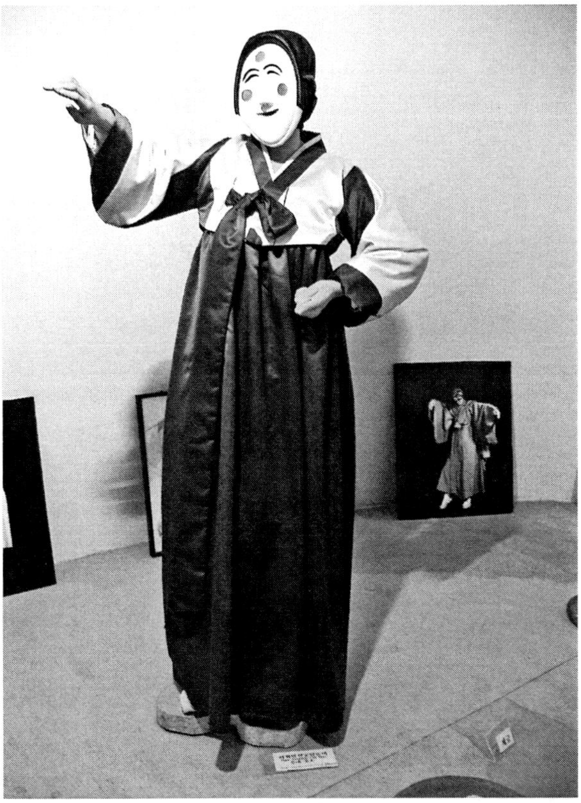

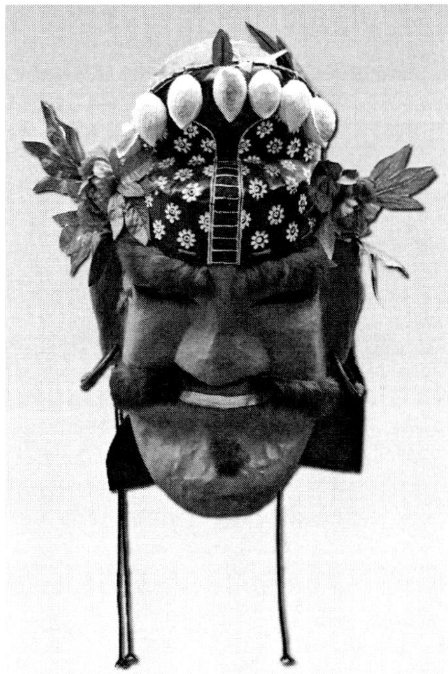

Exhibits in mask maker Kim Dong-Pyo's *Hahoe* World Mask Museum. Photographs *(top left—clockwise)* displays examples of the *Songpa Sandae Tal* masks. The character for the white mask and black hat is called *Songpa-sandae-nori* and he is a policeman of high standing during the Choseon Dynasty. In the play, acting as an unprincipled government official, he takes by force the other man's mistress. *Top right*—displays the *Yecheon Cheongdan Norum Tal* masks which appear in a dance that involves the interaction of the masked four seasons: *Kyeoul, Kaeul, Yeorum,* and *Pom* (or Winter, Fall, Summer, and Spring.) *Bottom right*—presents the *Cheoyong Tal* dance mask of the long-suffering but patient and forgiving foreign king, Choyang, who gradually wins the respect of his adversary. *Bottom left*—shows one of the *Yangju Pyeolsandae Nori* masks: the "Flirtatious Woman" dancing.

#121. Like the *Yangju Pyeolsandae Nori*, the remaining original mask characters represent typical village personalities such as a depraved Buddhist monk, an aristocrat, a bride, a scholar, a butcher, a scatterbrained meddler, an old widow, a servant, a lady, and a fool. The dance movements that correlate with these highly realistic masks are very simple, making the images even more human-like. They are carved out of alder wood.

The current *Hahoe* World Mask Museum exhibits masks representing both North and South Korea. My guide explained that the shaman rituals involving masked characters have historically been of major significance for the Korean villages and up until 1928 they were performed as often as every three years but sometimes ten years would pass between productions. Now versions of the shaman ritual are in tandem with other popular forms of masked dances and occur annually during the early month of January.

The museum has one section that displays the carving stages in creating a *Hahoe* mask, specifically Yangban the Aristocrat. It also showcases other examples from a range of categories of Korean masks and photographs of masked performances. Prominently displayed are the *Yangju Pyeolsandae Nori* masks. These folk masks are carved out of wood or papier-mâché. They are readily identified by the various scarf wrappings that hide the performer's face and frame the mask. There are thirty-two characters representing village characters such as the Acupuncturist, the Dark-faced Monk, the Pockmarked Monk, the Blinking Monk, the Aristocrat, the Servant, the Government Official, and the Female Entertainer. The various characters tend to be deformed and satirize the elite classes.

John Nunley in *Masks: Faces of Culture* tells of a typical *Pyeolsandae* story in the form of a masked dance about a lecherous Old Monk who becomes attracted to a Dancing Girl. When the Old Monk pursues her, a younger Bachelor protests and fights with the Monk, usurping the Old Monk for her attentions, and then belittles the unrepentant old man, who simply runs off with another Dancing Girl.[150]

The museum displays several other significant categories of masks. One category, the Tiger masks, has historically accompanied versions of the Tiger Dance throughout North and South Korea. Another category of shamanistic masks called *Bangsangssi* assists in chasing away evil spirits. These masks were traditionally buried near the grave of a recently deceased person or destroyed by fire. Consequently, new ones were always needed to continue the funeral rituals. These masks often included more than two eyes. The museum magnificently displays a category of masks called the *Yech'eon Ch'eongdan Norum T'al,* which appear in a beautiful dance that involves the interaction of the masked four seasons: *Kyeoul, Kaeul, Yeorum,* and *Pom* (or Winter, Fall, Summer, and Spring.) Several photographs of these masks underscore the beauty of this dance in action.

One of the most revered categories of masks are those from the *Ch'eoyong T'al* Dance. Using a folk tale that emphasizes the concept of ultimately repelling bad spirits, it conveys a "turn the other cheek" parable. It tells the story of a foreign king, Choyang, who tries to respect the sinister East Sea Dragon god by building a temple in his honor. After the king discovers the god's son cavorting (in human form) with his wife, he avoids getting angry and consequently gains the respect of the god. The god rewards him and promises that he and his sons will avoid Choyang's wife from then on.

Bill LeVasseur's Impressive Collection

Midway along a picturesque, steeply sloping street in northwest San Miguel de Allende, one can discover a magnificent collection of contemporary indigenous ceremonial masks.

Bill LeVasseur, who has spent the past two decades collecting these masks from all regions of the country, has become very familiar with the distinctive styles of the most noted mask makers. This private museum, entitled *The Other Face of Mexico*, exhibits over five hundred masks. The museum can be viewed only by appointment. LeVasseur advertises once a week in San Miguel's local newspaper, but most visitors learn about the museum by word of mouth. The museum features nine elaborately costumed mannequins, two of which display *Tigre* masks, three of which display masks for the Dance of the Deer and Dance of the *Pascola*, and four of which display various Pharisee and devil masks. LeVasseur is also the curator of the museum. His detailed texts provide remarkable information for serious aficionados of Mexican masks, while his arrangement of Mexico's wide range of mask styles, extending into several rooms, highlights major mask themes for less knowledgeable viewers. LeVasseur has no formal schooling in anthropology, Mexican history, or masks but, fully bilingual, he has researched all three topics for years and is now well known for his expertise. Universities in the United States as well as Mexico regularly invite him to guest lecture. He donates all proceeds from his museum to a local orphanage.

The collection took several years to plan and assemble. The museum became LeVasseur's primary focus after he and his wife Heidi built a Mexican colonial home with rooms spilling onto a large center courtyard surrounded by terracotta sandstone pillars. This gracious site has several outdoor living spaces that look out onto the courtyard and the city's historic district below and visitors can take in the spectacular Guanajuato mountain range beyond. Initially *Casa de la Cuesta* was to be their retirement home. (LeVasseur had been an advertising executive, and Heidi continues to be an accomplished artist and teacher.) But they soon realized that its grand size with six bedrooms could become a bed and breakfast. The website for this dream spot boasts of "spectacular sunsets as its specialty," along with abundant breakfasts offering both American and Mexican cuisine.[151] As guests enter the inconspicuous door on the street, they immediately see a dramatic corridor with twenty lit arches, each

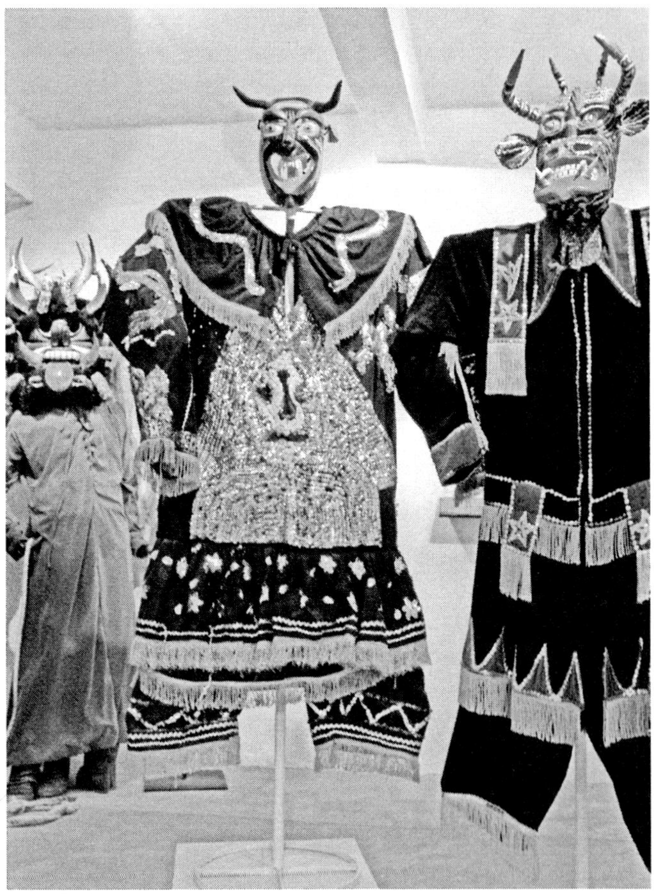

Several devil masks at the entry into Bill LeVasseur's Mexican mask museum, *The Other Face of Mexico*, in San Miguel de Allende.

holding a Mexican mask. Thirty-four winding steps later, the spacious courtyard with large lush plants, stone, tile, and sculpture welcomes them to a Mexican paradise, complete with paintings, indigenous textiles, handcrafted toys, *Catrinas*, *Calaveras*, and *Milagros*. The LeVasseurs also designed and built a large, fully equipped separate kitchen where students from cooking schools abroad learn how to prepare authentic Mexican specialties. The cooking space, the gallery of local art, and the mask museum are housed in a separate building in back of the bed and breakfast. School children regularly visit the mask museum and learn how to create their own masks. Their first visits with Bill and Heidi are often the first formal introduction to their Mexican indigenous heritage.

Bill LeVasseur's interest in masks commenced when he learned that by visiting a typical mid-sized Mexican city on the feast day of its designated saint, he could observe first-hand the accompanying celebrations which so vividly reflect Mexico's cultural spirit and unique blend of both Hispanic and pre–Hispanic customs. Often these celebrations involve masks. As he became increasingly familiar with these masked celebrations, he began to appreciate the skilled makers of the masks as well.

Annual celebrations such as Carnival, Christmas, Easter, Day of the Dead, Independence Day, Day of the Revolution, and Labor Day also incorporate numerous masked dances and ritual. LeVasseur divides the use of masks in these events into five basic categories: Historical Dramas (such as the Santiago enactments), the Christian Dances (triumphant celebrations of Christianity over paganism), Agricultural Dances (to encourage fertility or to celebrate the harvests), Occupational Dances (such as the Dance of the Fish in Guerrero) and Entertainment-oriented Dramas, (designed for amusement or for didactic social lessons.)[152]

LeVasseur acknowledges that the dancers he has encountered do not always know the exact significance of their dances or masks, but they usually know a story or two associated with each celebration. Many stories have evolved over time due to the interesting mix of pre–Hispanic and Hispanic associations. Less than three decades before Cortés arrived on the coast of Yucatan in 1519, Spain had expelled the Jews and the Moors. When a black Moor showed up with Cortés, the indigenous population assumed he was a god. LeVasseur notes that all of Mesoamerica considered black to be the holiest color. That concept along with the image of Spaniards possessing never-seen-before horses, steel swords, dogs of an unrecognizable breed, and gunpowder all suggested divine stature. Almost immediately from the beginning of Spain's arrival to the New World, Yoruba from Africa were brought over as slaves, who brought more dynamic cultural perspectives. Mesoamerican indigenous groups mixed with the African and Spanish populations and their cultural and spiritual stories and celebrations blended in a variety of ways. The Catholic Church encouraged the use of pre–Hispanic masked celebrations combined with Christian practices to encourage more rapid comprehension of Christian theology. Consequently, today one village can have a quite different understanding of masked celebrations than another village.[153] Yet masks fall into several major categories.

LeVasseur's museum prominently displays his masks primarily into six character groupings: Negro masks, Pharisee masks, devil masks, *tigre* masks, Old Men masks, and Day of the Dead masks (although several other mask and dance categories are identified as well.)

Negro Masks

Negro characters portrayed in various masked celebrations take on particularly exotic significance, partly because the African slaves tended to be overseers over the indigenous

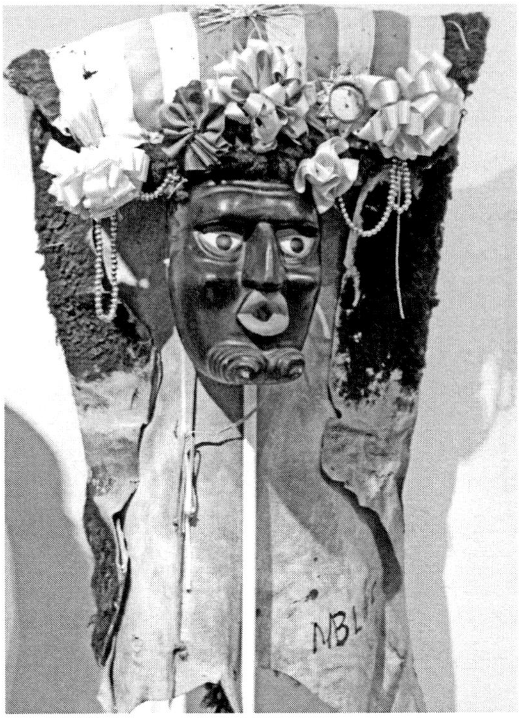

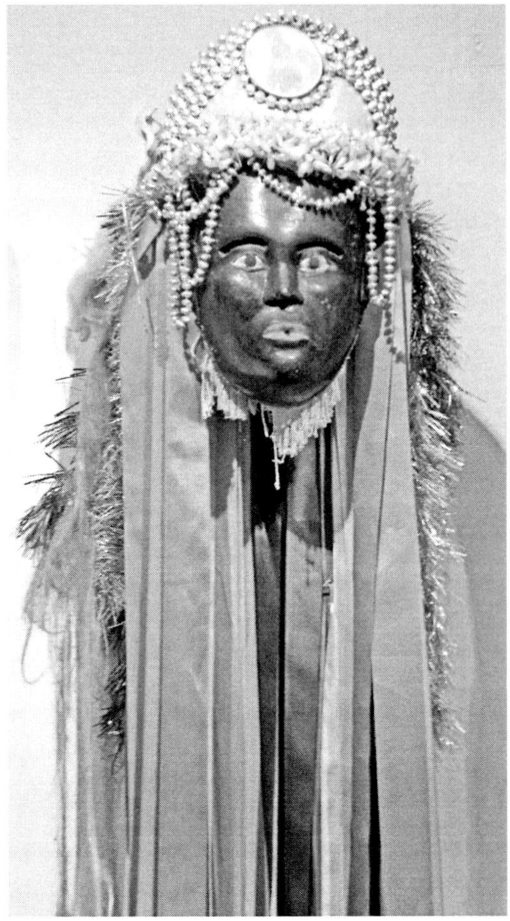

Elaborate versions of the exotic Mexican mask category known as "Negro masks" as part of Bill LeVasseur's Mexican mask museum.

inhabitants on the plantations and partly because African slaves such as the Yoruba had distinctively different religious beliefs from those of the Catholic hierarchy, making African Mexicans even more mysterious. The black masks are often elegantly decorated with brightly colored ribbons in a manner similar to some Catholic saints, also portrayed in masked celebrations. Indeed, LeVasseur says that "black" in the Purepecha culture (one of several tribal cultures still evident in Mexico today) is synonymous with elegant. African Mexicans were often treated as "status possessions" similar to the way someone today might look upon a Rolex watch. Even so, some masked celebrations involving African Mexican references curiously use white masks along with black masks (identifying all of them as Negro masks, the term that remains in use) and no one knows exactly why.[154]

PHARISEE MASKS

Pharisee masks dominate many village dance celebrations during Holy Week (Easter). The Catholic Church especially encouraged these masks as a way of demonizing the Pharisees (Jews) who freed Barabbas rather than Jesus at the time of his crucifixion. Pharisee masks often appear as horned animals with bulging eyes and long tongues. Often the Pharisee demons (in some villages they are called Jew masks) are presented humorously. When engaged in fighting with unmasked Christians, the Pharisee characters always lose. Mask maker Dalio Angel Perusquia especially enjoys making such Pharisee devil masks. When

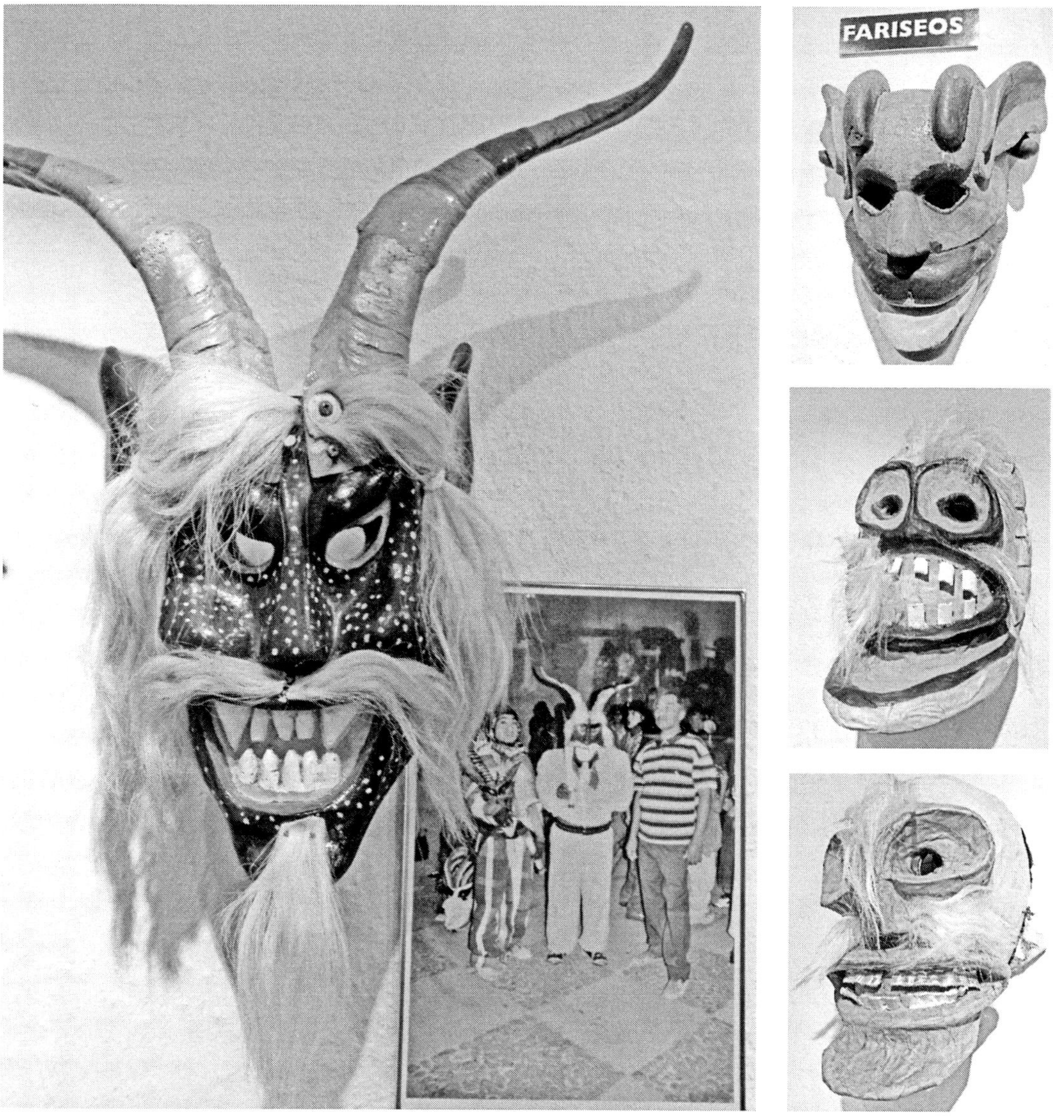

Pharisee masks as part of Bill LeVasseur's Mexican mask museum. Photograph at left is an exhibit of Dalio Angel Perusquia's Pharisee mask and a photograph of Pharisee community masker member wearing it during the Easter Holy Week *Pelea de Los Cuernudos* celebrations in San Bartolomé de Agua Caliente, Guanajuato.

he was younger, he occasionally purged some of his frustrations and anger by transferring his feelings to his Pharisee masks as he created them.[155] Other Pharisee masks are considered so sinister, however, that performers, particularly the Yaqui, Mayo, and Cora Indians, must destroy the mask in a rite of purification by either burning or drowning their masks at the river after the masked performance in order to be cleansed.[156]

Devil Masks

Mexicans also love to hate devil characters in mask celebrations. The devils appear in many versions. The late mask maker Juan Horta Castillo admitted that he identified with

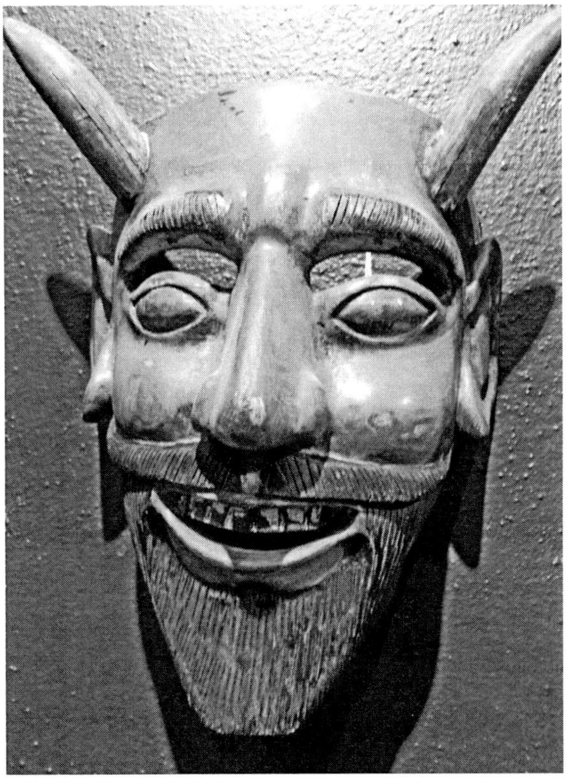

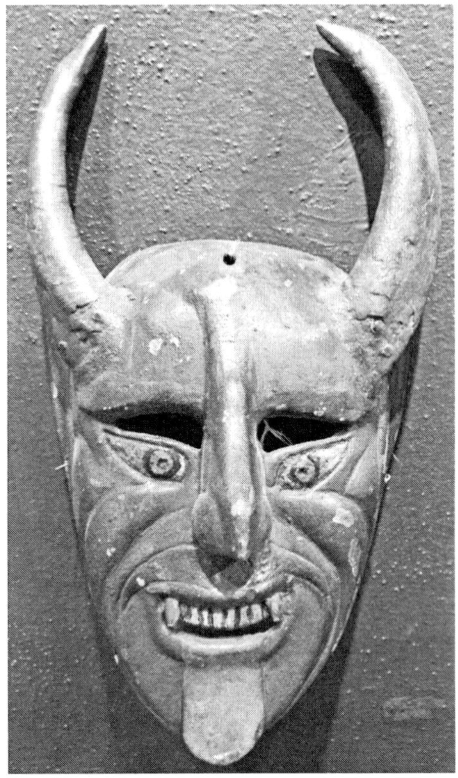

Carved wood devil masks exhibited in Bill LeVasseur's Mexican mask museum, *The Other Face of Mexico.*

devils much more than with the saints, whom he considered to be dramatically boring.[157] Catholic priests considered the pre–Hispanic deities to be demons and added horns to their images whenever they encountered them.[157] Some devil dances hearken back to myths that African slaves carried over to Mexico. Devils can wear elaborate costumes with feathers and sequins in pageant fashion or they can wear old tattered clothes and dramatic masks made of cardboard with long ears, horns, and horsehair. In some dances, the head devil wears chaps or leather trousers and carries a whip. Guerrero celebrates the Mummery of the Devil annually on September 16 when contestants dress like devils and carry whips. Prizes are given not only to those with the most elaborate devil mask, but also to those who have the stamina to crack their whips the most number of times consecutively. Occasionally seven devils will line up in dances that showcase the seven deadly sins. LeVasseur suggests that when the devil or *diablo* mask is used humorously, it has the potential to address sensitive personal scandals and social or political issues well known to members of the village. This unusual forum can break down and release tensions that exist within the community at large.

TIGRE MASKS

According to Karima Muyaes (whose parents assembled an extensive mask collection in Mexico City and supported several noteworthy mask makers for over half of the past century), the *tigre* masks invariably evoke qualities of strength and power.[159] There have

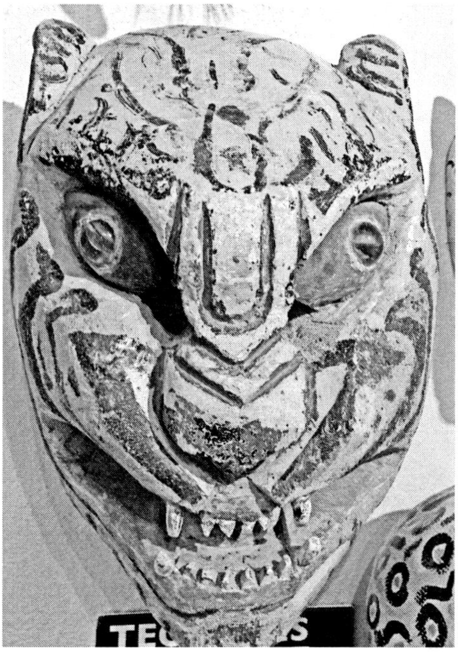

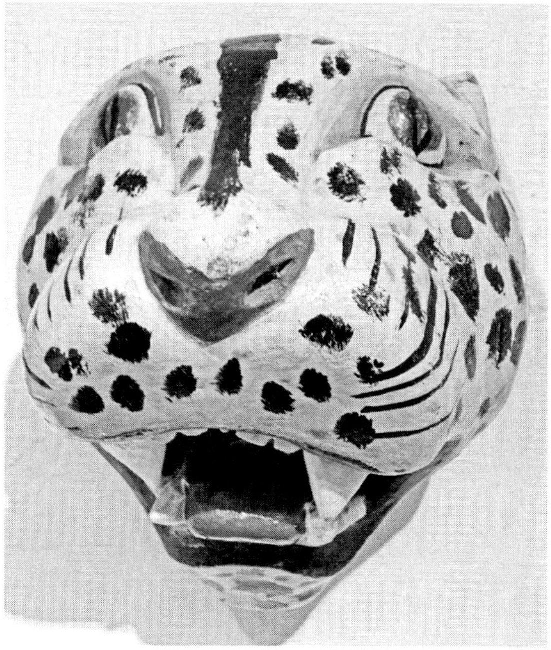

Carved wood *tigre* masks exhibited in Bill LeVasseur's Mexican mask museum.

never been striped tigers in Mexico similar to the Bengal tiger, but in colonial Mexico and in Mexico today there are what we would call spotted leopards, pumas (mountain lions), and black leopards which LeVasseur believes are also known as panthers. He suspects that the depiction of a striped tiger in masks and corresponding costume—and in fact, the use of the word *tigre*—probably worked its way into popular use with the advent of cross-cultural contact during the mid-colonial period.[160] The *tigre* masks as well as those of jaguars and pumas are much admired. The *tigre* can appear in the Dance of the Deer, sometimes acting as an aggressor with masqueraders in the dance, or even with spectators. Occasionally it protects the deer, which is thought to originate in pre–Hispanic times. The eventual death of the deer, a sacred animal, is synonymous with the spirit of the village that in time will rejuvenate. LeVasseur cites Markman and Markman in *Masks of the Spirit, Image, and Metaphor* when they note, "The thread running through every manifestation of Mesoamerican religion is the symbolic relationship between the underlying life-force and the natural world it forms and sustains. And for all this, of course, the mask is the metaphor."[161] Surely the *tigre* masks, above all else, suggest this life-force in nature. In the *Pocho* Dance, the convergence of hunting and agriculture is celebrated. Each of the masked *Cojoes* carries a rain stick and often ties fresh or dried palm leave, corn stalks, and bouganvillia flowers in his hat and costume to signify a good harvest. The *Cojoes* will often hunt a group of *tigres,* and some *Cojoes* always manage to escape. This outcome aims to maintain a perspective of equilibrium among the animal life in the region.[162]

Old Men Masks

Mexican masked celebrations seem particularly fascinated with old men. Hermit masks are usually fair-skinned, bearded elderly men who are isolated from the world and its temptations, dedicating themselves to prayer, meditation, and penance. LeVasseur describes them

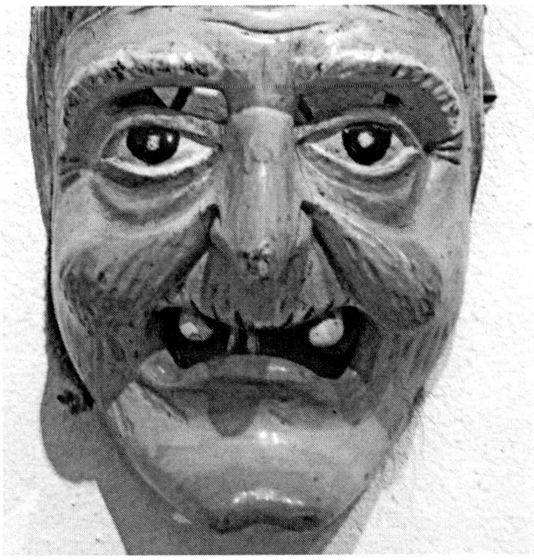

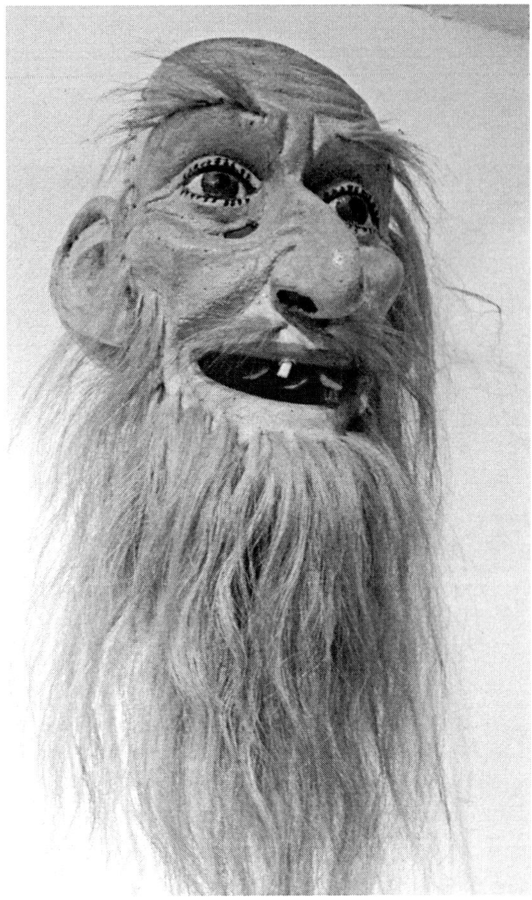

Old Men masks created by Manuel Valencia Chavez and Antonio Cervantes Delgado exhibited in Bill LeVasseur's Mexican mask museum.

as exhorting the *Pastorela* audiences to meditate on the drama about to be presented and to beware of the dangers of temptation. They represent the good, the wise, and the elderly. The expressions of their masks reflect both the vulnerabilities and the wisdom that come with age. The Dance of the Old Ones incorporates other masks from pre–Hispanic tradition: the *Huehue* (old men) who offer petitions and prayers during the sowing of crops and subsequent harvest for the fertility and protection of domestic animals and to prevent or cure plagues and epidemics. LeVasseur says that originally the dance was performed only by young men who had not reached sexual maturity. Today either two or four grown men perform the dance in honor of a community's patron saint to the music of flute and drum.[163] But perhaps the most well-known masks of old men are *Los Viejos*, who appear in the *Viejitos* dances, particularly in the state of Michoacán. They smile whimsically (some interpret their expressions as lecherous.) Most often they wear white pajama-style pants and tunics with serapes while young pre-adolescent girls, always unmasked with gaily decorated braids in multi-colored bows, accompany them in their complicated dance rhythms and patterns. The masks depict toothless or semi-toothless grins and long thinning wisps of gray hair strands.

DAY OF THE DEAD MASKS

Probably no contemporary culture confronts and celebrates the eventuality of death to the extent that Mexicans do. The annual Day of the Dead (*Dia de los Muertos*) festivities at the end of October connect with the ancient celebrations which remember and honor the ancestors in the realm of the dead. While some people might find the custom of parents and young children eating and sleeping at the grave sites of their loved ones macabre, Mex-

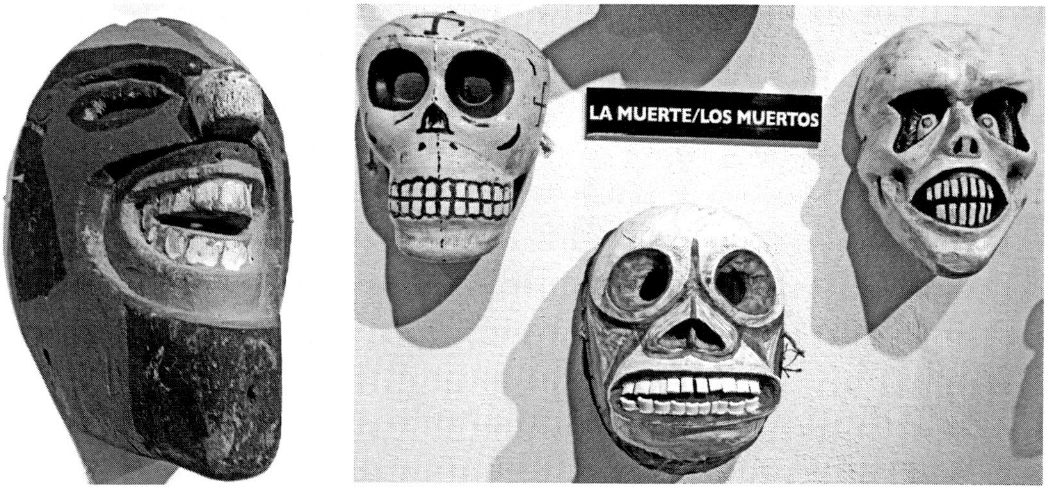

Examples of "Day of the Dead" masks that Bill LeVasseur has collected and exhibits in his mask museum.

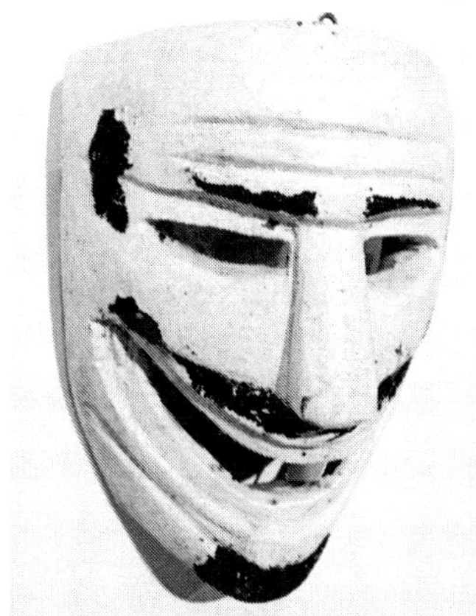

icans consider this practice to be a healthy way to remember them and an opportunity to communicate to their children their ancestors' stories and contributions. Other world cultures could learn much from this frank, frequently humorous and loving approach toward death. Day of the Dead celebrations bring a sense of community to families as they gather over potluck meals. Family relatives erect altars with flowers and food that honor the deceased and aid in creating closure and acceptance of their loss. The *Catrina* masks make humorous references to the fact that we all have "one foot in the grave" as soon as we are born. On the other hand, the masked beggars representing the dead who roam from house to house visiting their "living relatives" and pleading for food and drink recall more sinister aspects of death (although not even the children fear their visits.) These primitive-looking masks often display open mouths showing decayed teeth and gums or grimacing expressions. Sometimes they are smoking. They resemble disquieting images of death, regret, lecherousness, and pain. Occasionally one will be smiling, but in a bizarre way.

During the conquest of Mexico, the Spaniards were motivated by both gold and God simultaneously. That is, exploiting the New World riches, including gold, could justify the aggressive military conquest while the quest to bring new souls to God also brought eventual monetary support and allegiance to the Church. Therefore, any way that the Church could connect with the pre–Hispanic values of the Mexican inhabitants was considered acceptable. While the European Catholic Church did not use masks, priests in Mexico easily adapted to the power of community celebrations with masks, thereby inadvertently perpetuating their ancient connotations. At the entrance to his museum, LeVasseur quotes Maria Teresa Pomar in *Behind the Masks in Mexico*: "Mexican masks are admired for their intrinsic value but also they are linked with the fervor, the ethnic, and the vigor with which a town dresses itself in order to define itself— to show in a thousand faces of its masks its expressive capacities and its deep cultural roots."[164]

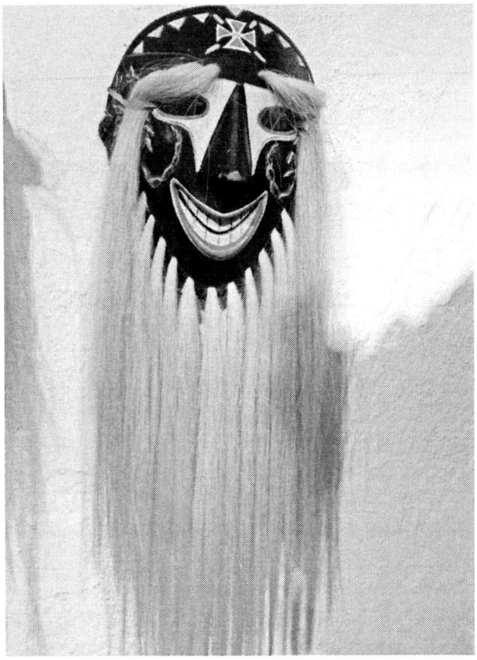

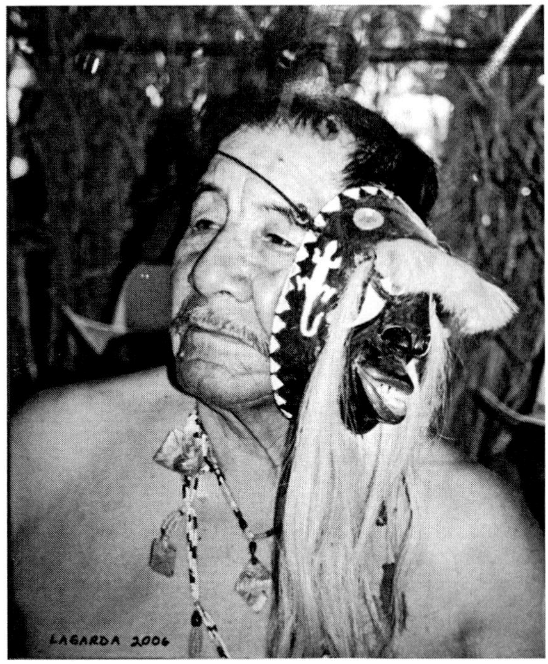

A sacred mask for the *Pascola* Dance. The *Pascola* performs as dancer, master of ceremonies, and community clown. He represents the ritual communication between the Mayo communities and the *huya aniya* (supernatural/magical world.) Photograph at right shows the *Pascola* performing as a human (outside of the sacred space where the actual masked dance is performed). Photographer: Bill LeVasseur.

On a separate note: Another private and very large mask collection is in Mexico City. It was assembled and maintained for half a century by Jaled Muyaes (a Lebanese-born anthropologist, painter, and sculptor) and his Mexican wife, Estela Ogazón. After their deaths, their daughters, Karima and Kena, inherited the collection and occasionally allow mask aficionados to visit by appointment, though it is not generally open to the public. The collection has no accompanying text as does LeVasseur's museum in San Miguel, but over three thousand masks are carefully hung and stored in categories according to style and function. Karima and Kena Muyaes can be reached at karimanuyaes@hotmail.com.

Southern Illinois University Carbondale Collection

To align with the 2005 International Mask Conference sponsored by Southern Illinois University Carbondale, its University Museum exhibited a wide range of masks representing global cultures such as Latin America, Africa, Native America, Nepal, Melanesia, and Thailand as well as contemporary masks possessing similar agendas under such headings as Defense, Sports, and Festivals.

The museum itself has an extensive permanent collection of masks, but a number of people and institutions across the United States lent masks for the 2005 exhibit, including the Abraham Lincoln Presidential Library and Museum, Dr. Patch Adams, Aldon Addington, Erasmus Justus d'Almedia, Marilyn Codding Boysen, Cedarhurst Center for the Arts, Mel Goot, Marvin and Marion Kleinau, Christian and Carolyn Moe, Ron Naversen, Schingoethe

Center for Native American Cultures at Aurora University, and Jeff Semmerling (mask maker and teacher based in Chicago). The entire exhibit featured over three hundred masks.

The University Museum's director, Dona Bachman, declared that she found the perfect person, Michael Hernandez, to curate this impressive mask exhibit. "He has the anthropological interest necessary for mounting such a detailed historical examination of masks," she explained. "Michael Hernandez and Ron Naversen coordinated the immense amount of masks loaned from a range of mask collections worldwide. Hernandez worked well with students and recruited many to assist with the research, painting and construction, and the creation of an educational area for young people." Not surprisingly, his decision to include a Ku Klux Klan hooded mask caused the most controversy within the academic community and provoked a range of critical comments from the public.

Hernandez mentioned that another aspect of the exhibit which aroused considerable consternation from the community was his display of masks under the heading of "Clowns." He proceeded to muse over his ability to effectively curate such an exhibit without initial feedback from audiences. "In the beginning clowns played an important role within the children's educational section of the exhibit," he said.

> In this section I wanted to explore the use of makeup in creating different personalities and emotions. However, during a visit to a local after-hours childcare facility, I was struck at the reaction both adults and children had to the images of the circus clowns and mimes. Most of the children would pick up the example images and quickly put them down, making comments such as "the man is ugly" and "I hate that one." Three of the children unexpectedly walked away from the images and completely stopped their participation in the project. One began to cry. The adults who were supervising the children's group also reacted unexpectedly. One of the adults asked me if there were images of clowns before I had even begun the discussion. She stated, "If there are clowns I do not want to see them." Another adult, after looking at the images, removed herself from the room. Later I approached her and asked if she was okay. "I always hated clowns. I remember going to the circus.... My mom told me that it was going to be fun and happy.... When we got there, these unhappy and evil creatures tormented me.... She [mom] lied."[165]

I discuss possible reasons for this reaction in chapter 6. The visceral qualities of the emotions we experience reside deep within us when seeing masks if only as exhibition objects. One cannot hope to fully define the mask or describe its essential characteristics and wide ranging, underlying objectives. Each of us responds to the experience of seeing a masked performance or seeing a display of masks from personal viewpoints. We interpret the mask's power for ourselves. The mask maker becomes a guide into another realm, but can only point the way. The viewer is beguiled with the mask's ability to richly suggest nuanced and multiple interpretations.

3

Mask Making Techniques

American Mask Maker Bruce Marrs

Mask makers who also perform, such as Bruce Marrs, initiate a more profound exploration into the characterization process. Midway in my career, I decided that I needed to revisit the world of the performer's creative process in order to better understand how I might contribute more as a stage designer. I had not reviewed the performer's creative process of creating a role since my college years, though much of my work culminates within the final interpretation of the performer. After team-teaching a course on the mask in performance I concluded that I took for granted the performer's exploratory process for interpreting characterization and began to ask myself what I might take from that process as a designer to create more depth of characterization.

My husband occasionally recites from W. B. Yeats' "A Prayer for My Daughter," "How but in custom and ceremony are innocence and beauty reborn?" The designer and performer should regularly revisit the traditional creative processes used in both design and performance as one way of revitalizing efforts to create character. The performer often ritualistically visits the process of creating a character, using a series of performer-specific exploration techniques in much the same way as a designer often uses a series of designer-specific exploration techniques.

While admitting that such a reexamination of the performer's creative process held tremendous appeal, I could not ignore the fact that I am not a performer. Ultimately the exploration of that process would demand that I return to the vulnerable state of confronting unfamiliar terrain in a classroom setting. Thus I approached the process with a mixture of trepidation and fascination. Somehow, the prospect of attempting to perform (and ultimately exploring the process of performing) seemed much more intimidating than it had in my college years, when I understood less well the characteristics of a good performance and blissfully had far less awareness of my own limitations.

I decided to sign up for Bruce Marrs' annual summer mask-making workshop which also introduced basic performance exploration techniques with the mask at Dell'Arte International School of Physical Theatre. His sense of humor and playful spirit helped me regain my balance and a bit of confidence. In addition to an examination of papier-mâché and neoprene mask-making techniques, Marrs spent an equal amount of time on the process of creating the character, often utilizing movement techniques, improvisation, ensemble work, and performance work with music. In addition to working with Marrs for two weeks, I studied *commedia dell'arte* performance techniques with Joan Schirle and Ole Brekke at Dell'Arte International as well.

Marrs emphasized the "zeroes" of the mask — that is, the essential states of the mask. He pointed out that all successful masks have more than one emotional state or essence — or zero. A mask is "dead" if it can only express one state of being. A successful mask should allow an expert performer to embellish a sense of dramatic tension with the mask and evoke several different emotional states. The mask maker and the masked performer strive to find several zeroes in the mask to make it come alive. They can take great delight in discovering and showing the "counter" zero as well.

We spent a great deal of time learning how to trust the power of the mask. "The mask loses focus when it moves too much. Work for economy of movement," he frequently reminded us. "Remember that we are vertebrate creatures. Actions in the body resonate into the mask. Consider the walk of the deer and its head. The actor becomes involved in non-specific actions when a movement momentum takes over or dominates the performer's presence. Avoid this 'modern dance' approach in masked performance."[1]

Sheila Kerrigan's book, *Collaborative Creativity*, held new meaning after taking Marrs' mask-making workshop. She describes the necessity for understanding and practicing body language skills and creative thinking skills in group improvisational work. Marrs demonstrated important aspects of his creative process as a mask maker/designer and performer by showing how to integrate these skills at the most basic level to achieve a more vivid characterization with the mask.

Bruce Marrs showed me how to more fully appreciate the challenges of the performer and how I might use the performer's vocabulary to help contribute to the performer's vision of character. I highly recommend this workshop and others offered by Dell'Arte International to designers of the mask interested in exploring processes of creating characterization from a performer's perspective. I now think of mask work in a completely different way.

Neoprene Masks

Neoprene is a synthetic rubber that simulates latex as a casting material. Like latex, it is non-toxic but it should always be used in a well-ventilated room. There are various rigidities on the market that dry into relative levels of hardness. Some levels cause the mask to crack while softer levels will stay very malleable. A medium rigid consistency (#521) works well for initial experimentation. A mask made out of this base will have a slight bit of flexibility. Spartan Adhesives in Chicago has a Chicago Latex Products line that stocks neoprene. It cures into a white color, but dyes and paints and pancake makeup can be mixed into it before it cures, making it potentially any color desired. It can freeze so you must wait before ordering it during cold weather.

The neoprene mask will need the positive plaster head mold and the negative plaster mold to hold the neoprene in its liquid state. First, Marrs offers some suggestions for creating successful plaster head molds that use plaster bandages as the negative cast:

Plaster Face/Head Mold from a Negative Bandage Cast

- Two six-inch-wide plaster bandage rolls can be used for casting faces of three people. Use plastic bags, tape, and Saran Wrap. Marrs prefers Johnson & Johnson Fast-Setting.
- After preparing the model, apply one layer of tissue paper with Vaseline.
- Apply damp plaster bandages starting at the chin, then forehead, and have the model have slightly open lips. Work around the lips and then do the forehead.

- Anchor the nostrils with a plaster bandage tab down the middle of the nose with vertical strips at the corners of the lip. (Use half-inch strips here.)
- Then start crosswise bandage strips across the face, including across the lips.
- Place four-inch squares on the outside edges of the lips to help strengthen that area.
- Do basically two layers of bandages and then do two diagonal, long, thickly twisted strips to form an X shape in order to strengthen the cast.
- When dried, gently pull off and check for pin holes. Fill in and also fill in nostrils with a double bandage.
- Think of the negative cast as a bowl and add extra strips around the neck or lowest points to even out the bowl. Pay attention to any vulnerable spots by adding more bandages.
- Pour plaster into the "bowl" face mold and when plaster dries, pull away the cast.

Sculpt the Clay Using Terracotta Clay

- Wet down the clay with a damp rag between sculpting intervals.
- Avoid symmetry in the clay mold. Symmetry can be very limiting. Where does one plane intersect visibly with another to avoid goggle eyes? The outside corners of eyes do not hang forward like goggles, but go back into the face. Ears can't be flat; pulled back somewhat, but not flat. Find planes to the lips and eyelids. These planes will accentuate and define the features of the mask when light hits it during a performance.
- The corners of lips stick up instead of in. Marrs states that lips are a mystery. The corners of the mouth go up or down, sometimes simultaneously. There must be two separate lips to have a realistic relationship. In classic beauty, the bottom lip terminates before the top lip does. Again, strive for asymmetry and repetition of shapes between facial planes. How does each plane relate to the face and to each other? Don't make envelope mouth corners. The corners of the mouth go into the face and do not stick out. The lips terminate into the face, not into the other lip. They rarely terminate in the exact same spot.
- The sides of the mold should be smooth.
- Play "fast and rough." Throw the clay around to get an expression. Try sketching the image first. Ultimately, however, a mask is not a drawing. Don't make pinched features into the clay mold. Keep all the features very three dimensional.
- A face has two eyes, one nose, two lips, with eyebrows, cheeks, a chin, and some character lines. Don't make anomalous features. Marrs admonishes us to avoid making "modern art." Don't let the style of the mask overwhelm the character.
- Don't make isolated features. Learn to integrate features instead.
- Don't make skirt noses. A nose has two nostrils and a center part between them.
- Masks tend to work best when the eye holes fit at the eye level of the performer's face.

Cast Plaster Mold of Clay Positive

- Seal the clay mold completely with clay tubing (so that a negative space will allow you to grasp and pull the dried plaster off of the mold).
- Pour Hydrocal plaster and wait for two or three hours.
- Gently and firmly pull apart the plaster negative mold when it is ready to be pulled from the clay positive mold.

- The plaster will have quite a bit of clay residue. Remove some of it with Q-tips swabbed in acetone. You can also pour a quick layer of liquid latex into the plaster mold. The latex will take out more clay residue when pulled out.
- Plaster molds need to be thoroughly clean and dry (thirsty) before pouring the neoprene, so let the mold sit for at least a day.

Pouring the Neoprene Positive Mask Mold

- Fill the negative plaster mold with neoprene. Tap the mold a little to release air bubbles.
- Wait about an hour and a half and pour out the neoprene. The neoprene that is left on the surface of the plaster will dry within ten hours and can then be pulled out. Trim the neoprene mask as desired before it hardens more within several hours. Cut out eyeholes and nostrils at this point.

Painting the Neoprene Mask

- Dyes or scraped powdered makeup or paints can be mixed in with the wet neoprene before it dries.
- Try sanding the neoprene before painting to rough the surface. This might ensure better paint adhesion. You might prefer to spray an adhesive spray onto the neoprene surface (or spray a fine mist of neoprene onto the surface — neoprene sticks to itself very easily).
- Marrs prefers to use acrylic paints because the plastic base of acrylic paints lessens the chance of it cracking on the mask.
- Consider a base coat as the main color of the mask, with highlights and shadow colors added.
- Work in rhythmic brush strokes, going in one direction.
- You can dry brush for color texture. You can do a translucent wash by mixing the paint with water, or finger paint by rubbing the paint onto the base coat. Try sponging paint on as well, just as a performer sponges on makeup for performances.
- Marrs believes that adding blue tones give depth and are often appropriate. Red tones suggest blood and can add an appearance of vitality to the skin.

Use Goop to Attach an Elastic Band to Either Side of the Mask

- Attach the elastic a fourth of an inch above the top of the ear — should be above eye level.

Papier-mâché Masks

- Tips on plaster negatives: Make sure your negative mold is deep, all the way to the beginning of the ear, down to the neck. Shore up the dip in the negative from the neck so you have a deep "bowl" in which to pour the plaster. Vaseline well, but thinly so that the Vaseline coating isn't a texture in the positive. If pouring from moulage (a plastic-based casting product) or alginate (a product used by dentists for casting the inside of the mouth), again make sure the mold is deep. It is good to put a wire hoop into the back of the positive as the plaster begins to set up. As plaster starts to get thick, scoop away from the hoop so that you can grab the hoop to remove the positive from a difficult mask. Make sure the hoop is level with the back of the positive so that the positive can sit flat.
- To begin, place the positive on a wooden board. Anchor down the positive with clay so that it doesn't move about. Use clay to raise the positive if necessary, and

extrapolate the clay line from the positive to the board so that the mask can have more depth. Shallow masks just don't work as well.

- Use oil-based clay or Plastilina (Plasticine) clay. Sculpt directly on the positive plaster mold. Don't cover the eyes as you will need to keep track of where they are so the mask fits you. Bring all perimeter edges to the perimeter of the positive mold. Most of the fit comes from the perimeter, and a mask that sticks out past your own face looks anomalous. Other places that must fit are between the upper lip and the nose. If the mask is to speak, try to keep mask surface off resonators next to the nose.
- Marrs repeats his favorite admonitions at this point: Remember to avoid anomalous features. A face has eyes, nose, mouth, cheeks, and eyebrows. Avoid the attempt to make modern art! Make your mask easy to believe.
- To papier-mâché, first Vaseline all plaster exposed, but not so much that the underside of the mask comes off all greasy. Use heavy-duty brown paper bags. Some white bread bags are also nice for alternate layer distinction. (With contrasting colors, you can discern when you need to start a new layer of flour and paste.) Tear away all factory edges from the bag as cut edges don't blend well. Tear the bag into pieces about ten to eighteen inches square. Soak in warm water for a few minutes. Take it out. You don't want to work with sopping and dripping paper. Cover the whole piece in pre-mixed wallpaper paste. (According to Marrs you will never go back to any other paste.)
- Cover the mold with five layers of bag tears. If you have trouble remembering how many layers you've done, use a felt-tip pen to cross hatch a layer or two, then rip and paste, or use a white bag or newspaper for alternate layers. Use a piece as large as will fit the curvature without wrinkling. You do not want any wrinkles. Cover the eyes so you can later cut away a smooth edge. Marrs reminds the novice mask maker to strive for good work. The sequential layers of paper should be rubbed well into the base. Make sure all layers are well bonded, and possible glue pockets are squeezed out. It is okay to do all five layers at once or a layer at a time. Sun dries papier-mâché best. A heater is a good alternative, especially if you have a fan. Wind dries better than a heater. (At least, wind in northern California works well.)
- Get the dried mask off before the clay underneath dries out. Don't leave it for four or five days or you will be in trouble.
- Clean out residual clay. Wipe off Vaseline if there is any inside. Cut edges and eyeholes and nostrils. Papier-mâché edges by folding a layer of wet, glued paper over the whole edge of the outside mask. Start at one end and go around until you have finished. This will give you an edge of seven layers. Dry out the mask.
- Spackle with regular new-mix spackle. You can use water to smooth it a bit. Use your finger. Don't use too much as you must later sand most of it off. Cover the whole mask outside layer. Dry. Sand with 100-grit sandpaper until mask has a marble look.
- Sand well. Often craftsmanship goes out the window at this stage. If you rough up the paper a bit, smooth after sanding with water and paste; rub until very smooth again. Let dry.
- If using house paints for inside and base coat, use eggshell luster latex paint. Semigloss is too shiny. Flat paint gets too dirty. Think in terms of three tone values. Your base is your medium value, highlight is your high value, and shadow is your

shade. Use fine art acrylics for fine painting. Add reds as you would in make-up, unless red kills the color scheme of the mask. Darken the mask towards the edges. It works well by adding depth to the mask. Remember painting techniques: dry brush, blending brush, translucent wash, finger paints, and sponge techniques.

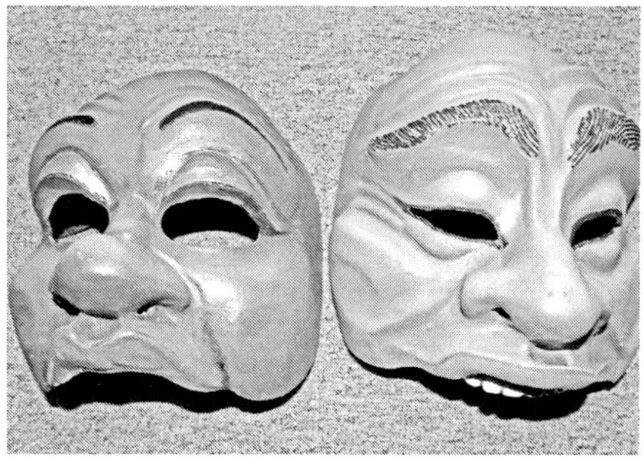

Examples of Bruce Marrs' neoprene masks.

- Paint the inside of the mask with black acrylic paint to seal the sweat away from paper that will otherwise melt the paper and glue.
- The strap is glued on with "Goop" or "Shoe Goo" found at most hardware and lumber stores. Remember that the corner of the ear is a fourth of an inch above the corner of the eye, so make sure that the strap's bottom edge is a fourth of an inch above the corner of the eye.
- Before considering the mask completed, get a trained outside eye to help you discover more personality aspects of the mask. Remember that a mask is made of luck as well as craft. If you are unlucky and the mask is not very lively, or requires more work than the gift it gives, admit it. See if it works on somebody else. If it is a dull mask, make another; get lucky the second time.[2]

Consider ways to crown or frame the mask. Does the performer's hair go with the mask for the appropriate personality and style? If not, get a hat, a wig, a cloak with a hood. Find the layer that connects the mask to the actor and the costume.[3]

Rob Faust's Leather Masks

Rob Faust, who has lived for the past decade in Canada, has developed a fine appreciation and expertise in working with leather masks and below are some examples of his mask work.

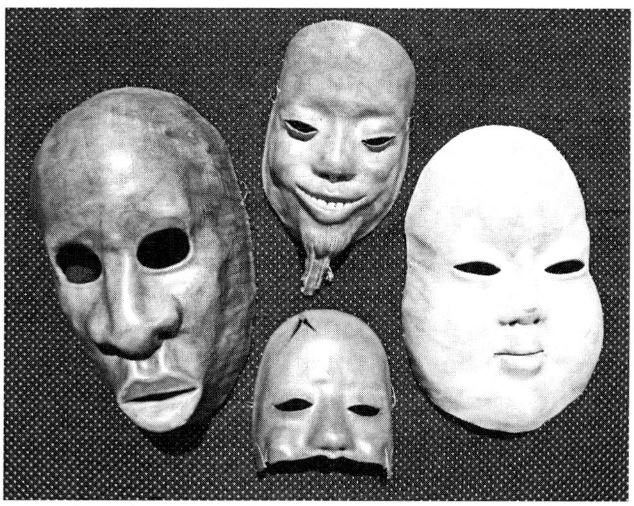

Several of Rob Faust's leather masks, clockwise from left—The African, Sage, Baby Buddha, and Cherry Blossom.

Later in this section, I will identify general techniques used in making leather masks and describe Faust's unique technique for using resin as the positive mold on which to shape the leather. But first, I'd like to summarize essential differences in leather mask-making techniques by several well-known traditional masters in this field. Brazilian Venicio Fonseca and Swede Torbjörn Alström, both introduced in this book, have created very expressive leather masks using the traditional method of molding and shaping leather over a wooden matrix carved in the desired shape of the mask.

Thurston James, in his book, *The Prop Builder's Mask Making Handbook*, suggests another process for creating the foundation on which to build the leather mask by using a positive Hydrocal plaster mold created in the likeness of the initial clay mold built on top of a plaster life cast of the performer's face. James' Hydrocal plaster mold is anchored with a block of wood which can then be used to pound the stretched leather onto it as the leather dries into shape. This saves time because the plaster mold is easier to cast than the wooden matrix is to carve.[4]

I took a leather mask workshop with Newman, a British expatriate, while he was living in Oregon. (Currently he resides in Bali where he assists Joan Schirle with the Dell'Arte International study abroad program in Ubud.) He has supplied masks to training programs at the Swedish National Theatre in Stockholm, the Globe Theatre, and Central School of Speech and Drama in London, *Cirque du Soleil* Saltimbanco in Paris and countless colleges and universities around the world from Mumbai to Montreal. Newman has invented yet another innovative way of creating leather masks using frozen Roma Plastilina #4 clay as the positive foundation mold over a plaster life cast of the performer's face. Newman's process has several advantages. His process eliminates the extra steps involved in casting a positive plaster likeness of the mask and eliminates the extra step in carving a wooden likeness based on that plaster positive.

Newman's method of working with a frozen clay positive mold as a starting point is much easier for students. We simply cast face molds in plaster and then sculpt the desired likeness for the leather mask with the Roma Plastilina #4 clay onto the face mold. The clay mold is then frozen before working with wet leather on top of it. The leather seams are not pounded onto an attached wooden base, but rather laced with sturdy waxed nylon sinew at the seam edges at corresponding opposite ends of the mask's back side. The lacing takes place in this manner around the mask base, keeping the sculpted leather appropriately stretched and taut until it dries into the desired shape.

There are essential considerations when making leather masks using plaster and clay molds. But at this point, we should explore the advantages of using leather for masks. Why have traditional mask makers preferred to work with leather for millennia? A leather mask offers significant advantages over other materials. Lighter in weight than a wooden mask,

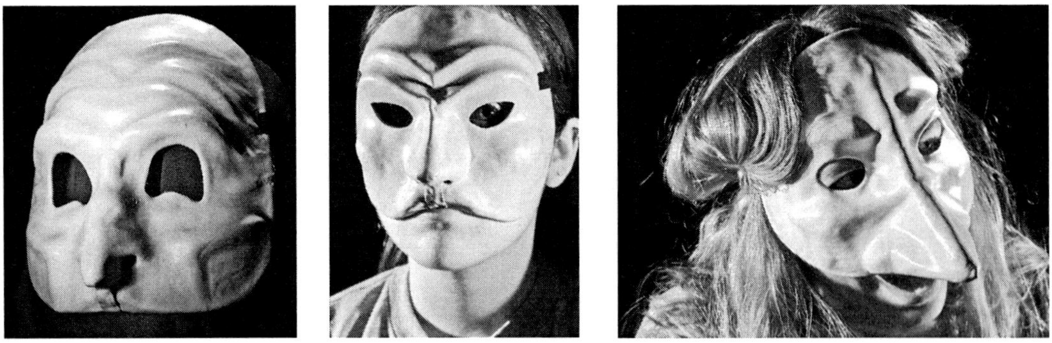

Leather masks created by students Emily Satterfield, Beth Anne Kirby, and Erin Doughtery at the University of North Carolina at Greensboro.

leather "breathes," making it more comfortable to wear in warm temperatures. Leather looks like human skin; it stretches with relative ease, and consequently offers more potential for a fluent expression. Unlike wood, leather does not attract termites and worms and does not break down for several centuries. It develops a lustrous patina over time. Some aficionados claim that the color of the elegant black *commedia* masks in Italian museums was actually the color of skin colors when the masks were created, but over time the color became darker and richer. The old adage rings true: "Leather ages like a fine wine or a fine woman." The scars and patina that leather eventually acquires are considered marks of beauty.

Selecting appropriate leather for a mask can be a subjective and daunting quest. The leather industry has no standard for grading leather quality other than the maxim that higher grades typically begin with "A" or "1." A lower grade of leather uses a more primitive process of tanning and has more holes and scaring. The best advice is to take a reputable leather dealer's advice. Ideally, one should visit the dealer to make selections because each leather hide is unique. Hides have irregular shapes, making it difficult to estimate accurate square footage for purchase. One should overestimate yardage to ensure that there will be enough leather for the desired number of masks. Top quality leather has good elasticity, shape memory, thermal insulation, and water resistance.

Cowhide and buffalo hide are considered the best leather for masks; some mask makers prefer to use belly leather. Leather masks are best when made from leather weighing between three ounces and seven ounces. Three-ounce leather is almost too thin, while seven-ounce leather is almost too thick. Thicker leather makes it much more difficult to achieve fine, nuanced facial features, though it will result in a more durable mask. A hide designated as "top grain" signifies that the top outside layer of the leather has not been split. This leather is ideal for masks. Split leather, leather that is split from the outside skin surface, has two "fuzzy" or suede sides. It is considered less supple and less durable. Leather in neutral colors tends to be less expensive than leather treated to appear as non-organic, exotic colors.

General Advice

- Consider the most appropriate plaster to use for each project. Regular Plaster of Paris is not recommended for the life masks that serve as the base for the positive clay mold fashioned in the form of the mask design because it isn't always strong enough. United States Gypsum Company, based in Chicago, describes Hydrocal White Gypsum Cement as a product that offers higher strengths than typical plaster products. It can be used for a variety of arts and crafts applications and it is especially intended for thin sections which require high green (early) strength to minimize breakage during removal from intricate latex molds. But Ultracal 30 is even stronger and only slightly more expensive. This product is super-strength gypsum cement and recommended for extreme accuracy and greater surface hardness. It has the lowest expansion of any rapid-setting gypsum cement available. Both of these products make effective positive life casts and appliance molds.
- The basic process for achieving a fine leather mask can be described rather briefly here in the next few pages, but bear in mind that achieving mastery over this process requires time and experience. First, refer to the other sections in this chapter with information by Bruce Marrs and Michael Meyer for tips on casting fine positive face molds.
- After you have completed a plaster face mold, carve the face mold with a band saw

so that the plaster after the top lip is cut away. The forehead might need editing as well. Full face masks are more difficult to sculpt in leather and the novice should not attempt them.

- Chip away plaster on the back side of the face mold with chisel and mallet to create sharp outlined edges. These edges will allow for the leather to crease crisply when it is folded back on itself to create the outside seams.
- Once you have edited the plaster face mold, hammer or screw a nail into the apex of the nose. This will help to anchor the clay mold that will be applied on top.
- Use Roma Plastilina #4 clay to fashion the clay mold that will indicate the exact mask design desired. The clay is very hard and a bit crumbly, making it more challenging to shape. Cut the clay up into "butter-size slices" and then gingerly, firmly apply and press onto the plaster face mold. Make a consistent layer all over the mold about a fourth of an inch thick. This initial layer makes the rest of the clay mold easier to apply and shape. Avoid bulbous-shaped noses because these are more difficult to sculpt in leather (though possible with more expertise.)
- Leather mask makers I have interviewed recommend fewer but highly exaggerated facial planes. Exaggerated, raised planes can catch the light more readily and convey clearer expressions to an audience.
- Shaping and sculpting the leather can be accomplished by using leather tools such as stamps, a rounded wooden stick called a *sticketta,* and a mallet. The outside skin surface of the leather takes on interesting textures, lines, and shapes that can make it resemble a human face more than the suede side can. Wooden clay modeling tools with rounded edges work well on leather. Leather can be cased and burnished. Avoid using metal tools which can alter the fine grainy texture of leather (unless desired), and avoid tools that have edges or points that are too sharp because they can puncture the leather when applied too forcefully.
- The leather should soak for at least ten minutes, but leaving it in water longer does not harm it and might achieve more consistent saturation. The leather must then air for thirty to sixty minutes before it reaches a point when it has optimum capacity for molding and shaping. Once it reaches this state, shape it for one to two hours before it gets too dry. If drying occurs, sponge the leather down, and work it a little longer. If frozen Roma Plastilina #4 clay is used for the positive mold, it might need to be frozen again after one or two hours before reworking the leather. (But depending on the design of the mask, the clay is so hard that it can often serve as a positive mold even without re-freezing.) If the clay needs re-freezing, place the clay mold and the enveloping leather mask in a plastic bag before placing it in the freezer. When taking it out of the freezer, let it thaw a few minutes before proceeding to sculpt the leather.
- Cut enough leather to allow a one- or two-inch overhang on the mold and extra length directly under the nose to allow plenty for the eventual "dart" (which takes up all of the excess leather after the rest of the area has been sculpted) that will be cut out with the edges juxtaposed next to each other to form a flat seam.
- When sculpting the leather, always start with the nose first and work out the excess leather around the face until the dart section is formed.
- Clamp this excess dart area until the other facial features have been shaped, and then cut out this section at the bottom of the nose. (The excess from the dart is not entirely cut away, but will eventually form a small flat seam extending from the edge

of the nose, down the lip, and back up into the nose cavity, forming a support section.)

- Skiving, or shaving the inside layers of leather, can add a more professional look to the mask. Wherever the leather has cut edges, skiving will make them thinner and cause them to lie flatter, giving a more elegant appearance. A double beveled 1/35-millimeter chisel and #7/20 or #7/25 curved chisel work well for skiving leather. Take care not to press too hard or skive too quickly. Placing the leather on a board when skiving will help to protect the blade.
- The seam around the entire leather mask should be clearly creased and then notched so that the curved seams will eventually lie flat.
- Skive these notched edges and hole-punch each notch. The notches will then be laced (with wax nylon sinew, purchased at leather supply stores) to stretch the leather firmly to the base of the plaster face mold.
- This is done by lacing the notches from opposite ends of the leather mask's seams at the base of the mold. Work around the base until all notches are laced. Take care not to lace too tightly.
- After the leather has dried, cut the lacing and lift the leather off the mold.
- Trim then glue down (with barge cement) the seam sections, saving the nose section remainder left after the nose dart has been cut out and trimmed.
- Glue the top portion over the top of the seam where the dart edges are aligned to each other (see photograph below).
- Then glue the extra length along the inside of the lip and up into the nose cavity.
- A long skived pig skin strip about a half-inch wide can go over the glued-down notched edge inside seam to give a nice flat, smooth appearance inside the mask. (Photographs next page. Torbjörn Alström avoids an over-flap where the seams line up at the nostrils, down toward the chin. He simply supports the back of them with a thin piece of leather.)
- Consider coloring the mask, particularly the lips and eyebrows, with leather dyes. Remember, however, that the beauty of the leather can be in itself sufficient if the mask design has effectively raised planes to adequately suggest facial features.
- Painting a layer of lacquer or rabbit glue to the back of the mask will make it more durable, though doing so makes it a little less comfortable for the wearer.
- Attach an elastic band by using Goop glue and apply the elastic band a little higher than the mask's eye line. Or make a slit in the leather and wrap and stitch the elastic through the slit. One can also grommet the elastic to the leather.

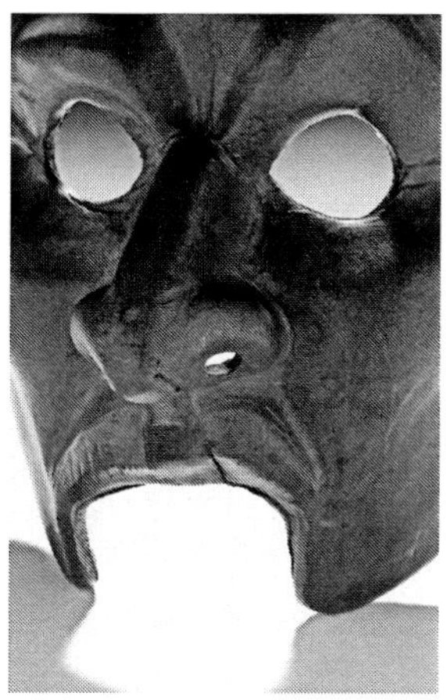

Make nostrils and eye openings slightly smaller than necessary, then dampen the leather and insert a pencil or round clay modeling tool, pushing toward the inside of the mask to get a smooth, finished opening. This mask has airbrushed leather dye on the lips. Note the seam that extends from the tip of the nose, over the lips, and back into the mask cavity. Photographer: Dan Smith.

Working with Leather Masks

Faust has experimented with leather masks, many of which are rather small in size or about seven inches long. When worn

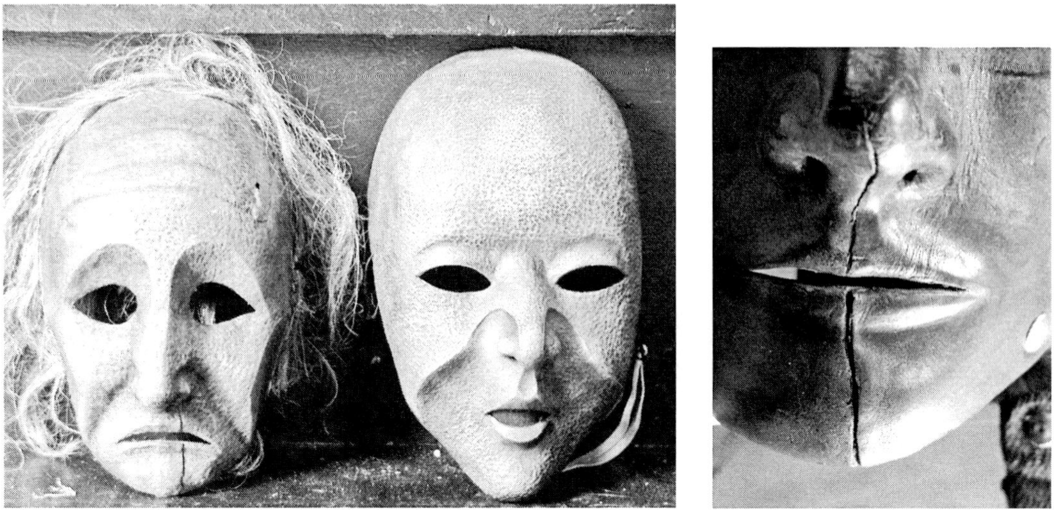

Torbjörn Alström has another method for joining seams where the excess leather is cut away.

these petite masks project a rather fantastical look because they are not in scale with the rest of the body. Faust uses the example of this leather mask called "Sage" to explain his process.

CREATING FAUST'S CHARACTER, SAGE, OUT OF LEATHER

First Faust created the mask called "Sage" by casting a plaster gauze face mold of a seven-year-old girl. He then made a plaster positive and sculpted teeth, cheekbones, and smile in water-based modeling clay. He offers the following suggestions for making such a mask. (Refer to Marrs' and Meyer's tips on casting plaster face molds in other sections of this chapter.)

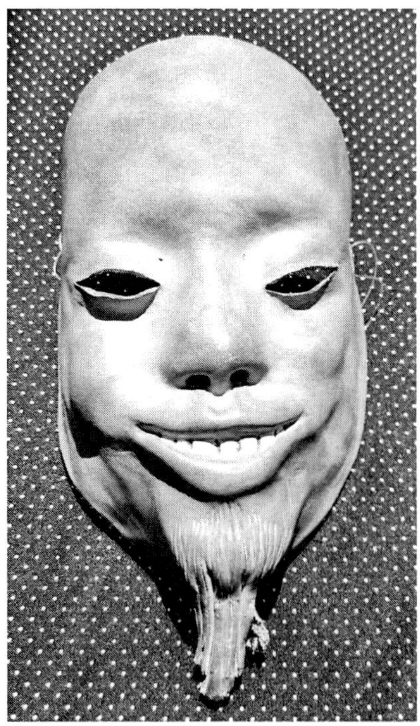

Rob Faust's Sage mask.

- With modeling clay, sculpt the character's features on the top of the plaster face mold. Fashion teeth (if desired) out of clay as well.
- Create a negative mold by applying damp plaster bandage strips around the clay mold. Apply several layers to make it sturdy.
- After removing the plaster bandages, brush a layer of fiberglass resin inside the gauze negative, which results in a strong positive fiberglass mold of the expression from the clay.
- Drill six very small holes into the low points of the fiberglass mold: at the top inside corners of the eyelids, the outer edges and bottom of the nostrils, and at the outside corners of the mouth.
- In order to shape the damp leather over the resin positive mold, use corks, nylon thread,

and leather patches. The sequence of these layers is as follows: corks, resin mold, damp leather, and leather patches to protect the leather mask as the nylon thread is pulled through each hole and tied to itself over the cork. That is, nylon thread is pulled through the holes in those six strategic places of the resin mold. The thread holds the wet leather in place at the pressure points where the leather corresponds to the resin mold at the bridge of the nose, the base of the nose, and the mouth. The thread, protecting the six areas of the leather mask with a corresponding scrap of leather on top of each hole in the leather is synched down to the resin mold by pulling tightly and is tied in triple knots over large corks on the back of the fiberglass mold.

- Always distribute the leather evenly so that working the excess to the edges will be possible on all areas of the mask.
- Punch holes in the leather approximately one inch beyond the outer edge of the mask-to-be, and synch tightly around and behind, the way a drum skin might get tightened. The corks allow for additional support for the fiberglass mold, so that it will be sturdy enough to press and shape the damp leather over top of the fiberglass mold. Faust prefers to use a wooden spoon or wooden dowels wrapped in thin leather as modeling tools, though other leather modeling tools also work well.
- Work the excess leather either around the back, or into the wrinkles for the character. In some cases there is no need to be too slavish in recreating the original expression seen on the clay mold. Let the leather speak to you as it lets you know what it is willing, and not willing, to do. The photo below shows how Faust actually achieved five different characters using the same resin mold, working the leather in different ways. The Sage mask's goatee was achieved by shifting the excess leather toward the bottom and shaping, cutting, and tying it to resemble hair.
- Pushing and stretching the leather requires substantial effort and strategic wetting and drying of different areas of the mask as the leather form evolves.
- After the general shape is there, trim all of the leather around the outer edge of the mask.

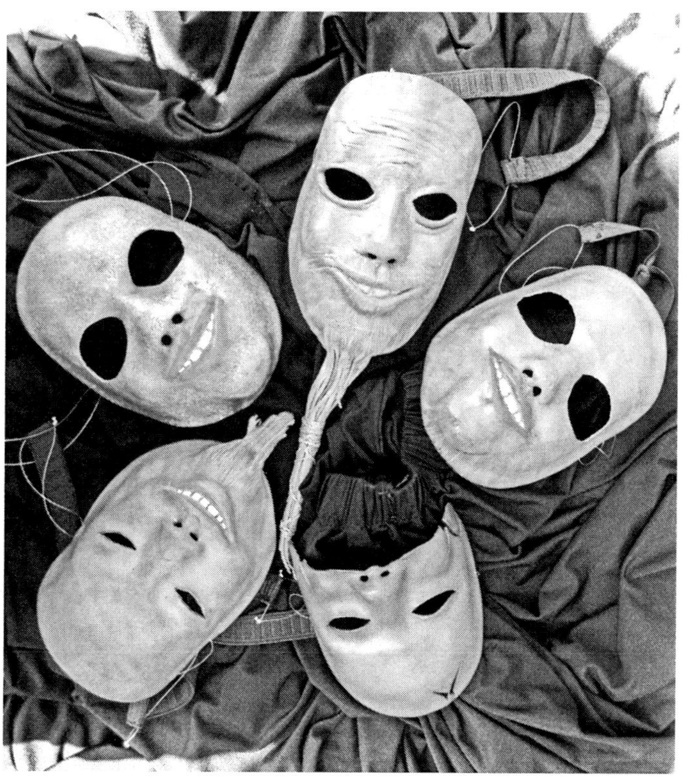

Rob Faust's characters created from the same resin mold.

Shaping intricate details such as leather teeth required perseverance and determination. Each tooth has to stay clamped with one finger or tool while the next ones are shaped. But, frequently, a leather mask functions better without intricate detail. So consider carefully the overall design before investing too much effort on features that will not necessarily show up for an audience.

- Faust likes to color his leather masks with Fiebing Leather Dyes. He achieves various skin tones by mixing and diluting various shades and staining the leather in order to make the mask seem richer and more translucent like skin. Even blue dye colors can add depth and interest for the tan tones. He also likes to use water-glazed white acrylic paint highlights.
- Once the mask is completed, Faust dyes and paints the mask. He does this first, before applying rabbit skin glue solution on rear of the mask, so that tiny spills and seepages of glue won't affect the absorption of the dye/paint job on the front. Faust uses a solution of rabbit skin glue and water, approximately one heaping teaspoon per half cup, to firm up the finished product while letting it continue to breathe a bit.

According to Torbjörn Alström (who received the support of a grant from the Swedish government to explore possible ancient materials and methods for making masks), ancient leather masks have not survived in Sweden even though leather shoes from the Stone Age have been discovered. He has demonstrated that his ancestors had the capacity to make masks out of bark and fish skin as well as animal hides using handcraft techniques and tools available in his region, but with no remnants of ancient masks in Sweden, he assumes

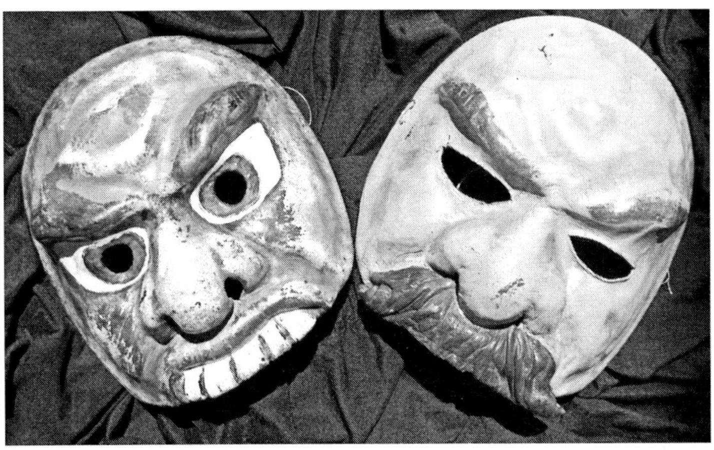

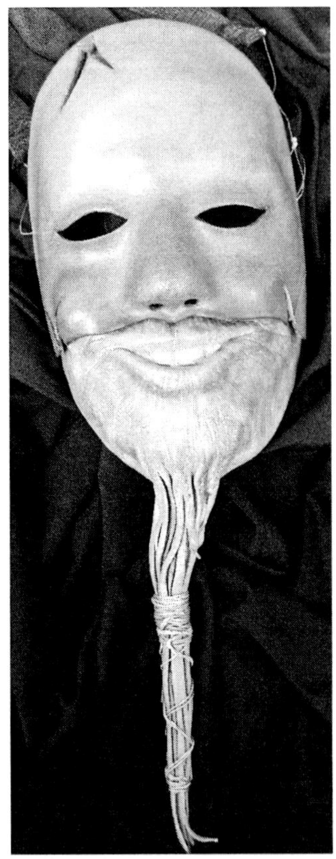

Left: **This photograph shows two different mask characters in Faust's repertory. Each used the same resin mold, but Faust fashioned the leather over the resin mold in different ways. On the left is the Wild Man, reminiscent of Balinese masked clowns with bulging eyes. On the right is the Coach. Faust made the moustache out of excess leather that was difficult to stretch. The leather inspired the rest of the character when Faust recognized its potential. He created Caucasian eyes by making almond-shaped slits instead of rounded slits.** ***Right:*** **Two masks in one—Faust's Cherry Blossom mask on top of his Sage mask.**

that they were used in temporary ways, perhaps created for certain rituals using bark or another short-lived material.

Aström suggests that each region developed mask styles and choice of mask materials according to the myths of the culture living in that region. These myths, no doubt, responded to the terrain of the land. If the spirits of the animals have significance for the myths in an area, then leather will be used to create the masks. Likewise, if trees are the important carriers of the history and myths of an area, then the wood from the tree will be used.[5] This hypothesis seems particularly relevant when we examine the very old traditions of carving wooden masks in Bali where there is limited land suitable for grazing animals, but its jungle terrain supports trees rather well. Master Balinese mask carver I. Ketut Molog demonstrates the fine art of creating intricately detailed masks in the following section.

Wood-carving Techniques

Balinese mask carver and masked performer I. Ketut Molog has presented other mask-making workshops that Dell'Arte International has arranged (currently annually) in Bali, Indonesia, for over two decades. The following detailed section on Molog's mask carving techniques is taken from Professor Ron Naversen's 2004 *Theatre Design & Technology* article, "Learning to Carve Masks in Bali," after taking Molog's workshop in 2003.

Mask Maker I. Ketut Molog

Ketut Molog is a forty-three-year-old master carver from the village of Mas, which is known throughout Bali for its many many fine woodcarving studios. Molog finished his formal education when he was twelve and began to practice carving when he was seventeen. His first source of carving wood was the family's firewood, which he had to protect from his mother who was trying to cook the family meals. This was in the early days of Balinese tourism and woodcarving was not yet a major profession. Bali is now famous for its woodcarving and exports thousands of carvings each year.

Molog was especially drawn to carving the *Topeng*, which is Balinese for masks. His love for masks began early as he experienced the masked dances and ceremonies integral in the numerous village, temple and house ceremonies that take place throughout the Balinese year. Much like the Italian *commedia*, these masks represent traditional characters, which are familiar to every Balinese. Molog could therefore practice his carving skills by copying masks of established characters and begin to understand the personality of the mask. Once he had begun to master the techniques of carving he was able to add his own style and interpretation to the mask's character.

With experience Molog developed a sense for which woods were appropriate for carving masks and began to see qualities inherent in each piece of wood that he could coax out for the mask. Molog discovered that he saw the mask more clearly when he concentrated on both the character and the wood. He continued to carve masks and was pleased that people began to buy them. When he was twenty-seven years old, Molog was proficient enough to apprentice under master I. Bagus Anom, whose family members have been celebrated mask carvers and dancers for several generations in Mas. Molog studied under Anom for four years, learning the finer aspects of carving and of mask characterization. It was under Anom's tutelage that Molog learned the importance of music and dance to the creation of the mask.

They often carved to the mesmerizing Gamalon music of the *Topeng* and *Wayang Wong* (*Ramayana*) stories. Anom is also a celebrated *Topeng* performer and through him Molog was inspired to take dance lessons to better understand the interrelationship of dance and the mask.

Eventually Molog established his own studio in his family compound and began training his own apprentices. One of his first apprentices, his son Kadek, is already a skilled mask carver. Molog currently has apprentices ranging from twelve to twenty-five years of age. The younger apprentices saw, split, and chop the wood into the basic mask shape. Molog, Kadek and the experienced apprentices carve the masks and Molog often refines the mask's final features. Molog's wife, Nyoman, and daughter, Comman, sand, stain and polish the "production quality" masks, which are taken each morning to the local woodcarving market to be sold to tourists and stores throughout Bali. Masks commissioned for performance are painted, decorated and purified in a ceremony whereupon a spirit is invited to inhabit the mask to aid the performer to become the character.

Topeng *Mask-carving Workshop (article by Ron Naversen)*

Less than four months after terrorist bombs in Kuta killed 202 tourists and Indonesians, I arrived in Bali to study mask (*Topeng*) carving as part of Dell'Arte's Study Abroad program. Despite the tragic event I looked forward to this opportunity. It was hard for me to believe that my six-week sabbatical proposal to study mask carving had led me to this paradise. I always thought artists and academics were supposed to suffer.

After several days of helpful orientation sessions to Balinese culture, language and customs by the Dell'Arte faculty, I was ready to begin my formal instruction in mask carving. I stepped off the *bemo* [Balinese bus] into the brilliant sun and stifling heat on the main street of Mas, a village famous for its many mask and woodcarving shops. I entered a winding alleyway leading to the family compound of my Balinese mask-carving teacher I. Ketut Molog. Molog's extended family and apprentices live together in this compound along with an array of dogs, chickens, ducks and pigs. Domestic activities blend with carving as the women come and go to market, wash clothes, prepare daily meals, feed the animals, dry rice in the sun, make daily offerings to their Hindu deities and sand and polish the finished masks. Men pass through the studio to and from the rice fields behind the compound, make house repairs, maintain the family motorcycles and carve their masks. It was in this domestic setting that I learned the fundamentals of carving and much about the Balinese way of life.

My first carving lesson was very different from my own teaching style in America. There was no syllabus with an outline of educational objectives, topic headings, evaluation scale, and absence policy. We had no introductory discussion about carving history or philosophy, no formal demonstration of tool usage and maintenance, no step-by-step outline for learning basic carving practices progressing towards more complicated techniques. Molog simply asked what kind of mask I would like to carve and we began. I would learn by actually carving a mask; first by observing Molog's technique and then by attempting to copy it.

Looking at the many elaborate masks that hung on the walls of his studio I selected one with simple facial features. I didn't want to take on more than I could handle on my first mask. My mask work prior to this had always been an additive process modeling from clay, plaster or papier-mâché. Now I was dealing with a subtractive process where I thought any mistake was irrevocable and permanent.

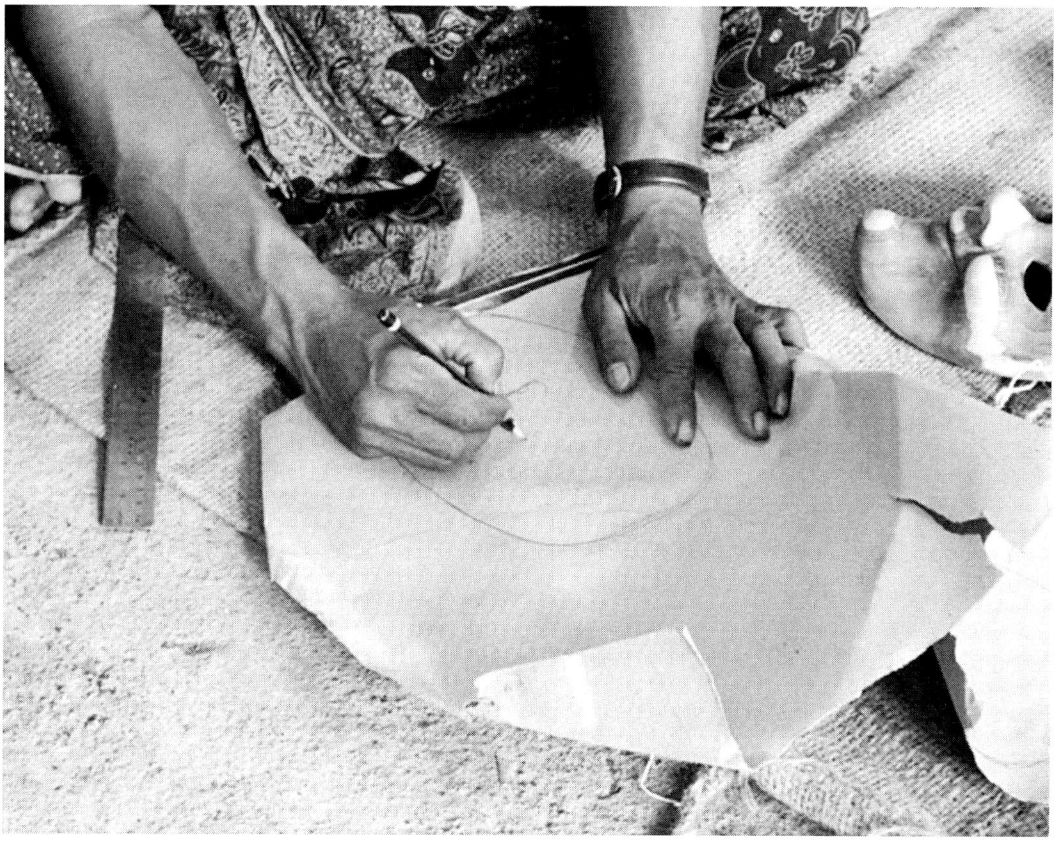

Tracing the outline of the mask at Katut's studio in Bali. Photographer: Ron Naversen.

We began by tracing the outline of the mask I was to copy onto a piece of paper, cutting out the pattern after folding it along the centerline to make sure it was symmetrical. The position of the eyes and mouth were also sketched on the paper for future reference. Measuring the pattern, Molog selected a log about eighteen inches in diameter from his woodpile. A favorite wood for mask carving is *pulai*. *Pulai* is a straight, fine-grained, cream-colored wood, which is carved while still green and soft. The *pulai* hardens as the mask dries becoming lighter and stronger.

[Note: Nigerian and Mexican mask makers told me that they prefer to work with aged wood rather than "green" wood that Naversen identifies as the preferred wood for Balinese mask makers. When I asked him about this discrepancy, he responded,

> I think this is probably due to the nature of a particular wood. *Pulai* and red alder (used by Pacific Northwest Native American mask carvers) are best carved green when it is softer, more flexible, and denser as it still has much water. As the wood dries it becomes lighter and harder which is good for the mask performer. Both the Pacific Northwest and Bali are wetter climates so that may affect the wood carving qualities because they won't dry out so quickly. Drying too quickly can make the wood split. Some Mexican masks I have are carved from a palm wood which is very very soft and may need to dry before it can be carved effectively. I suspect Nigeria and Mexico are drier climates and so wood naturally dries more quickly. I personally have not found a dry [aged] wood that I like to work with—it is so difficult.][6]

We used a two-person handsaw to cut the block to the height of the mask, allowing an extra half-inch at the top and bottom for safety. An old axe head was inserted into the cut to prevent the edges from pinching the blade. The cut log was then measured so it could be split into three individual blocks, each of which would become a mask. The back of the mask is oriented towards the harder heartwood so the facial features can be carved into the softer sapwood. This way the circular growth rings correspond to the rounded features of the face. We began the split by using the axe head to cut a half-inch-deep line across the wood block. More axe heads were driven into this cut, creating a split into which a thicker wedge of wood was driven to completely split the block.

We placed the mask block on a wood block about fifteen inches in diameter and about three inches thick on one edge and four inches on the other. This slightly raked block allows the carver to position the mask at different angles while carving. Molog then demonstrated how to use a small axe or *timpas* to clean and level the back of the mask block. The *timpas* is the size of a hatchet with a nine-inch handle, five-inch head and two-and-one-half-inch-deep blade that begins its bevel about one and a half inches from the edge of its slightly curved blade. The most unusual feature about the *timpas* is that the head is offset from the handle twelve to fifteen degrees, which allows the carver to maintain a straight stroke while making cuts into the block's side. Molog made a few quick, deep, unerring chops whereas mine were hesitant, shallow cuts that often missed the mark. Once I missed the mask entirely and chopped into the wood block. Molog smiled and explained the block was there to protect the concrete floor from the apprentices. This was the first inkling I had of Molog's gentle sense of humor.

Once Molog was satisfied that the back was flat, he traced the paper outline on it and demonstrated how to rough out the corners at the top and bottom and then round the chin, cheeks, and forehead to start bringing the face into relief. Roughing out simply means to quickly cut away the bulk of the waste wood before starting to define and model the carving. This process is also called grounding or wasting. Molog demonstrated on one side of the mask and had me copy on the other side. He would watch my progress, offer suggestions and occasionally reposition my hands and guide my stroke. Molog then used the paper pattern to locate the eyes and mouth on the face of the mask. He chopped a straight cut directly

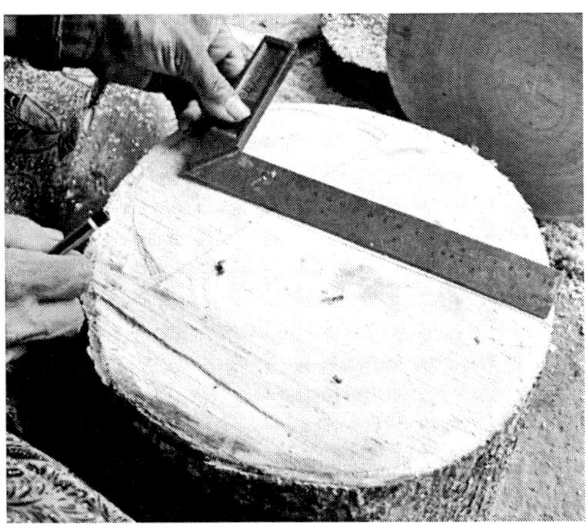

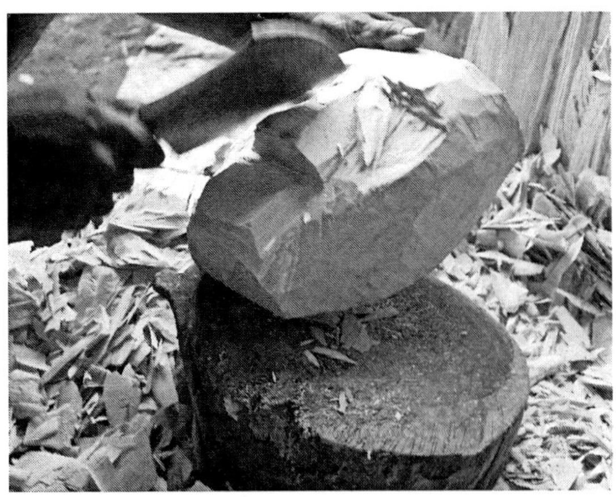

Left: **The cut log is measured in order to split it into three individual blocks for three separate masks.** ***Right:*** **Molog defines the eye socket. Photographer: Ron Naversen.**

beneath the nose and then an angled cut from the top of the lips to make a notch. Then Molog made a diagonal cut to define the left side of the nose and another cut along the top of the left eye to define the socket. Giving me the mask and *timpas*, Molog indicated it was my turn to copy these cuts on the other side of the mask. Again my strokes were hesitant and less efficient than Molog's, who continued to give helpful suggestions.

Later I learned that many Balinese carvers would often switch to a small axe called the *kapak* to rough out the features in greater detail. However, Molog had found that his *tamu* students were less comfortable wielding an axe and preferred to move to the more controlled chisels and gouges. Molog felt that the added expense of the *kapak* wasn't justified in our initial training.

Besides the *timpas* we received a wooden mallet, six flat chisels and seven round-edged gouges as part of our carving set. Our mallet or *pongotok* was made from a dense native wood. The handle was about eight and one-half inches with a head about four and one-half inches long, two inches wide, and three inches high. The flat chisels or *pahat*, ranged from a quarter inch to one and one-half inches wide across their cutting edge. The rounded gouges, or *pengacap*, ranged from an eighth of an inch to one and one-half inches wide at the edge. These tools were cut from recycled industrial saw blades by a local blacksmith and then sharpened by Molog using a wet stone. Both the chisels and gouges were beveled along a single edge. The *pahat* typically functions with the beveled edge up while the *pengacap* alternated as we cut either convex or concave gouges into the wood.

On one side of the mask Molog demonstrated how to use the larger *pahat* to slope the forehead, cheeks, and chin down to the sides and back of the mask. Next he showed how to use the smaller *pahat* to cut the valley between the nostrils and cheeks and flatten the notch between the nose and lips. I copied, less skillfully, on my side and once a rough facial structure emerged we moved to the curved *pengacap*. Molog demonstrated how to cut valleys into the brow and cheek, blending them into the eye sockets, the bridge of the nose to the cheeks and the skin to the lips and cheeks. We then turned the *pengacap* over to gently round the raised areas of the nose, nostrils, cheeks, lip, and chin into softer hills and mounds.

Perhaps the most difficult aspect of carving was learning how to hold the wood securely

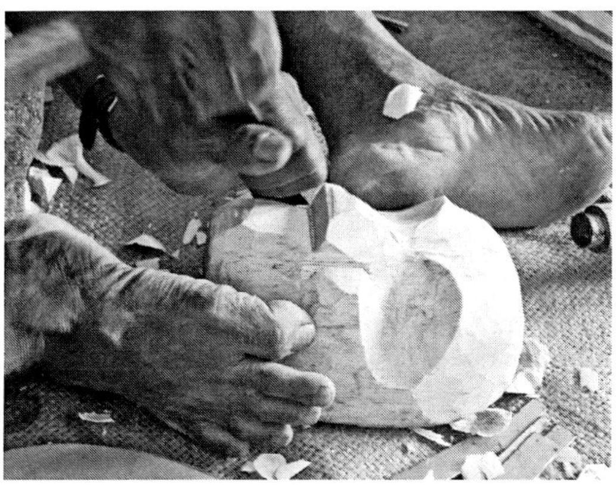

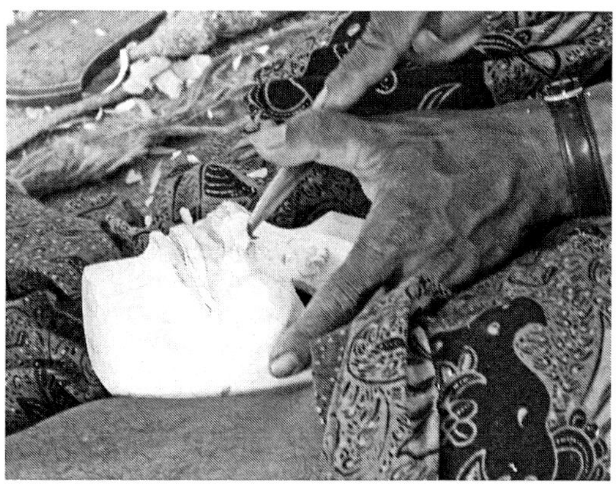

Left: **Molog uses a *pahat* to cut the valley between the nostrils and cheeks and flatten the notch between the nose and lips.** ***Right:*** **The *pengacap* is gently turned over to round the raised areas of the nose, nostrils, cheeks, lip, and chin into softer hills and mounds. Photographer: Ron Naversen.**

in place while one hand wields the *pongotok* and the other manipulates the chisel or gouge. The Balinese carver solves this problem by using his feet as the vice to hold the wood. Molog and his apprentices were extremely flexible and their facile, almost prehensile, feet and toes allowed them to grip and rotate the mask quickly and efficiently. While the other students and I could hold the mask between our feet for short periods we could never hold it as securely or rotate it as easily as the Balinese carvers. In Western carving tradition we secure our wood to a worktable, but I've since discovered that this method doesn't allow the quick repositioning of the mask to facilitate the carving strokes or to check the balance and symmetry of the mask. The *tamu* students also needed cushions to sit on for long periods where the Balinese could sit cross-legged for hours on end.

An interesting note about the use of feet in mask carving is that Balinese cosmology reveres the head as the purest part of the body while the feet are considered polluted or unclean. Therefore, since the feet touch the wood in the carving process, it is necessary upon its completion for a priest to ritually purify the mask before it may be worn for any religious ceremonial performance.

With each mask I carved I became more aware of how important it was to continually rotate the mask and approach the cut from the appropriate angle depending on the type of cut that was desired. Ideally a cut across or at an angle to the grain is best. The cuts I found most difficult were end grain cuts at the crown nose, lips and chin. Cutting into the end grain will often split or chip the wood. I also learned how to make stop cuts in the wood by cutting down into the wood severing the grain. This serves as a break or stop for a subsequent cut coming towards the stop cut.

Before the facial features are cleaned with knives the mask should be hollowed to fit the wearer's face. Hollowing is the process of digging out the waste in the back of the mask. The mask is turned over and placed face down on the wood block or on a nest of wood shavings to help protect the high relief features of the nose, chin and brows. The larger *pengacaps* are used to gouge a divot in the center back of the mask. This divot is then popped out and the sides are continually cut back, creating a bowl-like depression. The bowl is made larger and deeper until the sides of the mask are about a half-inch thick. Knives are used later on both the outside and the inside edges to refine the features of the mask and reduce the wall thickness to one-quarter inch. Balinese carvers will actually use the *timpas* or *kapak* to start the hollowing process, allowing them to quickly chop large cuts from the back before moving to the *pengacap*.

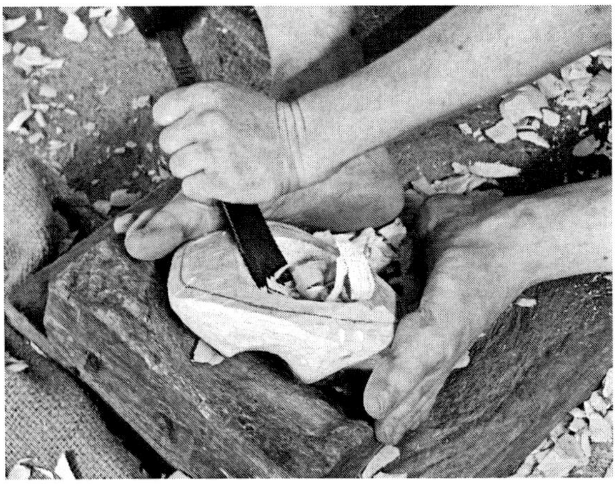

One hand wields the *pongotok* while the other manipulates the chisel or the gouge. Photographer: Ron Naversen.

Care must be made during the hollowing process to keep from cutting through the mask. I found that the *pulai* is translucent if carved too thin. On the occasion when I did cut too deeply Molog showed me how to carve a slender piece of *pulai* to fill the hole and then glue it in place using the Balinese version of Superglue. During the hollowing process the thinner edges of the mask

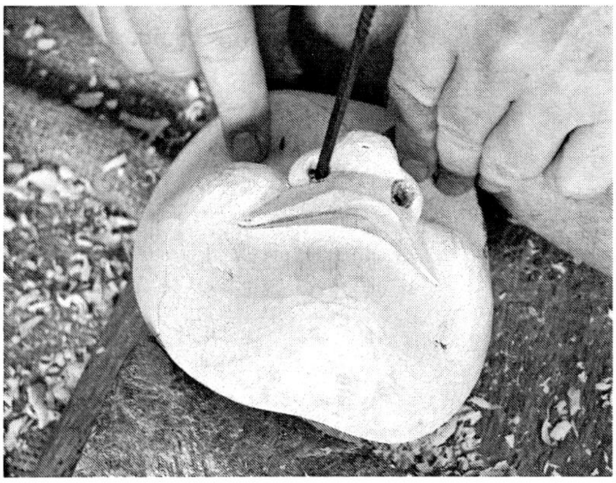

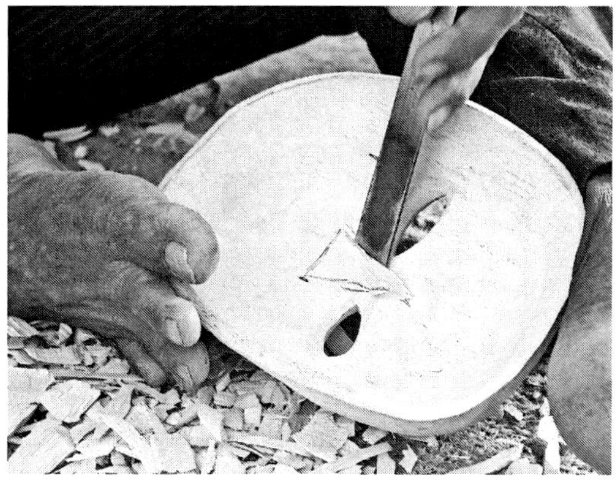

***Left:* The nostril holes are made by rotating the $\frac{1}{8}$" *pengacap* to cut a small circle from the front to the back of the mask. *Right:* The back of the nose is then excavated with a medium *pengacap* to accommodate the wearer's nose. Photographer: Ron Naversen.**

may occasionally split or crack. The carving students were understandably crestfallen if one of our masks split, but when this happened Molog would laugh and produce his bottle of Superglue, which securely welded the edges back together. While shopping for masks at other studios I would occasionally see the tell-tail discoloration of Superglue along a thin line on the back of the mask and knew that even the master Balinese mask makers occasionally had to fix some of their masks. So, I learned that not all carving mistakes are irreparable!

Once the mask is sufficiently hollowed, the eye and nose holes are cut through to the back of the mask. After sketching in the eyes, different sized *pengacap* are used to make a stop cut along the circumference of the eye. The wood inside the eye socket is excavated and the process is repeated until the *pengacap* punches through the mask. The nostril holes are made by rotating the one-eighth-inch *pengacap* to cut a small circle from the front to the back of the mask. The back of the nose is then excavated with a medium *pengacap* to accommodate the wearer's nose. I noted that American noses generally needed more excavation than the smaller Balinese noses.

Several knives are used to clean wood from behind the eye and nose, smooth the features of the mask and carve fine details. Included in our carving set were two sizes of straight knives or *pamutek* and two curved tipped knives called *pangot.* Both knives have a single beveled blade edge, but the *pamutik* only has a blade on one side while the *pangot* have double-sided blades and tips that curl up away from the blade. Both sets of knives have long handles, which the carver employs in a levering action using the thumb as the fulcrum or pivot point. This way the knife blade can either be drawn towards or pushed away from the carver, allowing the carver to select which direction is best according to the wood grain. Molog carved the handles for our knives, which were made of the same recycled metal as the chisels and gouges.

The *pamutik* are used to clean the flat and convex surfaces and make straight incised cuts into the wood. The *pangot* are used on concave surfaces with the curved tips particularly useful in excavating the smaller crevices and undercuts around the nostrils, eye sockets and lips. The *pangot* are also invaluable for excavating the nose and eye sockets and cleaning the gouge marks in the hollowed back. Molog's skill with these knives was formidable. He could make long graceful cuts to add wrinkles, define the curving lips, flare the nostrils and

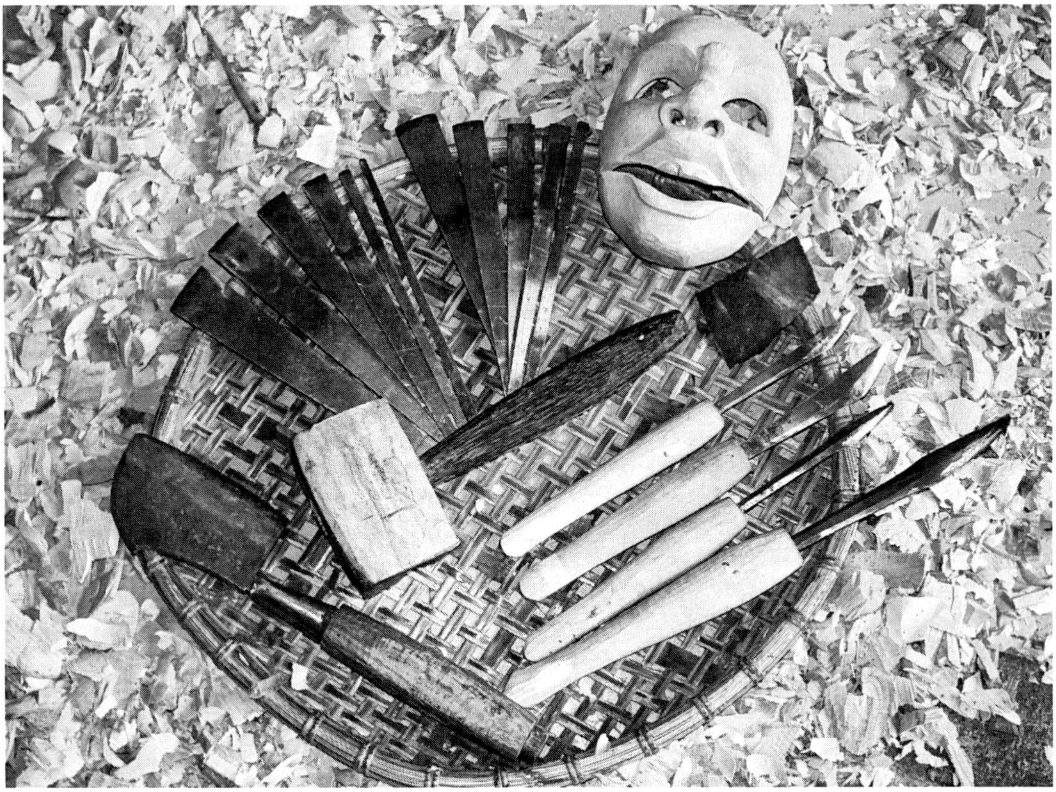

Balinese mask carving tools. Photographer: Ron Naversen.

round the teeth. My knife strokes were short, choppy slices that I hoped the sanding process would soften and blend.

The *pulai* wood is still soft and wet when the carving is complete so the mask is allowed to dry for several days before being sanded. Because Molog cleans his masks so well with his knives he only requires a single two-inch-by-two-inch piece of 80-grit sandpaper to finish the masks. The sandpaper is curled into tubes and folded into points to get into difficult cracks and crevices. While the mask surface needs to be smooth, it shouldn't be overworked, muting the details.

Although at this point I'm focusing primarily on carving techniques, I should briefly mention the meticulous painting and decoration that these masks undergo once the carving is complete. The traditional white priming paint is made from ground calcified pig bone and mixed with fish-based glue. This paint is mixed to watercolor consistency and requires fifteen to twenty layers to effectively base coat the mask. The mask is sanded every fourth or fifth coat to smooth the surface. Traditional pigments for base coats are obtained from a variety of shells, insects, fruits, plants and beans, including coffee. Traditional black is made from the lampblack of burnt coconut shell. Contemporary mask painters use convenient acrylic latex house paints, which are still thinned to a watercolor consistency, requiring multiple applications and sanding between coats. The irises, wrinkles and facial accents are also applied in several washes of thinned gray-black paint. Store-bought synthetic brushes are used for the base and prime coats, but for detail painting Molog makes his own tiny brushes by attaching goat or monkey hair with thread to a carved handle.

These masks are further decorated with mother of pearl for teeth, goat and monkey fur for mustaches, eyebrows and beards, braided horse manes for hair, and gold leaf and jewelry findings to indicate royalty.

I carved five masks while in Bali. On the first mask I would estimate that Molog carved 75 percent while I did 25 percent. My second mask was 60 percent Molog and 40 percent me, and on the third mask these percentages were reversed. My fourth mask was 25 percent Molog and 75 percent me and on my final mask I did 100 percent of the carving. I was both surprised and honored when Molog offered to take me on as an apprentice. He thought that in several months I could become a skilled mask carver in my own right. It was tempting to stay in paradise and continue to hone my skills under Molog's tutelage. But I had other obligations and I was anxious to return home and share my experiences with my students, colleagues and friends.

Now that I am back in the States I have continued to practice my carving. *Pulai* is not available in the states and red alder (almus rubra) is suggested as a comparable substitute. Alder is also carved while green, but changes from a cream to a reddish color while drying. Unfortunately alder doesn't grow in Illinois so I have it shipped green from Oregon.

Mexican Mask Makers' Suggestions

Mexican mask carvers Dalio Angel Perusquia, Manuel Valencia Chavez, Manuel Abeiro Horta, and Antonio Cervantes Delgado shared a range of tips on wood carving and painting techniques. Each mask maker identified personal preferences for wood selection, ways of preparing the wood, and ways of getting an appropriate texture and color to the final rendering of each mask. Ron Naversen's article (immediately preceding this section) gives a more detailed description of the exact process and types of tools he studied under I. Ketut Molog in Bali. That basic process seems similar to the process most mask carvers worldwide utilize. Here I describe some of the nuanced differences in the overall process of mask carving by these individual Mexican masters as a way of demonstrating the range of individual artistry inherent in each mask maker's approach.

First, Manuel Abeiro Horta, like his father Juan Horta Castillo, frequently receives inspiration for his masks while dreaming. He acknowledges the importance of snakes as often seen in his masks, saying, "Snakes are good luck in dreams. To dream about snakes is to dream about money. Though I'm nervous about snakes in real life, I like to incorporate them in my masks."[7] Bill LeVasseur's mask museum displays masks with similar connotations of prosperity and fertility; masks with *chintetes* (scorpions, snakes, lizards, and frogs) decorating the cheeks, nose, and forehead. According to LeVasseur, "These masks, still seen in the Huezquistles Dance in Guerrero, are thought to have pre–Hispanic origins for the purpose of petitioning the rain god Tlaloc for a good harvest as the dance clearly suggests procreation and fertility. Other masks in the same region depict female masks with *chintetes* who depict La Malinche, the Indian consort of Hernán Cortés."[8]

All four of these mask makers mentioned the difficulty in finding appropriate wood. Earlier in this chapter Ron Naversen notes that he prefers to use "green" wood (freshly cut) because, as I. Ketut Molog says, it is easier to carve. However, Perusquia and Chavez say that they learned early on to dry out the wood before carving in order to prevent eventual cracks. Kasali Aganbe Ogun and Kolawole Adeola in Nigeria give similar advice, saying that they allow the cut trunks of trees to dry out in back of their studios over time before attempting to carve them. One assumes that these differences in opinion must relate to the type of wood being carved. Perusquia notes that he likes to use trees that have already fallen,

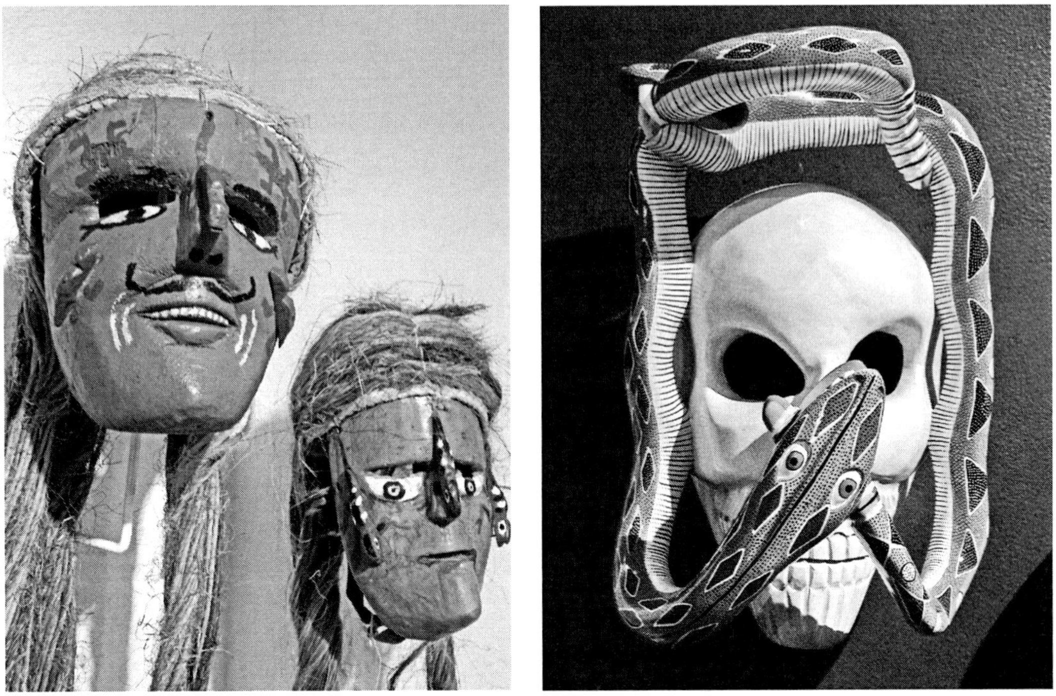

Traditional *La Malinche* masks with *chintetes* (lizards and snakes) as decoration in the first photograph alongside a photograph of Jean Horta Castillo's contemporary mask.

but he cuts into the trunks of trees only during a full moon so that the wood will not host worms and termites.[9] (Perusquia showed me a worm-eaten mask which had been cut from a trunk at a time other than at the full moon to make his point. This factor was also mentioned by Delgado and Chavez, though no one really understands why. It is a traditional belief that seems true by trial and error but with no scientific basis.)

Dalio Perusquia and Antonio Delgado both mentioned that they receive inspiration from studying the base of a tree trunk, where the thick roots form. The name of this root is *ahuehuete* and it comes from a type of cypress wood. Perusquia showed examples of these sinuous roots at his studio and then showed examples of masks in process that utilized aspects of these roots to help form the basis for horns and beards on the masks. Noses also often morph from root sections in his work, as well as bestial ears.[10]

All of the mask makers said that they prefer to use *colorin*, a type of lightweight balsa wood that is relatively easy to carve and easy to wear, even though it is technically considered a hard wood. This wood is known as *patol* in the Otomi language and *zompantle* in the Nahuatl language. But this rare wood is illegal to use nowadays. So they must find it dried and aged on the ground. Delgado says he can still find it in his home town in Michoacán. He also enjoys working with the wood of the avocado tree and says that he allows this type of wood to dry for several months before beginning to carve it. He added that pine wood doesn't need to dry out. As long as he cuts the mask according to the grain of the wood, it will not crack.[11] Juan Horta Castillo's wife Endina Ramos Horta mentioned that Juan and she would boil really large masks in water for several hours in order to keep them from cracking, but his son, Manuel says that boiling is not necessary for standard-size masks.[12] Delgado also likes to work with *aele,* a type of ash wood that he says can be found near small water streams near his childhood home, but he admits that it too is increasingly difficult to find.[13]

The primary tools mentioned by all of the Mexican mask makers resemble those identified for carving Balinese masks as mentioned by Ron Naversen. The tools can be divided up into four major categories, the ax or *hachasuela* (a small ax), the chisel or *formon* (it has

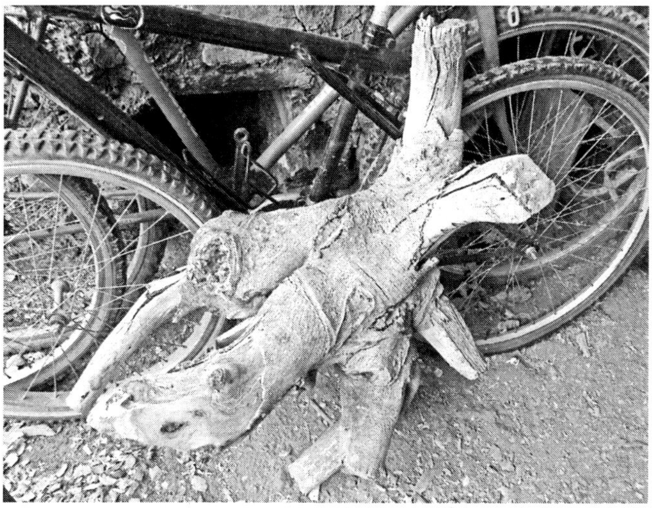

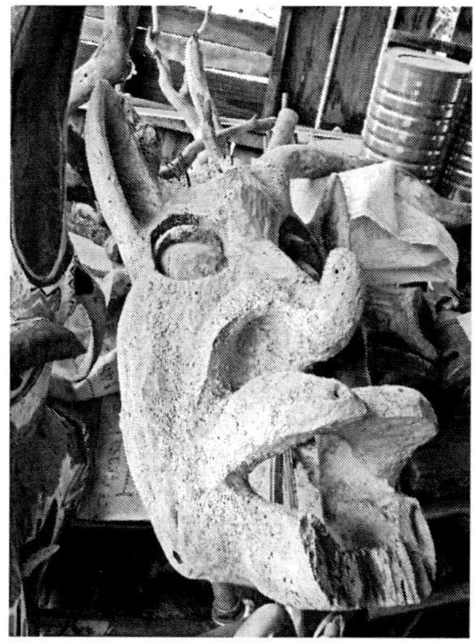

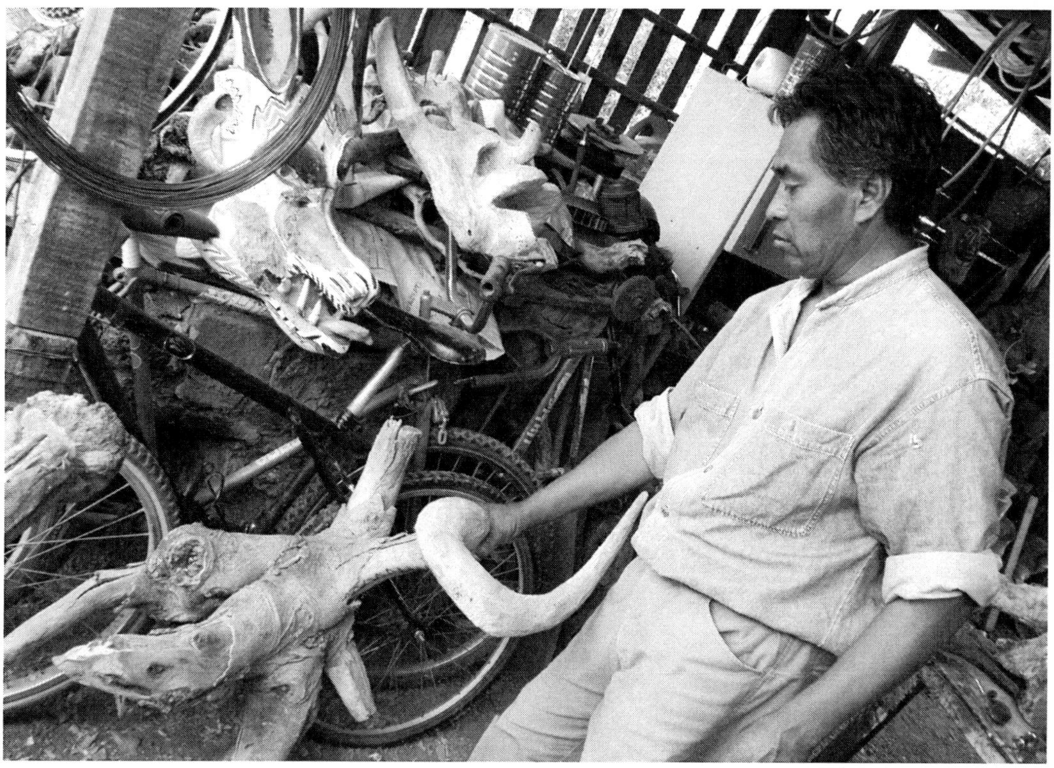

Dalio Angel Perusquia shows how the tree roots can inspire the mask's design at his studio in San Bartolomé de Agua Caliente, Mexico.

a flat, slanted blade), a carving knife having different blade shapes such as curved, flat, or in a V shape called a *gubias* or *gurbias*, and a tool that sands the wood called a *rayador*.[14] Perusquia and Valencia occasionally use electric drills to speed their work, but Delgado and Horta do not. Chavez gets his hand tools from a hardware store in Mexico City, whereas Perusquia and Chavez get their hand tools from iron workers in Pátzcuaro.

Hair for the beards, eyebrows, and moustaches for the old men masks and hermit masks as well as horns for the Pharisee and devil masks are usually acquired from slaughter houses. Chavez mentions a slaughter house that he favors in Cheran.[15] Cow tails and horse hair from tails and manes are preferred, though hair from goats is also used. For extra vitality, the mask makers like to use manufactured glass eyes sold in stores that sell them for dolls and saint sculptures in Mexico City. Delgado prefers to use the whole iris, not just the front half of it, which creates a greater reality.[16] Delgado acknowledges that he wants most of all to achieve correct facial proportions in his masks. He first makes a clay model, carefully studying the expressiveness of the face, to ensure that he achieves his vision. Then he concentrates on making an exact copy as he carves the wood. "If I carve too much on one side, I have to fill in the other side with glue and sawdust, which I avoid using because it weakens the mask." (When asked about the proportion of this glue and sawdust paste, he simply responded that he mixes it until it is thick enough.)

They each had developed processes for painting their masks. Manuel Abeiro Horta uses five layers of sealer (similar to a white paint primer for walls) in order to make the wood very smooth. He then uses two layers of acrylic water-based paint (usually air-brushed) and then a final coat of air-brushed lacquer.[17] Delgado also prefers to use acrylic water-based paints. The first coat is a white layer which he also calls "a sealer," comprised of white powdered pigment and white glue similar to Elmer's glue. He then adds one layer of paint.[18]

Alicia Martínez Álvarez is a mask maker and artistic director for her theatre company in Mexico City, called *Laboratorio de la Máscara* (The Mask Laboratory). She established the company fifteen years ago and it has enjoyed frequent support by FONCA (National Fund for Culture and Arts). She is not a mask carver, though she sculpts clay and uses that technique as the basis for creating masks in resin, leather, and bronze. When necessary, she collaborates with commissioned mask carvers after describing the mask style and characters she needs for a particular production. She acknowledges her propensity to recycle materials and considers recycling to be a basic philosophical component for her theatre company.

Álvarez says that she gets her best ideas while dancing. "My ability to move allows my ideas to flow. I can better organize my thoughts this way. I also need a clean, well-organized studio when working. But ultimately I do not deny the importance of living; I believe in making time to see friends, to read, to travel. In this way I am open to the world around me. The world feeds my soul and I am able to respond as an artist."

Álvarez works with any material that seems most appropriate for the production but prefers to make her masks out of resin. She molds the shape of each mask using Plastilina modeling clay and then makes a negative silicone mold of it. She makes a paste mixture made from fine sawdust and white glue diluted with water she paints onto the inside of the silicone mold. Once that is dried it becomes the positive mold and then paint a resin called "Standar" combined with fiberglass. This resin mixture, once dried, is rather fragile and can break easily if hit, so the supporting layer of the sawdust and glue paste underneath this resin mixture makes the mask quite sturdy. Occasionally if it breaks, she will spackle more of the sawdust paste into the resin's crack. She likes to sand the mask several times and then finally uses a stone agate to polish and refine the final texture. She paints with

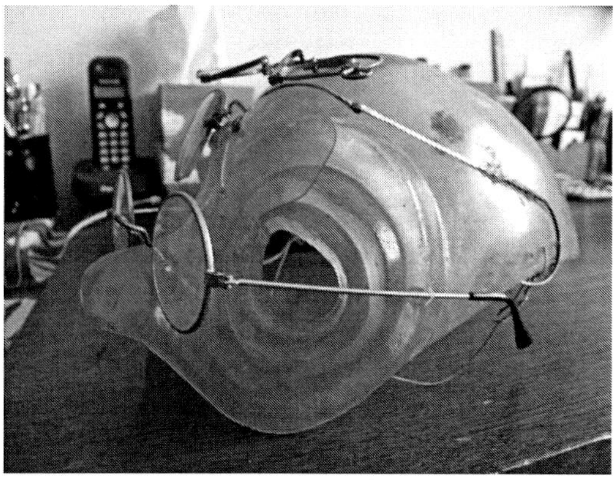

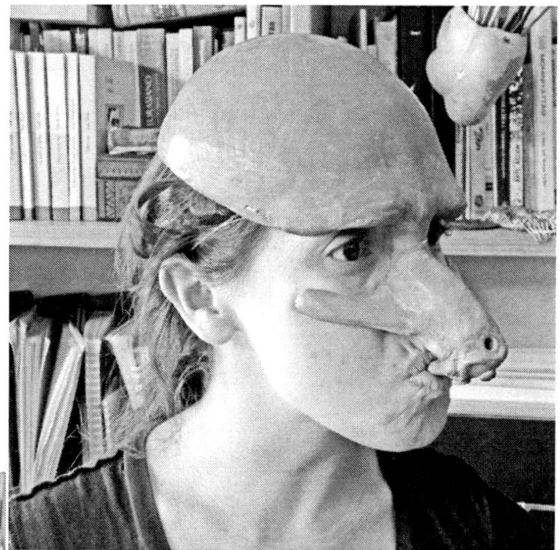

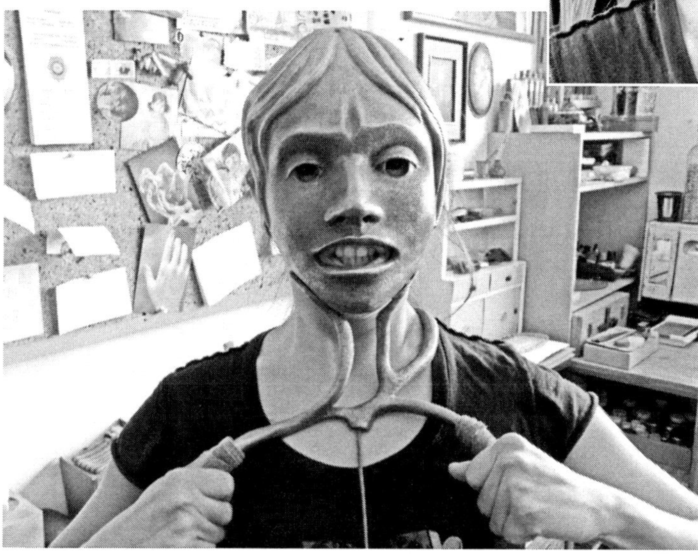

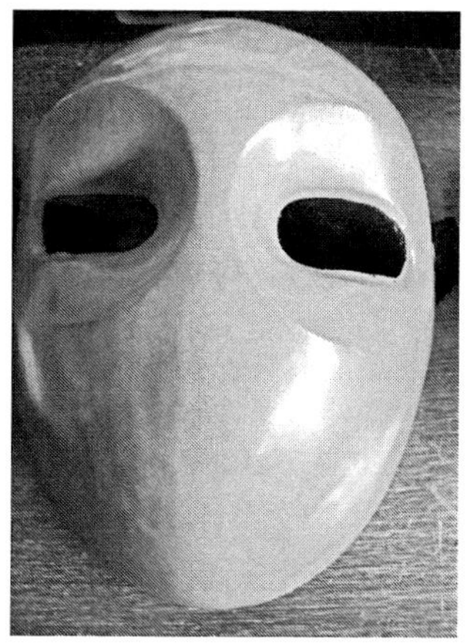

Top left: **Álvarez's resin mask used in *Ubu Roi* (2006), produced by her theatre company in Mexico City, *Laboratorio de la Máscara*. *Right:* Álvarez created the resin whistle mask for *Demonios* (2007), a concert for myths and rites. *Bottom left:* She created the hand-held bronze mask as well for a première play entitled *The Pendulum of the World* (2007) which Álvarez considers a particularly theatrical transformative event. A bare room, two actresses, four masks, a huge lump, a stone, a pot, and wood chips are the elements that give life to Antigone and her emblematic tragic story. The performer, Norma Duarte, can use the bronze mask in multiple positions. *Right:* This leather neutral mask, created by Etienne Champion, is frequently used by Alvarez's company members in preliminary rehearsals at *Laboratorio de la Máscara* in Mexico City.**

pigments diluted with water and glue or sometimes uses an air brush. This process achieves a look of porcelain.

German Mask Maker Michael Meyer's Prosthetic Appliances

At the age of fifteen German expatriate Michael Meyer apprenticed for seven years as a makeup artist or *maskenbilder*, a term that affirms expertise in cosmetology, makeup, wig making, traditional mask making and mask making using foam and latex prosthetic materials. The first three years he concentrated on hairstyling and then he spent two years as a professional hairstylist in France and Germany. His final two years involved learning skills in makeup and mask work. He became interested in the field from having watched his father, who was a props master in the German film industry. "I grew up with the idea of building things and working on small gadgets, repair, and mold work. I visited my first film set when I was ten years old and saw special-effects makeup artists. I knew at that age I wanted to develop my skills and artistry in this field. I loved fantasy films." Meyer says that he was paid by the government-supported Hanover State Theatre throughout his apprenticeship and passed the Union Exam afterwards.[19]

He considers his training excellent, which covered not only practical skills but also courses in literature, history, specialized arts, and color theory. Fluent in English and French as secondary languages at an early age, his apprenticeship allowed him to learn from a group of twenty-five full-time professional makeup artists, collectively holding hundreds of years of experience. "We all learned from each other," he says. "Many projects were one-of-a-kind, requiring innovative approaches and new materials.

"And the atmosphere, while seriously focused on creating spectacular effects, seemed very informal. German audiences traditionally respond enthusiastically but also quite critically to theatre productions. Even the children can be very opinionated. This atmosphere encouraged theatre work with high standards," Meyer recalls. "Even so, backstage there was a certain amount of goofing around that made the work intense but enjoyable. It was a crazy environment and very improvisational in seeking solutions." Having experienced film and stage work in the United States as well as Germany, Meyer thinks that theatre work backstage in the United States seems to approach projects more seriously though perhaps, consequently, a little less creatively. He attributes this situation to his belief that American audiences prefer more traditional versions of theatre and American artists respond accordingly. He also admits that budgets have become increasingly tight (even in Germany), making artists everywhere less inclined to experiment.[20]

Meyer's circuitous route to North Carolina included wig, makeup, mask, and prosthetic work for well over 100 opera productions in Germany at Hanover State Theatre and several dozen operas at San Francisco Opera. He considers his greatest stage triumph to be his Blue Angel transformation for San Francisco Opera's *St. François.* Designer Andrea Schmidt Futterer wanted an androgynous, naked, one-winged blue angel. The performer had to lean out a window at a forty-five degree angle, which required a custom flying harness. The performer had to appear as this Blue Angel so the harness had to be hidden under a custom prosthetic suit created by Meyer to project the androgynous look. Everything had to be lightweight, very streamlined, and custom fit so that the performer was not restricted in her singing capabilities. It took the team from the costume stop and Meyer about six weeks to accomplish this magnificent effect.[21]

"I was not surprised to end up in the United States. I had always dreamed of working in the American film business. I aspired to be another Stan Winston or Rick Baker. I especially loved Baker's work on Eddie Murphy in *Coming to America*; making him like a triple Eddie Murphy into a Caucasian, in the barber shop scene. Wow, it was brilliant!" Meyer exclaims. "I've always loved the artistry of this work. It is such a high. When a character changes appearance within a split second, I think, that is the seduction and challenge of this profession for me. It is truly magical. Immediately the actor adds more vitality to the effect and the result is often something quite different from what I imagined, but it all happens in an instant when the audience sees the final product."[22]

Certainly the medium of film offers the most recent landscape for masks. Positions in the film industry for special effects in makeup perpetuate the mask maker's continued quest for transformation in our era. The artists and artisans in these positions draw attention to the art form in bold new ways and have the potential to reach significantly higher numbers of audience members beyond those who gather to view mask effects in small village performances and intimate stage settings. Additionally film positions in special effects offer financial support rarely received by most local traditional mask makers today.

Since coming to the States, Meyer has worked as a special-effects makeup artist for several films, including *Eyeborgs*. (This 2008 action thriller set in the near future presents robotic eyes that are essentially distinctive masks consisting of one eye that operates like a camera.) "Mask making does not pay a great deal if you work on one mask for weeks and weeks and some of my prosthetic works takes weeks," he admits. "However, if I do it for film, the compensation is quite fair and my teaching career adds a certain level of economic stability."[23]

When asked about his creative process in approaching the challenges of contemporary mask work in film, Meyer acknowledges that he "has to be inspired on cue, on the count of four. But I try to pace myself so that I'm not in a mad dash at the last minute."[24] The "hurry up and wait" mentality required on film sets often demands instant solutions and a wide range of knowledge about the ever evolving materials and chemicals available to the special-effects makeup artist. Production sites invariably have intense deadlines with large sums of money at risk, requiring optimally efficient use of time and effort with careful advanced planning and implementation of correct solutions. Contemplation or quiet meditation on a film set becomes an impractical luxury.

"I have a good data base of materials, but I am always searching for new materials that handle better, last longer, and work easier. And admittedly I don't always feel I achieve the perfect solution during film production. In my world, the end product is rarely perfect. I want to stay true to traditional materials but theatre and film are based on illusions so I will use the best materials for the effect needed, even if it requires synthetic materials and chemicals. Of course I am always striving for perfection, but achieving integrity and honesty and technical skill of a character in film is difficult to achieve under such intense collaborative conditions. Occasionally I will find that I have discovered a better solution, but two years later."[25]

Above all, he acknowledges the importance of collaborating directly with the performer: "I talk quite a bit with the performer. The performer has a lot in conjunction with the director to say to me. I get my concept ideas from the director and designers but finally the actor's ideas are most crucial for deep insights into the character. I can often change my approach while collaborating with the performer. Developing multiple approaches for a character is not unusual for me. While I cannot always achieve perfection in transforming the performer into the character, I feel that my work is most effective when my art and the art of acting are in unison. Then I know I've done my work properly, especially when the actor appreciates my work. If, as an audience member I do not see the art of my masking, then I have done my job. I want the storytelling to dominate."[26]

Meyer emphasizes the importance of maintaining the performer's safety and health. "This consideration is perhaps not so critical for traditional mask makers, but for special-effects makeup artists in the film industry, this factor is paramount. Many materials out there have the potential to be hazardous or even toxic when used incorrectly."

When asked about the extent of his use of mythological and archetypal influences in his designs, Meyer admits that these elements probably indeed surface in his work, especially Wagnerian elements, but in vague, subtle ways.

> I don't want to replicate a specific image that has already been created. And this is the tricky part, with so many fantasy creatures in theatre and film these days, how does one maintain originality? If I need to replicate a cat image, the only ingenuity required is the selection of the appropriate materials to use. I can do such a work on auto-pilot. But a character or force with more spiritual or psychological dimensions will take more effort. For me, a sketch book to visualize ideas or exploration with a lump of clay becomes a meditation in itself. The exploration just starts to develop and a really good mask can come out of a divine state of looking for appropriate clues. My fingers work without thinking too much about it exactly. I let it happen and then see if it "works." The process of this type of exploration can take as little as ten minutes. Then the refining (editing) samples come later, preferably a day or so later with a fresh eye. I need to stay flexible at that point. If the initial idea is not working, I need the courage and discipline to start the process over again.

Meyer mentions an exercise he often requires of his students. He asks them to create a witch, but it can't be green. It can't be a stereotype from *The Wizard of Oz*; no long nose and chin. "I want your witch to be instantly recognizable as a witch," he tells them. "And I want to be truly scared in an unusual yet universally recognizable way." He expresses surprise at the level of consternation this challenge causes for his students. "They can easily take several weeks on their own to develop their ideas, rejecting many preliminary ones before arriving at an appropriate solution. Yet invariably each student's design becomes very different and interesting. It is an exercise in seeing how far one can go with a blank page."[27]

Successful Prosthetic Appliances

Prosthetic appliances are three-dimensional sections of synthetic material used to create facial effects and exaggerations for human and animal characters. They require a positive plaster facial mold (or other body part) and a negative plaster mold for the shape of the appliance desired. These appliances can be made out of latex, foam latex, neoprene (as discussed earlier in the chapter), or a high grade of gelatin. They are then glued on the performer's face and specially treated to take various types of oil-based and alcohol-based makeup. Prosthetic appliances became popular in the late twentieth century for both theatre and film production. They are especially helpful to dramatically age a character, or change a performer's features to look more like his/her character, or to create exaggerated abstract or animal features on the face. Such prosthetic appliances can be created fairly quickly and present a new way of creating masks that are relatively easy to perform in. Michael Meyer has created a wide range of prosthetic appliances for a number of film and theatre productions in Germany and in the United States, where he currently lives. He has taught at University of North Carolina School of the Arts for almost a decade and has offered numerous prosthetic appliance workshops at his campus and at professional organizations abroad. What follows are Meyer's preferences and tips on techniques for creating, applying, and coloring these appliances on the performer. The brief summary that follows (intended as merely an overview) indicates the complexities of this field. A mask maker who uses prosthetic synthetic molds to create a range of realistic and abstract human features must have considerable skill and training. S/he must devote careful attention to ordering appropriate materials and making informed choices about products that rapidly evolve with the demands of the film industry.

Casting Positive Face Molds and Negative Prosthetic Appliance Molds

Face Casts

- Use alginate mix with water. Alginate is a medical material developed for dentists in taking molds of their client's mouths.
- There is no such thing as a perfect recipe. Vendors offer a range of recipes and one needs to experiment with each brand to decide on the best ratio to achieve the best consistency for each specific appliance project.
- Meyer likes his alginate thicker than most recipes and orders frequently from Burman Industries in Los Angeles.
- There are five or six different alginates available, perhaps even more.
- Meyer prefers alginate that takes four or five minutes to set. He takes two minutes for the front of the face and warmer water accelerates setting time.
- Take a cast as fast as possible.
- Never take a face cast in the room by yourself. A cast is generated most efficiently with two or three assistants.
- Have the model sit up, never have them lie down.
- Have noise level at a minimum.
- Remove piercings.
- Shaving is optional. With silicone, however, the model can't use a beard.

Silicone Molds

- For a "body double," smooth on using a big caulking gun. For a face, squeeze on face and avoid getting it into the hair at all times. Use petroleum jelly or another barrier cream on hair and eyebrows.
- Silicone is expensive but you have a durable mold — it can stay thick forever. One $35 cartridge can make one face mold.
- Silicone is a two-part material (base and activator). Use a specially designed caulking gun to mix both elements. Caulking gun costs $75 and using it makes for a nice arm exercise. They have caulking guns that are air-powered.
- European dance companies seem to have a greater propensity for masks and prosthetics. Meyer frequently used silicone in these types of productions and tends to prefer it for projects that require a great deal of action and durability.

Paint Choices for Silicone, Latex, and Foam Molds

- The coloring agent called Pax is a blend of Pros Aide (a prosthetic glue) mixed with acrylic paint to obtain a paint medium that bonds well to latex and related prosthetics. It will flex with the movement of the prosthetic and does not rub off or crack. It is not, however, appropriate to apply over silicone.
- RMG is good for latex products because it is based on castor oil which does not break down latex. Regular makeup can be applied over RMG to give the appliance more color depth if desired. It is also called rubber mask grease and comes in a wide variety of colors.
- Airbrush colors such as Skin Illustrator sometimes appear too smooth to look natural, but all brands are alcohol based. If Skin Illustrator is airbrushed in the traditional way, it can be combined with spatter effects and regular painting techniques for a more natural look.
- KY Jelly works nicely for shine, like for bald heads.

Face Cast

- To protect hair, saran wrap at the hairline around the front of the face. Even better, use an inexpensive non-latex bald cap for the full head.
- Silicone molds require the use of a vinyl bald cap for about $20.
- Sulfur from some foods or outside sources such as an egg salad ingested by the performer immediately before beginning the mold process might contaminate platinum cured silicones (face casting silicones), which can result in the silicone not curing completely. Meyer recommends performing a small cure test on the model's skin before starting the cast.

Ask the Model About Following Considerations

- Is s/he claustrophobic?
- Does s/he have allergies? What type?
- Might the person be intoxicated? Even a glass of wine for lunch or prescription medication can cause negative reactions.
- Develop sign language in advance of procedure.
- Explain process: application and cure takes five to seven minutes; plaster jacket takes about seven minutes; the total procedure should take about fifteen minutes of the model's time. It takes longer to prep the model than to take the cast.

Face Cast

- Place plastic bag over model to protect the model's clothing.
- Place another, overlapping.
- Tape down the plastic with arms outside of it.
- Bobby pin hair back.
- Use Saran Wrap (a long piece tightly around head and ears) and tape it all tightly. Or apply a bald cap.
- Fluff up the powdered alginate from bag or can.
- Start with about a third of a can of alginate for face. Experience will tell you the exact amount necessary.
- Have someone solely responsible for keeping alginate out of nostrils during the entire process. Use wooden sticks or straws.
- Always put alginate into water quickly to dissolve all lumps to a creamy consistency. Use the manufacturer's recommended recipe and adjust from there for a firmer, or more liquid consistency. Generally speaking, use a third more water than alginate.
- Push alginate into eye sockets first, and keep about a half-inch thick.
- Acucast sets in three or four minutes. Meyer orders the twenty-pound bag.
- Use a twelve-roll box plaster for several casts. It usually takes four to six rolls for a face cast.
- Use two layers of plaster bandage at once for finer areas (one strip then double), and four to six layers total. Put a ridge over the nose where most weight of plaster is.
- Take three to four bandages to form a rope around the cast. It won't deform when you take it off. Reinforce across the face.

Full Head Cast

- There are many ways to do a full head cast. Approaches vary with the make-up artist. Try starting at the back then go to the ridge at the ears and around the head. Vaseline the ridge and then start the front of the face.

- Don't use a hair dryer, as it causes a chemical reaction — use no heat, remove, take off Saran Wrap and tape.
- Meyer orders plaster from Atlanta and has it trucked in. He uses Ultracal 30. It sets up in thirty minutes and takes one and a half hours to partially cure, and twenty-four hours to totally cure.
- Meyer orders six to eight bags (in bulk) each time to compensate for shipping costs.
- Plug up nostrils with plaster bandages.
- Roll up the plaster in a ball and cover the nostrils, then flat strip.

Plaster

- Fill the bucket a third full with water.
- Use Ultracal 30. Davens@davensceramiccenter.com sells and delivers it.
- Measurement must be estimated according to when mounds begin forming as initial amounts are poured. Meyer likes to measure the plaster by looks, adding plaster to the water until the water is saturated and a small plaster mountain forms above the waterline. Too high of a plaster-to-water ratio will weaken the mold, but too little plaster will take too long to cure. Once enough plaster is poured, wait and let it set a little to reduce air bubbles. Also avoid them by stirring gently, not aggressively.
- Two ways of filling the mold with the plaster:
    1. A "splash coat" forces the plaster into the fine crevices. Then pour a slow, steady stream of plaster.
    2. For small molds, you can just start filling in.
    3. Blot off the film of water at top of mold with paper towel.
    4. Be careful not to leave bags of plaster outside. Even if sealed, they can go bad due to humidity issues.

Sculpting Tools

- Tools are somewhat important, but you can basically use spoons, hair pins, brushes, etc. Craft stores usually have a standard set available.
- A good prosthetic will feature short and thin edges that will blend perfectly into the surrounding skin; therefore, it is important that you sculpt your edge with the utmost care. Meyer likes to brush that edge with his sculpting tool from the sculpted part toward the plaster positive to assure this thin edge.
- Use a brush to get the petroleum jelly or rubbing alcohol into crevices in order to smooth out the sculpted surface before adding texture.
- If you don't texture, it will be shiny on stage.
- Use organic sponges or texture stamps in combination with other sculpting techniques.
- Heat up the clay with dryer, then don't press as hard.
- Burman Industries sells a good set of sculpting tools. Meyer uses silicone-textured stamps.
- Preserve the edges; don't go further than what is sculpted.
- Create a really sharp edge; the flashing should be a sixteenth to an eighth of an inch away from the nose or whatever part is being sculpted.

Flashing

- Flashing is a process to create a void in the mold to accommodate possible material overflow and a defined edge to your prosthetic.
- Use flashing to create the hollow space that goes up until that edge.

- Flatten clay and cut a strip that has a 45-degree or 30-degree angle, and goes toward the nose (the longer edge is on plaster facing the sculpted mold).
- Stay away from sculpting one-sixteenth to one-eighth of an inch from the clay mold then add more mounds of clay next to the flashing about a third of the way out on face.

Keys

- Add keys to refit the mold. Keys are used so that the two mold parts (positive and negative) will remember their perfect fit.
    1. Triangular keys are used for noses and small pieces.
    2. Keys are drilled into the plaster positive.
- Recut the flashing edge to make certain it stays sharp.
- Use at least three or four symmetrical keys so the mold doesn't wobble. Don't go deeper than the length of the conical part of the drill bit.

Contain the Plaster

- Do a clay wall and vertically surround the part to be cast, including your flashing and your keys. Make the clay at a sharp angle where it meets the plaster.
- Use texture blocks on the clay mold to break up the Vaseline, or try a soft sponge. Don't forget to use Vaseline to release the exposed plaster parts so that the two parts won't stick together. Vaseline is a good choice. Be careful not to apply the Vaseline too thickly and blend it with a texture stamp into the sculpted area.
- Make clay circle keys then drill before the clay wall.
- Make the clay wall no higher than necessary. It becomes more fragile. Start by applying a splash coat of plaster to your sculpture and let set for a bit. Add the thickening plaster mixture to build up the mold to about one and a half inches thick. The thickness will vary based on the size and application of the mold.

Materials

Silicone Appliance Molds

- Use a rubber bowl for a face, and use 400 grams of silicone with 40 grams of catalyst and 28 grams of fast catalyst. Standard mixing ratio is one part catalyst to ten parts base. Meyer recommends referring to the manufacturer's recommendation. Use any pancake makeup powder for easy skin coloration — you can mix multiple colors scraped into the mixture together to control shades.
- Nothing sticks to silicone except silicone itself. Consequently, don't use a glass bowl because glass is a silica product.
- Silicone never breaks down and is very skin-like, yet it is more expensive to use than some of the other prosthetic materials.
- You can use silicone in place of plaster for appliance molds with deep undercuts. Meyer orders it from Silicones Inc.

Urethane Foam Latex Appliance Molds

- Krylon and Burman Industries sell this. It is also known as Cold Foam.
- Foam Urethane is made up of two components: A and B. The ratio for Parts A and B are 65 grams of B to 35 grams of A (look for the manufacturer's specific recommendation.) When mixed, it starts foaming and expands seven to eight times the

liquid volume, so a small nose appliance does not require much. Try a 3.5-gram base, Part B to 1.5 gram Part A which is the activator.

- Always pour Part A into Part B.
- Scalesonline.com sells a Triple Beam Balance (OHAUS #750) which can accurately weigh Parts A and B.
- You can get severe skin reactions from Parts A and B, so always wear gloves.
- Once it cures, it is like car seat upholstery foam but less dense.
- Mix it outside or in a spray booth. Wear personal protective equipment.
- Meyer advises using a respirator with organic cartridges, but a small prosthetic appliance can be done in a classroom environment.
- It works best to drill holes into the positive face cast so that the excess foam can be displaced as it dramatically expands inside the face cast and negative appliance molds once they are strapped tightly together. Drill the hole on the face cast at its deepest point (probably the nose) with a 15/64 bit, starting slowly and going with more force until you get to the bottom. Be certain to use petroleum jelly (or Vaseline, which is less toxic and makes the foam harder) as a release agent inside the hole as well as on the face cast and negative appliance mold. The displaced excess ensures that the prosthetic is sculpted with nice thin edges. It will be more lightweight. Burman Industries sell mold straps, or you might try a heavy duty electrical tape.
- Experiment with twelve-ounce paper cups. Fill the mixture only a third full to allow for expansion. It will cure in about twenty minutes.
- Let it air for a day after it is completed. It can still release some gasses so you want it completely cured before making contact with skin.
- When Parts A and B are combined they normally expand seven or eight times their liquid volume. When combining the chemicals, the room temperature should be 75 to 85° F. A colder room will not let the combined chemicals fully expand and a warmer room will expand it too much. Humidity also encourages expansion and too much humidity will not allow the mixture to cure.
- The activator helps to open the foam pores but too much can make the appliance mold stiffer. Too little can make the foam softer but it will not expand as much.
- The plaster negative mold needs a release agent (which comes with the foam urethane chemicals as a separate order or included in a kit form, depending on the vendor) in order to easily pull the appliance mold from the plaster mold surfaces. This release agent is basically a wax suspended in a solvent. Vaseline works very well since it can potentially make the appliance mold stiffer while curing. Car wax or floor wax can serve well as release agents.
- Powder down the inside and outside layers of the urethane appliance as you pull it out of the negative plaster mold.

Latex

- Meyer prefers latex that is milky white. Ben Nye sells thicker quality latex that is good for build up. Meyer prefers Kryolan latex for very thin fine edges. It dries and will look milky.
- There are potential allergic reactions (due to the protein in it)—a severe reaction can be frightening—so call 911 if the technician or performer can't breathe. One can also be allergic to latex sponges.
- Do a latex test in advance to be safe. Use a Q-tip and place a small spot of latex on

the skin. Meyer prefers to use the inside of the elbow. If itching or redness occurs contact a medical practitioner or in severe cases dial 911.

- Allergies can develop even later in life, so it is wise to be mindful of the potential. (For those who are allergic to latex, Michael Davy Film & T.V. Plastic Products sells a slightly more expensive "latex-like plastic" called Water-Melon. It has several advantages over latex. It can be dissolved with alcohol rather than acetone remember that almost nothing that is skin safe will dissolve latex — and it can be brushed, sponged, slushed, or sprayed. Like latex, it can be tinted using Water-Melon tinting products. It works well to encapsulate gelatin appliances.)
- Ammonia in the latex smells bad but is not toxic in the small amounts found in latex and the ammonia maintains the liquidity of the latex, which is an organic solid from the rubber tree.
- Some makeup books recommend stippling but avoid hairy areas because there is no totally safe solvent for latex. Acetone is known to be a carcinogenic but is okay to use it in small amounts over a short, infrequent period of time. (Some nail polish removers contain acetone.) But don't use any more than you have to. Meyer uses acetone in small amounts to blend the edges of vinyl bald caps.
- Coat the inside of the mold and face cast with a couple of layers of latex and let cure, and then pull this latex out to help remove extra clay particles. Use a Q-tip for small crevices and allow to thoroughly cure. Next, paint or slush eight or ten layers of latex, making sure that each layer dries before the next application. Ten layers can work well and strong enough for smaller appliances. Don't reuse Q-tips after you've used it briefly. The curing latex on the Q-tip will tear other latex when touched. This characteristic most often applies to slush latex molds, used for stage use rather than film.
- Powder down the inside and outside layers of the latex appliance as you pull it out of the negative plaster mold.

Gelatin

- For gelatin, glycerin, Sorbitol, and gelatin powder, it comes as a complete kit or already prepared. Meyer orders it from FX Warehouse.
- This is the safest material for prosthetic appliances. It is even safe to eat. (Unless you are a vegetarian, in which case you don't want to eat it because it is an animal product.)
- However, gelatin can develop mold quickly, so use peppermint oil (found at local pharmacies) to keep it from happening. Do not ingest the gelatin once the peppermint oil is in it. It becomes toxic at that point.
- Have a gelatin that has a Bloom rating of at least 235. This refers to how saturated the gelatin rating is; a higher number indicates better elasticity and stability. Generally you need a 300 rating for at typical cast. (Gelatin from the grocery store has a Knox Bloom rating of 225.) A Knox Bloom rating of 335 is the highest.
- Gelatin must be heated up to get the right consistency, so it is possible to burn yourself. Never let your gelatin boil, the batch is useless after that.
- If the cooled gelatin becomes "gooey," it might not have a mixture that contains enough gelatin.
- Try mixing a batch with the following ratio: 200 gram gelatin, 500 ml glycerin, 500 ml Sorbitol, 120 ml water. (Less water will make the gelatin harder.)

- Use two drops of peppermint oil to act as a preservative.
- Add the water and gelatin together. The mixture will become one big lump that swells. Let it sit for 45 minutes to an hour. Add the other ingredients in a double boiler with high heat to slowly dissolve and blend everything for an hour or so. Do not stir the gelatin too much or it will get too much air in it. A wooden icicle stick works nicely. When the gelatin is ready, it will have a layer of foam on top of it which must be scraped off. That part won't gel well. It will get too hard.
- You can add food coloring or small amounts of scraped colored makeup powder to achieve various skin tones or blood colors. Meyer suggests trying Ben Nye's PC33 Ciné Light Beige but every project requires a range of skin tones. The food coloring in the gelatin tends to stain the skin.
- To get a blood effect with gelatin, use a fourth of a cup red food coloring with just a drop of blue food coloring. When the gelatin cools down it gets stringy — which can enhance certain blood special effects.
- Store the batch easily by pouring it into ice cube trays or baby food jars. These can easily be heated in a microwave to pour into future negative appliance molds. When microwaving gelatin cubes, do it in five intervals, only taking fifteen seconds for each interval to gently heat it. This process takes about three minutes but don't boil the gelatin or it is lost.
- A small appliance such as a nose will take half a cube or as much as a baby food jar can hold.
- Petroleum jelly works well as a release agent.
- You can either pour the warmed, liquid gelatin into molds or Meyer prefers an injection process, though it is a bit more complicated and requires multiple syringes.
- Like the urethane foam latex process, it works best to drill a hole into the positive face cast so that the pressure of the syringes will get the gelatin to escape out of the release holes once the face cast and negative appliance molds are strapped tightly together. Before strapping them together, drill the hole on the face cast at its deepest point (probably the nose) with a $\frac{15}{64}$ bit, starting slowly and going with more force until you get to the bottom. Be certain to use petroleum jelly as a release agent inside the hole as well as on the face cast and negative appliance mold. The displaced excess ensures that the mold is filled completely. Burman Industries sell mold straps, or you might try a heavy duty electrical tape.
- Body heat warms up the gelatin to give even more depth of translucency and an authentic appearance of skin. But if someone is very heat sensitive or sweats a lot, gelatin can't be used very easily. Companies that sell gelatin appliance products have zinc oxide available for ordering to help control body sweat. It is the primary effective ingredient in antiperspirants and sun block lotions.

Bald Caps

- Meyer orders bald head molds from Krylon. There is only one size for bald caps.
- These molds work well with Krylon's GLAZAN liquid "L," which is a chemical product that mimics the characteristics of latex in terms of stretch and durability, but is chemically dissolvable with acetone to blend edges.
- Use a disposable two-inch brush to brush the chemical along the hairline with strokes from hairline toward center of bald cap, covering the entire head in multiple layers. Build up four or five layers and let thoroughly dry in between layers.

Applying Prosthetic Facial Appliances

Helpful Products

- Spirit gum is very harsh and one must use rubbing alcohol for removing it. Meyer prefers to use Telesis 5 from PPI (Premier Product Inc. found at www.ppi.cc). Tellas 5 is a medical adhesive based on silicone and can be used with hairpieces and latex, silicone, gelatin appliances. It holds up well against sweat and comes with an inexpensive remover called Super Solvent.
- Pros Aid or Bond-Off is acrylic glue but it is difficult to remove. Use isopropyl myristate and hot towels. Isopropyl Super Solv (99 percent) from PPI takes it off fairly well.
- When gluing the appliance to the face, tear the latex edge at the flashing, never cut it, so that the outline will blend more easily with the face.
- Glue the body of the appliance to the face first, then take extra care to get the edges securely down by rolling back the edge and applying the glue. Then roll the appliance to the outside edge with the brush handle. If a wrinkle develops, there isn't any recourse.
- Another way to get the edges flat is to use Pros Aid and Cabosil (from Burman Industries). Cabosil is a powder that mixes into a paste that becomes a little thicker than Elmer's glue. Spackle on the edge of the appliance, then stipple lightly to get rid of the edge. Super Solv from PPI can remove it easily.
- If glue gets in the performer's eyes, immediately remove appliance and flush the eye at the nearest eye wash station.

Coloring Prosthetic Appliances

- Latex and foam latex needs rubber mask grease (RMG) makeup with a castor oil base. Other oils can break down the latex. Krylon has a good RMG product.
- Thin down RMG with alcohol before applying it.
- After RMG is applied, use an oil-based makeup rather than a pancake makeup.
- Foam latex can be sealed by (1) stippling latex over it, (2) using DUO (eye lash glue) which is a thin form of latex as a stippling product, or (3) using Pros Aid over it as a coating.
- If foam latex has a layer of latex as a release agent, it doesn't need sealing, and gelatin does not require any sealing
- Prosthetic appliances generally show up lighter under stage lights, so use slightly darker paint or adjust paint as rehearsals progress.
- Meyer starts by painting a layer of red on the prosthetic appliance to simulate the blood flow of the skin. He stipples big freckles of red.
- Most makeup and paints work best by lightly stippling onto the appliance or face. A sea sponge dipped in alcohol can be used to dilute RMG to get more irregularity in the skin tone. Respond in terms of color as needed.
- To add more life to a flatly colored appliance, do a final application of Skin Illustrator Paints (an alcohol-activated makeup), diluted a little with alcohol on the sponge and then stipple lightly into shadows which can give more translucency. There is no need to powder Illustrator Paints.
- Gelatin takes an alcohol-based makeup which is applied in washes of color. Meyer likes to work with Skin Illustrator's flesh-tone line which can be bought at http://graflobian.com or at www.ppi.cc. The solvent is 91 percent alcohol.

- Bald caps should be placed on the plastic head after powdering to keep it from sticking to itself. Use Telesis 5 to glue it. It does not need to get tacky; it dries quickly.
- Cut a dart up to the ear cavity and stretch the latex as you glue and clamp. Use a Q-tip to apply acetone at the edges to dissolve the bald cap material. It is possible to refine the edge with a second round of this process.
- Glue it down around the ear. It comes out of hair with the solvent.
- Store the bald cap in a Ziploc plastic bag with a cotton ball soaked in alcohol.
- Airbrush applications are very trendy because they give a fine translucency to the skin. Airbrushing works especially well in intimate theatre spaces and for film work requiring close-up shots. Airbrushing alcohol-based paint works well on all prosthetic appliances, but take care not to have the paint sprayed in mid-air too close to the performer's nose and eyes. Television performers love to use it but it isn't very healthy to breathe large amounts of it. Also, every flaw in a prosthetic appliance is magnified by the airbrush paint. The paints are very expensive.
- There are many different types of airbrushes on the market. Expect to pay twice as much for the compressor as for the airbrush and you should use an organic filter respirator for big projects to clean out most of the harmful solvents in the airbrush paints. Meyer prefers a brush called IWATA ECLYPSE with double action as a good brush for general use. Graflobian.com carries it.
- Finally, Meyer adds a disclaimer that all recipes and advice are given in good faith and people should experiment at their own risk.[28]

The range of traditional techniques described in this chapter and still practiced by traditional mask makers offers some perspective on the more recent innovative methods developed by mask makers such as Alicia Martínez Álvarez and Michael Meyer, which require more expensive synthetic materials. Bruce Marrs prefers to use neoprene, another relatively recent development in mask technology, even though he is also quite proficient with papier-mâché techniques. In some instances, especially when mass production is required, the synthetic materials and molds offer more efficient ways to create the masks. On the other hand, the traditional wood carving, leather molding, and papier-mâché methods offer unrivaled handcrafted beauty and distinctive characterizations as well as significant comfort for the performer. As Álvarez asserts, each method offers advantages and disadvantages according to the project at hand.

4

Insights of International Mask Makers

Mask Makers as Commercial Artists and Collectors

Frequently traditional mask makers sell copies of their work to tourists to supplement their income. The acquisitive tourist can find masks at markets worldwide. *Koukeri* masks (mummer masks) can be found in Eastern European villages, especially during the mummer celebrations. Day of the Dead Everyman masks in Mexico and parts of California; Korean and Japanese masks at traditional sites of ritual performance; Carnival masks for sale during the boisterous celebrations of New Orleans, Trinidad, Cuba, Brazil, and Venice indicate a thriving trade for the "tourist" mask. These commercial masks usually emphasize the mask maker's imaginative use of artifice rather than defining unique portraits/personalities that can function in a successful performance for a specific situation and performer. Of course, masks for commercial purpose can possess their own integrity, although the quality of craftsmanship and expressiveness usually depends on how much the buyer will pay.

A substantial number of mask makers I interviewed supplement their income considerably by selling replicas or versions of their work to tourists or to universities teaching masked performance techniques. A current list of web sites for these mask makers can be found at the end of this book.

Nigerian mask makers Adeola, Adebisi, and Kasali Ogun all sell tourist masks in addition to their ritual masks. Trinidadian masmen Griffith, Geraldo Vieira and Vieira Jr. typically sell many masks for tourists preparing for Carnival street celebrations.

Other mask makers I interviewed who regularly sell exceptional "tourist/educational" masks on demand include Newman, Canadian Xstine Cook, American Bruce Marrs, Balinese Anom and Dawig, Northwest Canadian-Tsimshian Victor Reece, Japanese Noboru Yoshikawa, Nigerian Kolawale Adeola as well as Mexican mask makers, the late Juan Horta Castillo and his son Manuel, Manuel Valencia Chavez, Dalio Angel Perusquia, and Antonio Cervantes Delgado.

Brief Quotes and Photos from Selected Interviews

These quotes present issues related to the motivations and techniques for mask making, past mentors, methods of collaborating, materials for making masks, archetypal/mythic images, ways of centering/focusing/discerning visual forms, as well as issues of integrity inherent in style and presentation.

Nigeria: Kolawole Adeola

"Early on, I had no job, and poverty encouraged me to seriously train for this profession. But my great-grandfather's masks were beautiful and famous. Often people would ask me to replace them after termites had destroyed them. So I learned at an early age how to appreciate the act of copying fine work to the best of my ability, and this training provided a solid foundation for excellence as I developed my own abilities to create more original work that comes from my heart. Now I rarely work for money. I can afford to work for God because my successful masks create sufficient income to care for my family. But if I need inspiration, I don't go to books or pictures. I have all the inspiration I need when I remember the masks of my father, my grandfather, and great-grandfather. Then I go directly to the wood to be carved, and I see my head [mask] in the bush [forest]."

Kola thinks that he does his best work in the early morning hours. "I need to get up early and drive far away into the bush, away from noisy cars and away from my children demanding biscuits!" he laughs. "For me, 8 to 10 A.M. is the ideal time to carve the head. My brain is cold and fresh and I can fully concentrate. I also prefer to do important finishing work at this time."

The challenges he faces as a mask maker seem daunting. "Too often we are forgotten in the bush. Too often our ancestors are forgotten. There is very little patronage nowadays. I make a decent living but many do not. Nigeria does not generally promote the carver as an artist and is not inclined to promote African heritage to the extent that it needs promoting. Prominent mask makers from the past are in museums, but the world seems to show little interest in the current generation, which seems less likely to stand on accomplishments of our ancestors. Our children don't see the value of carving without proper promotion. Also we mask makers generally lack appropriate documentation. We generally lack good cameras to protect and record what we are doing."

Nigeria: Agbede Adebisi

In accordance with tradition, his *Egungun* mask is reverently stored in the attic of his home or resides in the highest place within the highest room in his home.

"My greatest challenge comes when attempting to acquire appropriate materials. The brass is very expensive and sometimes I must compromise by mixing lead with it. Only the clay from Benin works best to create the molds."

Nigeria: Kasali Akangbe Ogun

"A successful mask must show strength and the elements within and around the mask must tell stories. The work needs integrity combined with beauty suitable for showing its *odu* or ideal spirit. The mask must be frank and yet dynamic. I'm not talking necessarily about scale, but it must have a strong, dynamic face. The carving must be led by Olodumare [God] just as one's life is led by Olodumare." Kasali's artistic son, Adekunle Akangbe Ogun, hopes to continue his father's work.

Northwest Canada, Tsimshian: Victor Reece

"I want others to understand the importance of my grandmother's voice. Keeping her stories alive through the masks I make and perform in is important for my own family, my

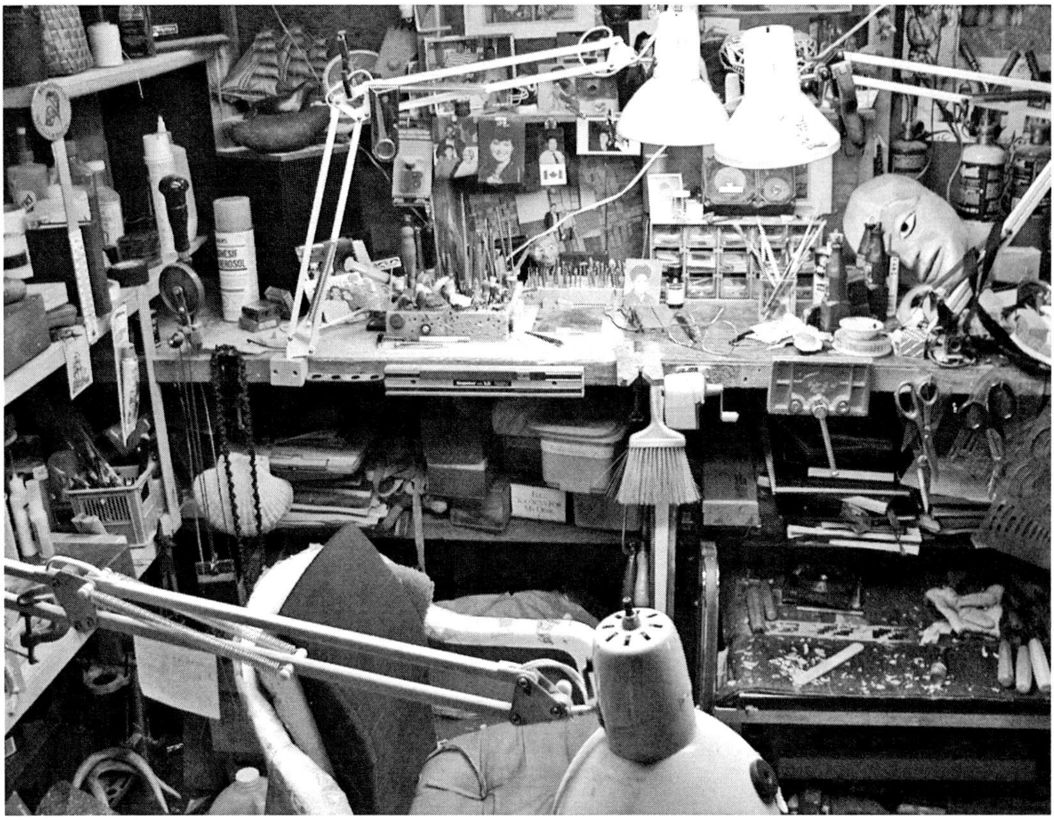

Victor Reece's mask studio on Pender Island, British Columbia, Canada.

own community, and for the global society as well. I express my culture and my grandmother's voice particularly as a carver of masks and as a storyteller. For me, carving and storytelling are very compatible. When I go off to tell stories I don't have to stop carving. I can tell stories even as I carve."

"A Hopi belief states that things change during any conflict arising from the merging of two or more cultures. When things change, the people who rise from the ashes of what is lost are the artists. Today, with so much change, there is room for many artists, particularly mask makers."

Calgary, Canada: Xstine Cook

"I like to tidy up when getting ready to create my masks. I'm not very organized but I like a clean space. I like to clean a space to make a mess. It looks like procrastination but it works for me as a process for preparing my concentration." Xstine, the founder and Artistic Director of Calgary Animated Objects Society, designs costumes, puppets and masks. She frequently directs and makes short puppet films in addition to serving as curator-producer for the International Festival of Animated Objects. She is also a co-founder of Green Fools Theatre, of which she was co-artistic director for thirteen years.

"I work with the intention to honor Aboriginal peoples of North America, to acknowledge the power and teachings in their stories. [Victor Reece served as an important mentor

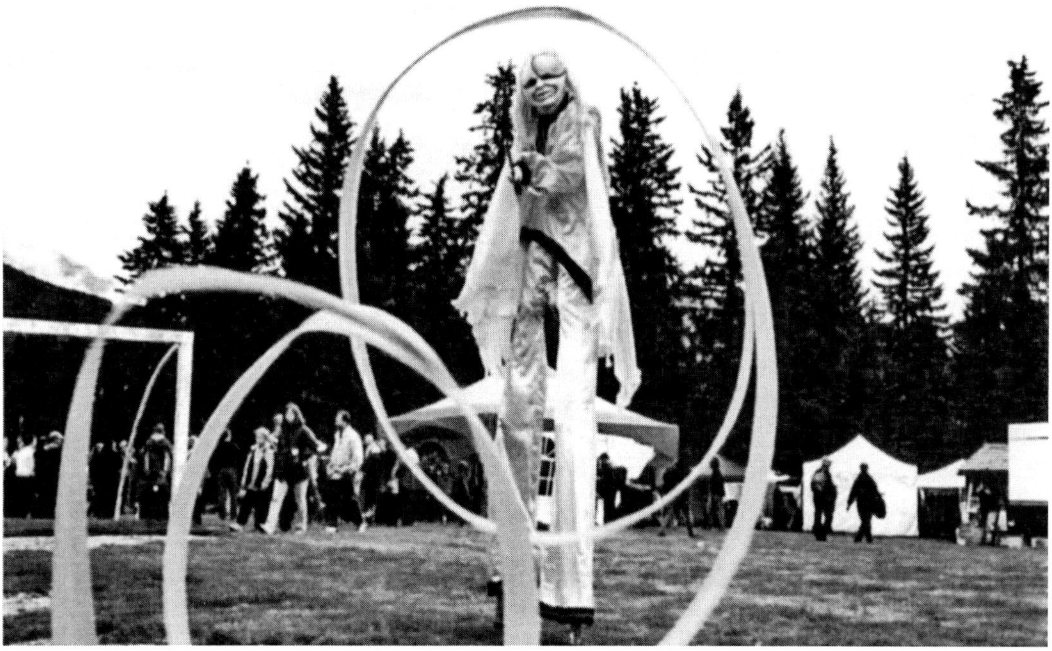

Xstine Cook's "Four Directions" mask was created for a solstice celebration at the Canmore Folk Festival in Alberta, Canada. Performer: Xstine Cook.

for her.] Canada's First Peoples lived in harmony with this land for thousands of years without causing global warming or making anyone go extinct."

"Spirit of White Buffalo (see page 2A) is a 12' tall puppet we built with elders, artists, inmates, youth, bike freaks and engineers. She was created for all people. Her message is a call to live in balance, peace and unity with all nations, the human nations, the animal nations, the plant, fish, tree and insect nations. The Spirit of White Buffalo is about bringing people together in a good way. It was appropriate to take an Aboriginal story like the white buffalo into the jail system because of the disproportionate number of incarcerated Aboriginals. Many of these people have been completely cut off from their culture, their languages, and their families. Residential schools were not something that happened in the distant past. Art has the power to transform and change people's lives and gives them the gift of visualization and the power of intention."

Toronto, Canada: Rob Faust

"There is nothing better than a human face. There you have theatre. You mustn't wear the theatre on your head like a big hat. The theatre is you and I. It doesn't exist without us. It is that simple ... and good theatre requires careful attention to simplicity. What I do is pretty simple but not simplistic. I have no plot or play—I'm just playing. The themes I choose just let me play. I do mask theatre; the masks drive it. I need to get out of the way with the masks. My characters don't change. Their masks are the essence of each character."

"If brevity is the soul of wit then everything is too long these days. Less is more. My masks can't be too fast or too close. My masked performances can't be too long. I know I am most successful when I can incorporate effective editing into my work. Another version of this technique is when you find what you want to say while you are saying it. You start with a sketch or a scribble or a gesture and then perfect it. The resulting artistic effort — when successful — somehow catches our dreams as they free-fall into visibility and takes us to a place where we are all connected. This altered state explains forces within us and is the prime motivation behind mask work. It explains why so many cultures believe mask work, like music, is a universal language."

Bali: I. Made Suryasa

"The mask must not only look good, it must also have the ability to receive and house the spirit. If one is lucky, the mask and performance will have 'taksu.' If the timing is good and the wood is good, I create a beautiful house to invite the spirit of mask into. Then it is automatically powerful. 'Taksu' is similar to 'charisma.' Ron Jenkins [*Subversive Laughter*] has referred to it as 'stage presence' and Joan Schirle [Dell'Arte International performer/teacher] refers to it as 'soul.' My preparation for work as a mask maker or as a masked performer comes when I calm my mind with breathing. My mood doesn't necessarily push me; my breathing encourages proper concentration."

"I like to have several projects going on at once so that if I become frustrated with one, I can leave it to work on something else that keeps my energy engaged. I love performing the Old Man in *Topeng* Dance. My performances are directly connected to the masks I make. I try not to (simply) dance. I try to behave from my inner part to bring out the character — this is beyond technique or culture. My performance becomes Suryasa's Old Man character."

Bali: I. Bodus Anom

"I don't like to work with sketches or photos. In art one must be free. I sketch in my mind and I respond to the wood. The wood speaks to me. I'm never satisfied with my masks. I always want to make something better. Yet I live with a feeling for each mask. My wife sometimes asks why I sell my special masks too low to people unable to appreciate them. I agree with her, and sometimes raise my price to certain people like that. I can never make another mask like the one I already made. Every mask I make is unique."

"Because I am also a dancer, Balinese music and dance are now inside me. It is always with me along with the Balinese stories as I create my masks. I like to chop and carve the wood to the rhythm of Balinese music."

Bali: I. Wayan Dawig

Dawig prays and meditates every morning. His teacher of mask carving was a holy man and Dawig believes in the power of the spirit of the altar (found in most Balinese homes) for his mask making. He is specially known for his sacred *Barong* masks with versions of cat, tiger, or pig influences depending on which region the mask will reside in

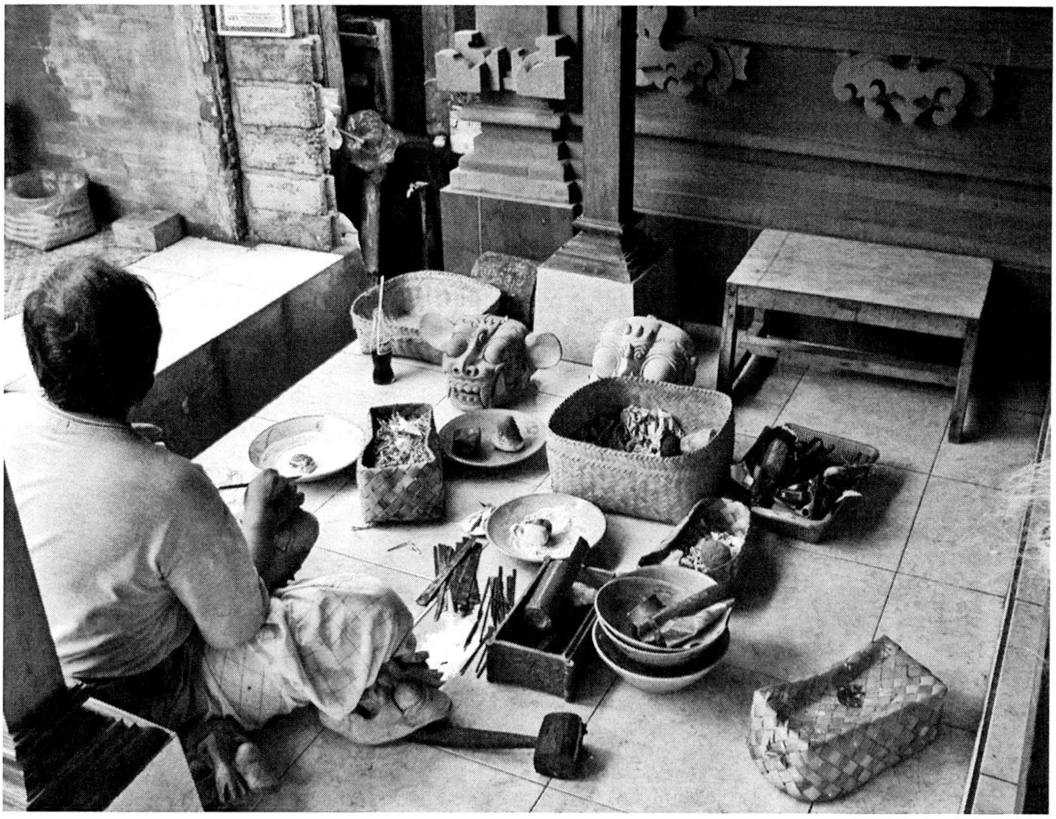

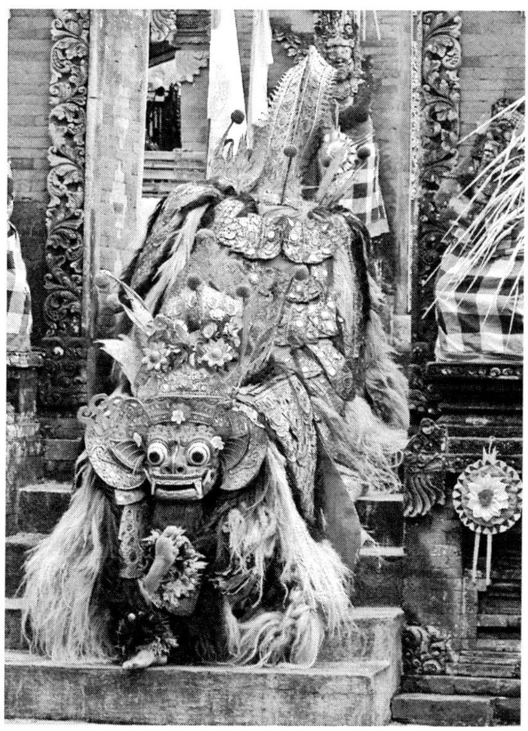

Above: **I. Wayan Dawig's outdoor mask studio at his home in Bali.** ***Left:*** **His elaborate** ***Barong*** **mask, influenced in this case by cat imagery.**

when completed. The *Barong* mask is a good luck/protector mask performed by two people in the Chinese dragon manner. Many other Balinese mask makers like Dawig use a special paint/lacquer made of white crushed pig bone and a glue derived from boiling sharkskin and buffalo hide. He sometimes uses over thirty coats of this special paint in order to get a strong, smooth surface color.

South Korea: Kim Dong-Pyo

Kim, a self-taught mask carver, has become very wealthy over the years, particularly with the factory he established to sell versions of the traditional *commedia dell'arte*-styled *Hahoe* half-masks to tourists in the Andong region. He made so much money that he decided to give the ownership of his factory to the factory's workers. He used his profits to create an important museum of Korean masks. He specializes in performing the female masked characters Pune (the flirtatious widow) and Kaksi (the silent bride) from the *Hahoe* collection, and he performed for Queen Elizabeth in 1999.

"My best time to make masks is between 10 P.M. and 2 A.M. because I can fully concentrate with no interruptions from my museum curatorial activity or family. I like total silence or sometimes low music while carving my masks. I escape into a more harmonious world. Sometimes I feel like a monk with my lifestyle — or perhaps like a vampire! The face and personality of the mask are in the wood and I try to dig out the internal mind of the mask with my carving. Each mask has its own spirit. You have to see the entire moment of the masked performance and the spirit of the mask, or you don't see the mask at all."

East Coast, U.S.A.: Orangeena

Orangeena has been an award-winning professional puppet maker in New York City for twenty years. In her spare time she enjoys performing for New York audiences. Orangeena was recently seen on the cover of *Blade*, a local New York gay publication and in the Style Section of *The New York Times*. Her last performance was entitled *The Passion of Orangeena* (as she was presented in her "fourth trimester of pregnancy"). "Ogee's not been with anyone for way over a year. Bummer, so I don't know exactly how this pregnancy thing happened. And no, I don't think anyone whispered in her ear."

West Coast, U.S.A.: Bruce Marrs

When asked how he initiates preparation or meditates in preparation for making his masks, Marrs responded, "This question reminds me of Krisnamurti's considerations about the notion of meditation —'One meditates, one finishes meditating, and then is not meditating?' I am never not an artist, and the bank is never empty. Well that's probably not true. I'm often stupid and dull. But I think my own interest is almost always at work. When I begin a mask, I know that I have begun already, long ago."

West Coast, U.S.A.: Donvieve

A well-known teacher of mask making in northern California, Donvieve believes that the act of making masks has remarkable potential for healing. "When things don't go well in a conflict, put on your self-portrait mask during the debate and see how much better you see yourself and your own values in third person. Try wearing your mask at home ... at dinner, for example, and see what comes up. My husband and I had such fun with this experience that I created a portrait mask for him as well. We now frequently perform in our 'Flo and Flim' masks for local groups." Donvieve is also a dancer and costume designer for her one-woman (often masked) performances.

West Coast, U.S.A.: Joyce Radtke

Radtke, herself a breast cancer survivor, assists others coping with catastrophic illnesses by using mask making as a process to help them find inner strength.

One of her protégés, Ed Duddleston, has been living with AIDS for fifteen years and found Radtke's mentorship inspiring. "While I worked with the clay, I could harness my own spiritual energies," he says. "I sort of let go and trusted my inner spirit to make my inner guide mask exactly what it needed to be. The process of coping with a life-threatening illness (like the process of making a mask) takes you on a journey. You have to go where the journey takes you. You can't fight it. The journey is exactly what it is supposed to be. If AIDS hadn't come into my life I might still be working fifteen hours a day waiting to retire before identifying my most important life-issues. We rarely get a chance to put 'a face' on our spirituality as I did with Joyce Radtke's guidance. The journey of making a mask is a sacred experience."

Trinidad: Marlon Griffith

"I do not like static costumes. Basically I design by trial and error. I believe the children not only develop a sense of *mas* while participating in these bands, but they also learn about myths, folktales, and even medicinal remedies for herbs. *Mas* has become so commercialized that you rarely see the sort of spontaneity that used to be its primary characteristic. Only with children's *mas* do we truly carry on our Carnival traditions while also allowing the stories to evolve with the new perspectives of child-like wonder."

Trinidad: Geraldo Vieira

The son of Portuguese immigrants to Trinidad, Geraldo Vieira's gigantic mask designs have won in the King of Carnival category at least seven times since 1971, and he frequently wins other competition categories as well. Geraldo Vieira smiles as he fondly quotes his late wife: "Geraldo, we could have purchased a fine house with all the money you've spent on your Carnival creations!" But he feels that he has maintained his autonomy and full creative range by not accepting backing from a demanding patron in the typical manner of Carnival financing.

He oddly insists, however, that he is no artist: "I'm not moody or temperamental enough to be an artist — I am an engineer, an artisan. I want to see my creations come alive. I start with a small idea and then I think of the geometrics and the logistics of the idea. Hardly anyone can beat me in structure. I often use pneumatics and even radio waves and robotics for remote controlling the movement of my characters. I am a pattern maker by trade, and I can produce the machine that makes the molds. Technology is the greatest thing in the world. I can design, construct, decorate, sculpt, mold, paint it — and sometimes I even masquerade it. Next year I will be the oldest masquerader in the history of Carnival to win the King Costume. I'm sure of this!" In 2006, he proceeded to accomplish this feat.

Trinidad: Geraldo Vieira, Jr.

Two of Vieira's recent mobile spectacles, *Aladdin's Last Ride* (2004) and *Trouble in de Bamboo* (2003), both designed by his son, Geraldo Vieira, Jr. (who won the Carnival King title in 1996 performing in the *Rainfest* mobile), possess humor and pathos. Aladdin, a figure of death, rides into hell as a king on a huge griffin controlled by robotics. Aladdin (performed by Vieira Jr.) seems to be having a grand time. A closer look at the blue devil in *de bamboo patch* reveals that he is eternally pestered by ants that are the real devils. The ants move seemingly at will, controlled by "radio waves." Both moving mobiles have several "masks" that interact with one another. Earlier versions of spectacle produced in the mid-nineties, *Splendoria* (homage to the dawn and sunset) and *Rainfest* (homage to the rain), easily compete visually with the environmental themes found in Peter Minshall's characters in *River* and *Song of the Earth*. For over seven years, the junior Vieira has designed or crafted work for Trini-Revellers, a major *mas* camp, and also for Carnival events in Barbados.

Trinidad: Sheldon Clemdore

Sheldon Clemdore credits Geraldo Vieira with mentoring him as he developed into a first-rate masman. Clemdore started making costumes and masks at age eleven and describes himself as "a total *mas* camp (mask factory or studio) because I'm so multi-task-oriented." He has a wide range of skills such as fabric painting, wire-bending, and sculpting (for which he has a particular talent). Vieira taught him how to make molds for plastic and foam products. Now he makes molds for commercial uses such as lamps, furniture, and three-dimensional sculptures for storefronts, movie houses, and the island's international airport.

He believes the mask traditionally inspires the dance. "I see the whole costume and mask and then I begin to feel the personality or spirit of them. My performance and mold mask-making work is very intuitive. I edit ideas quickly and evolve the character's essence to the point where it can live through me." He assisted Vieira Jr. and Vieira with the mask molds for their 2004 *Aladdin's Last Ride* and their 2003 *Trouble in de Bamboo* (both won in several competition categories). His mask for *Trouble in de Bamboo* required twenty-seven molds for the eyes, teeth, jowls, and ears. Several parts of both Carnival masked mobiles moved with hydraulics, presenting Clemdore with a more complex challenge.

Clemdore talks about the need for more community awareness in his country. He wants to establish a community center where he can inspire underprivileged children and uphold and continue the best aspects of *mas* tradition for them the way Vieira has done for him.

Italy: Donato Sartori

"I like to cook! Before I start my ideas for a project, I need a period of investigation to take a look at the script, rehearsals, research — to try to get the 'smell' of the project. At one point I know when it comes — I start cleaning or I cook for twenty people. When that moment comes, I know the next day I can begin work in my studio for as long as the project requires. It is difficult to describe but I have to reach that 'zero point' and then I go in one certain direction with my exploration. I leave the organization of my business side. I work in another way with no planned schedule."

Brazil: Venicio Fonseca

"I had a gut feeling but no technical experience. Some years later, I encountered Donato Sartori who understood the language of the theatre mask — the language of dramatic expression of the mask. I still remember Donato Sartori's comment about one of my early masks. He pronounced it 'beautiful but rigid.' After my encounter with Sartori, I realized that art doesn't come just from talent and intuition — talent fades and you need technique. The technique is the base that allows the talent to walk — explore. Technique is important but then also one must be able to forget it and have courage in developing new technical experimentation."

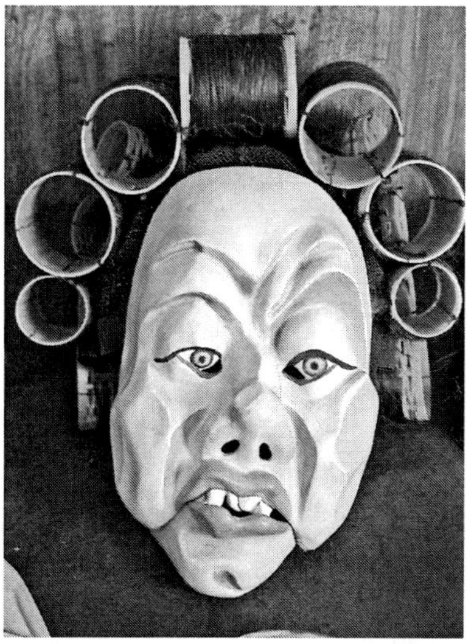

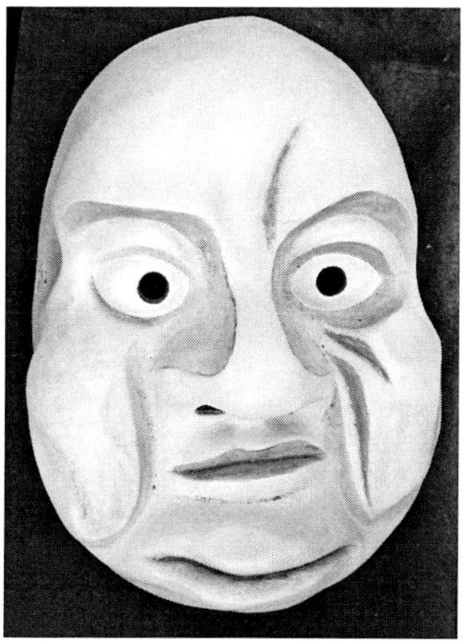

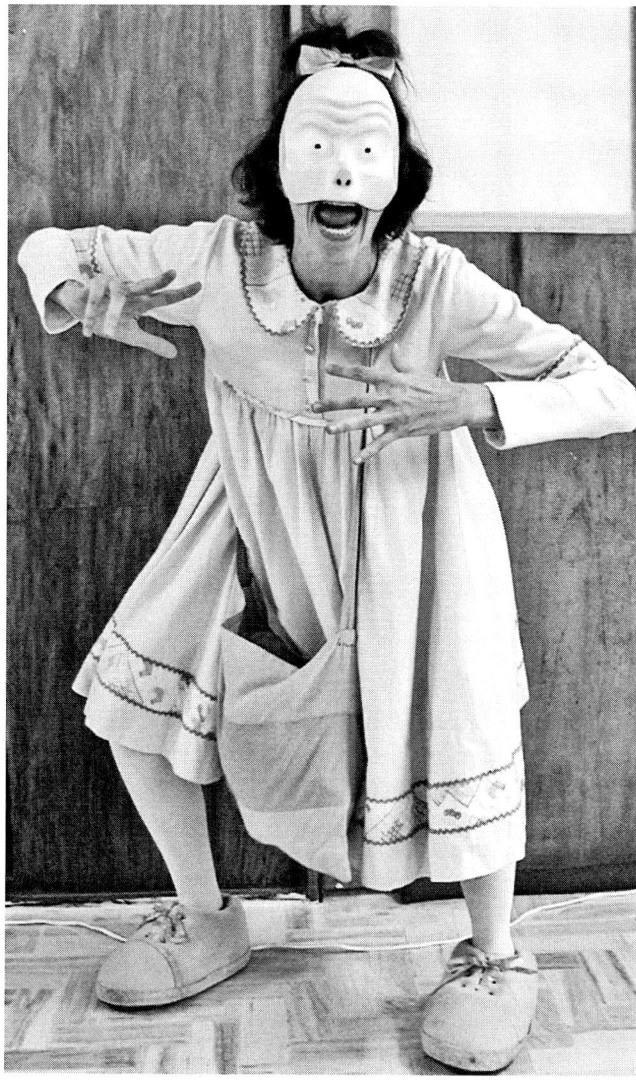

Top left: **Expressive mask made of paper and *tela* (Portuguese word for a large webbed cotton gauze). The character is "Maria dos Bobes" of the production *Lecture-Spectacle: The Mask in the Energy of the Actor* by the *Grupo Moitará* in Rio de Janeiro. *Bottom left:* Expressive mask made of paper and *tela*, used for training at *Grupo Moitará* in Rio de Janeiro. *Right:* Half mask made of paper and *tela*, character "Pipi" of the production *Rinfinfin no Medelin* by the *Grupo Moitará*, Brazil. Performer: Erika Rettl.**

Venicio Fonseca believes that the mask must not be too caricatured. "If it is smiling all the time, it is funny but after two minutes, the situation is different. The mask is an apparition—it has only one emotion. You need to counter the mask. The pigeon flies because it has opposition in the air. In all of life there is an opposition. The mask must have a dialectic quality."

Fonseca works very closely with his partner, performer Erika Rettl, in creating masks for original masked performances for their theatre company *Grupo Moitará* based in Rio de Janeiro. He believes that masks [three-dimensional masks worn on the face] are rarely worn at Carnival except on a stick because "people are too vain — they want to show off the glamour of the costume and claim it for themselves — rather than hide behind a mask."

Mexico: Juan Horta Castillo

"The wood speaks to me and I start. First I watch the wood, consider various types of personality and the block of wood gives me an idea — though it is up to me to sell the idea with the creation of the image. Sometimes I have a dream and I get up to work and that mask has to be finished with the idea from that dream." Castillo has especially enjoyed performing in devil masks, admitting that he relates more easily to the devil than to the saints.

His masks were selected by *Ballet Folklorico de Mexico* and featured in their worldwide performances. His work is a part of the permanent collection at the Mask Museum in San Luis Potosi, Mexico, and has been featured at Anaheim Museum, the Art Institute of Chicago, and Brown University, among others.

Mexico: Manuel Abeiro Horta

"It is natural instinct for each new generation to change but tradition is so strong here that I hope to maintain the traditional integrity of my masks. If someone asks me to create an unusual mask, I will try to include aspects of tradition in it. My father used to get angry when other mask makers in Tocuaro would copy his masks. So he would tell them to look at his devil masks and then 'go to bed and dream your own dreams.' My father was orphaned when he was ten and started making masks when he was twelve. This was the same age that I started carving masks. When my father started making masks fifty years ago, he used ash from the fireplace for painting his masks. By the '60s he used paints from the store. Today, I use five layers of sealer (white paint used to prime walls) which goes into the pores of the wood for a super smooth look. Next, I use an airbrush to paint two coatings of color. I then spray a lacquer finish."

"Snakes are good luck when they appear in dreams. To dream about snakes is to dream about money. Though I'm nervous about snakes in real life, I like to incorporate snakes in my masks."

Manuel presents mask making workshops annually in Chicago and Boston.

Mexico: Dalio Angel Perusquia

"Mask making is a very personal act for me. My masks come from within. I'm very aware of my ancestry. I usually take a long walk up the nearby hill before beginning my masks. There is a place where I can clear my mind. Before I did that, I found it very difficult to concentrate. I require total silence while carving. I think about what the colors of the mask will be and what the costume will look like as I carve. I especially love to dance in my masks but even when I make them for others, they reflect my own moods. My wife's great-grandmother encouraged me. Also I hung out with other dancers and was honored to be the youngest dancer at age twelve. I didn't copy anyone and borrowed tools from other mask makers to teach myself how to carve."

"I remember using old leather shoe tongues for my devil tongues. I only cut a tree for my masks at the full moon because afterwards termites cannot penetrate and eat the wood.

But nowadays I try to avoid cutting trees altogether to respect the environment. I try to use fallen trees; many of them come from electrical power companies that cut them to make way for telephone lines. I get horns from slaughter houses. Initially I used different minerals from various types of soil in the mountains mixed with water to get different shades of color. The colors were softer than those coming from paints that I now buy in local stores." Dalio's son Fabian is also an exceptionally skilled mask maker.

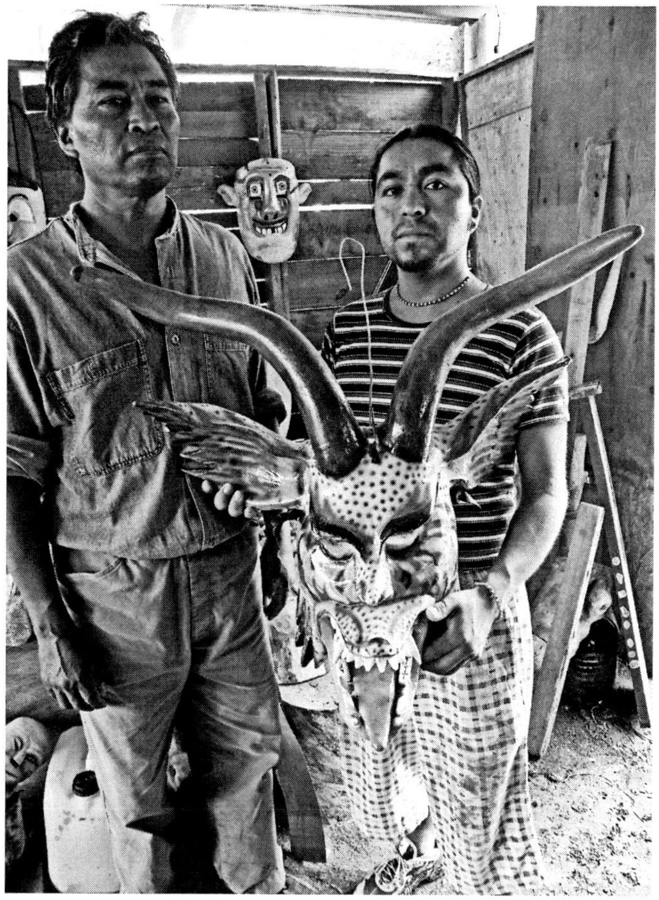

Dalio Angel Perusquia and his son Fabian show one of their intricately carved and painted contemporary Mexican Pharisee masks. The Perusquias specialize in these Pharisee masks. Their town, San Bartolomé de Agua Caliente in Guanajuato (and other towns as well), reenact the Passion of Christ during Easter Holy Week, including the *Pelea de Los Cuernudos* (the fight of the horned ones) in which masked Pharisees (Jews) fight unmasked characters known as *Barrabases* (Barrabas). The unmasked Barrabas characters always usurp the masked horned Pharisee characters.

Mexico: Alicia Martínez Álvarez

"Early on I studied visual plastic arts, painting, sculpture, print making. I saw a production of *Midsummer Night's Dream* that incorporated masks and dance and it deeply affected me. I've always loved dance and realized that my work in visual arts was not enough. I could explore all the areas of art that I loved by doing theatre with masks. In that way I could bridge my passions for art, dance, music, and theatre. But even if a dancer is not wearing a mask, the dancer has the spirit of the mask in the performance when using especially exaggerated gestures."

Álvarez performed at Dell'Arte International School of Physical Theatre in 2005. The students who worked with her collectively explored the traditional pre–Hispanic and post–Hispanic Mexican masks: Bartolo, the Old Man, the Devil, and Death and their potential interactions with "a woman." Entitled *To Die of Love,* the production effectively used a theatre setting rather than the typical village festival setting where these folkloric and mythic masks originated, much to the delight of northern California audiences.

"The mask inspires everything else, the costumes, the scenery, the dance, the text, and the music. It initiates the primary dialogue between the actors. The mask appears and then defines the direction. Thanks to this dialogue, I have few failures with my performances.

Experimentation with potentially appropriate materials for the mask may not work, but the idea of the mask invariably works. The mask succeeds if it has vitality, if it has a synthesis of its essence with that of the performer, and if it says what it needs to say."

Mexico: Manuel Valencia Chavez

"I've been making masks for over forty years. My father and grandfather made masks. When I was twelve, after coming home from school, my father would send me off to cut wood or to hollow out his masks. I did the grunt work. Then a couple of years later, he handed me a block of wood and said to make my own mask. It was a little deer. I enjoy listening to music while I work."

"I think that my performance and dance skills help me to make masks of high quality, not just my carving skills. I never do 'quick and roughs.' I have a special prayer every day before starting. I ask God to protect me from failing, to assist me in making a beautiful mask, and that the mask benefit my family. For me, a successful mask is one that has vitality and stands out on a wall or in a crowd. It should feel comfortable for the person wearing it. I try to please my customers but above all, I like to perform in my own masks. I often make my own costume."

Manuel Valencia is highly respected and well-known for his masks in his village, known as Sevina. He organizes the annual festival to celebrate the *Purepecha* Race, which takes place in mid–October.

Mexico: Antonio Cervantes Delgado

"I was too poor to have toys. My poverty inspired me to make my own when I was nine years old. I had only an elementary school education but loved carving so I audited evening classes in clay modeling, sculpting, anatomy, shadow, light, and volume after working days in a glue factory. My teacher was Tomas Chavez, the brother of the famed Mexican artist Jose Chavez Morado. He accepted me immediately at the school when I showed him some of my carvings, even though I didn't technically qualify to attend. But I felt good at the school because I had the talent and the capacity to learn. Tomas taught me a great deal about anatomy and also about patience. I make small holes in my masks, add glue, and insert hair strands with a nail into each hole. I get the hair from horse tails at the slaughter house. I get my glass eyes from a doll-making store and tools and water-base paint from a hardware store. I apply one layer of sealer which is a white powder paint and white glue, and then I color with latex water-based paint. Finally I spray a lacquer finish. A simple mask takes two days while a complicated one can take four or more days. Correct proportions of the facial features are very important to me but I only use photographs to inspire me, not to copy. All my life, I have only wanted to make masks."

In 1982, Antonio Delgado won first prize in Michoacán for his black devil mask and won a national FONART prize in 1990. At eighty-four years of age he still makes masks.

Japan: Noboru (Touryu) Yoshikawa

"I usually begin to focus on creating my mask by listening to public radio or sometimes karaoke music. I don't rest or wait for inspiration. If I have an order I work it out right away. The finish of the mask has to be especially well-timed. I prefer the traditional use of natural fibers and layers. Sometimes I work in the middle of the night if the proper finish requires it."

Yoshikawa often makes traditional versions of *Noh* masks but he specializes in his own design of a mask that represents his region's dragon spirit. Local masked dancers mimic the dragon with undulating movements and gestures, simulating the rolling mountainous terrain. The dragon spirit serves the god of the mountain as a protector of all the inhabitants surrounding the mountain. The dragon mask often has horns to create more ferocity in addition to movable lively eyebrows and mouth as well as popping eyes.

Japan: Iwasaki Kyoun

I interviewed Iwasaki Kyoun when he was eighty years old and a couple of years later he died in 2006. He did not start making masks until he reached his forties. His earlier years were fraught with the tensions and poverty of Japan in the aftermath of World War II, near Hiroshima. "What has always inspired me to make another mask is the happiness I feel when one is completed. Each mask I make, even if it is a mask in the traditional *Noh* style, becomes unique with my hands and heart. I especially enjoy the carving, the painting, and the final finishing touches. I love to perform in my masks and work regularly."

Sweden: Torbjörn Alström

"I suppose I wanna be God. I want to make what he made even better or, in agony, destroy what he made—well, honestly, this is true. Just understanding that leather could be used for such a sculpted object, I was thrilled. I just had to learn how to do that. The leather, the material itself carries so much within itself—of life and sensuality, but also more frightening things like power and violence." When asked how he manages to sleep after one of his horrific performances with his "Everyman Grotesque Mask," he responded, "I sleep very well. I get all that shit out on stage and feel like an athlete feels good after a good workout."

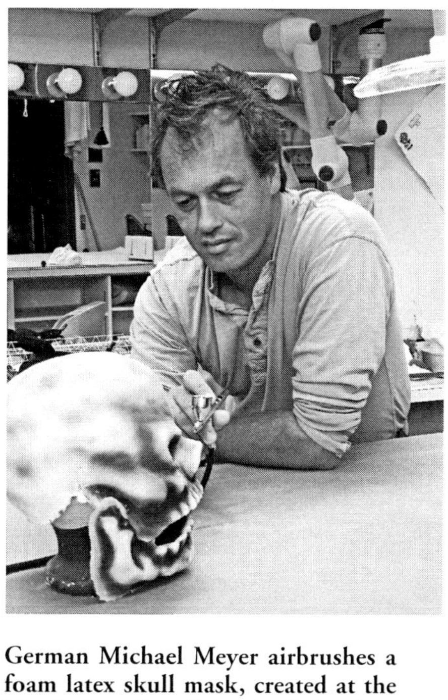

German Michael Meyer airbrushes a foam latex skull mask, created at the North Carolina School of the Arts mask studio in Winston-Salem, North Carolina, U.S.A.

Germany: Michael Meyer

When asked about his creative process in approaching the challenges of contemporary mask work in film, German expatriate Michael Meyer acknowledges that he "has to be inspired on cue, on the count of four. I try to pace myself so that I'm not in a mad dash at the last minute." The "hurry up and wait" mentality required on film sets often demands instant solutions and a wide range of knowledge about the ever evolving materials and chemicals available to the special-effects makeup artist. Production sites invariably have intense deadlines with large sums of money at risk, requiring optimally efficient use of time and effort with careful advanced planning and implementation of correct solutions.

"I have a good database of materials, but I am always searching for new materials that handle better, last longer, and work easier. And admittedly I don't always feel I achieve the perfect solution during film production. In my world, the end product is rarely perfect. I want to stay true to traditional materials, but theatre (and film) is an illusion so I will use the best materials for the effect needed, even if it requires synthetic materials and chemicals. Of course I am always striving for perfection, but achieving integrity and honesty and technical skill of a character in film is difficult to achieve under such intense collaborative conditions. Occasionally I will find that I have discovered a better solution, but two years later."

"While I cannot always achieve perfection in transforming the performer into the character, I feel that my work is most effective when my art and the art of acting are in unison. Then I know I've done my work properly, especially when the actor appreciates my work. If, as an audience member I do not see the art of my masking, then I have done my job. I want the storytelling to dominate."

Meyer emphasizes the importance of maintaining the performer's safety and health. "This consideration is perhaps not so critical for traditional mask makers, but for special effects makeup artists in the film industry, this factor is paramount. Many materials out there have the potential to be hazardous or even toxic when used incorrectly."

5

Influences on Mask Making for Contemporary Masked Performances

The Legacies of Amleto and Donato Sartori

Work in Response to Europe's Renewed Interest in Commedia Dell'arte

It is necessary to recall the range of French mime Jacques Lecoq's contributions to physical theatre to gain a better sense of mask maker Amleto Sartori's mid-twentieth-century impact upon the renewed interest in the Italian masked performance style of *commedia dell'arte.*

After having spent two years in Grenoble as an actor with the company *Les Comédiens de Grenoble*, Jacques Lecoq returned to Paris, where he taught at the *Education Par le Jeu Dramatique* School, founded by the great actor Jean-Louis Barrault. There he met Gianfranco De Bosio, director of the Theatre of the University of Pardua, who invited him to Italy to teach theatrical movement.[1]

In 1945 Lecoq founded a theatre company in Paris that emphasized physical training and gesture, but by 1948 he moved on to Padua where he stayed for eight years. Here he was invited to teach movement, and he continued to stage mime and physical theatre performances. By this point he had established a reputation of systematically analyzing physical theatre, in part by using various types of masks to aid in revealing body and gesture potential. He identified motivations for movement as the basic source of dramatic tension. He is perhaps best known for the adage, "Everything moves." Yarrow and Chamberlain write that, according to Lecoq, "Shapes can inspire movement. External qualities can inspire somatic impulses in precisely the same way as a mask."[2]

Lecoq met Amleto Sartori in Padua, and from that meeting sprang a long collaboration and friendship that ended only with Amleto's death in 1962. Having worked in France following the methods of Jacques Copeau, Lecoq had learned the use of the mask *du calme*; this was actually a mask copied from the Japanese female mask, the Ko-o-mote, of the *Noh* theatre. The actors made these masks themselves in a fairly primitive fashion. When Lecoq told Amleto about these masks, the sculptor created the extraordinary neutral mask that today is used in important theater schools. In Padua, a town with one of the oldest universities in Europe, Lecoq encountered and learned about the *commedia dell'arte* and discovered the theater of Angelo Beolco ("Ruzante"), also born in Padua, a key figure in the development of *commedia.* Lecoq and Sartori collaborated for many years with Giorgio Strehler, director and founder of the *Piccolo Teatro* in Milan, which still today, sixty years after it was founded, tours with the *commedia dell'arte* and its masks in prestigious theaters worldwide.[3]

By 1956 Lecoq had returned to Paris where he set up his renowned *L'École Internationale de Théâtre Jacques Lecoq* which still continues and boasts of having such famous alumni such as Ronlin Foreman, Steven Berkoff, and Julie Taymor.

Carlo Mazzone-Clementi was a childhood friend of Amleto Sartori in Padua and had served as Lecoq's assistant during Lecoq's eight years in Italy. Mazzone-Clementi became a key player in the transference of interest in *commedia* from its roots in Padua on to what became Dell'Arte International School of Physical Theatre in Blue Lake, California.

Arne Zaslove, Lecoq's first American student in Paris and supported by a Fulbright, eventually taught at the University of Washington and served for several years as artistic director at Bathhouse Theatre in Seattle. He describes himself as Carlo Mazzone-Clementi's first disciple just as Mazzone-Clementi considered Lecoq his greatest teacher.

Zaslove remembers that "Lecoq would always say that Carlo WAS *commedia*!" He points out Mazzone-Clementi's complicated relationship with his father, a "strict military man and fencing coach who drilled Carlo" when he was just a boy.[4] (Carlo was an accomplished fencer, according to Dell'Arte's Joan Schirle, who knew and worked with Carlo after his arrival in the United States.) One can easily imagine the ensuing tensions between two such contrasting son/father personalities, one possessing the spirit of a clown and the other possessing the spirit of a disciplined soldier (ironically the sort of disciplined spirit that *commedia* requires of the artist to balance with spontaneity).

Joan Schirle, Founding Artistic Director of Dell'Arte Company and School Director has performed and taught at the Company/School since 1975. She describes Mazzone-Clementi as part of the mid-twentieth-century nucleus of artists (along with such theatre directors, playwrights, and performers as Strehler, Lecoq, Fo, and Marcello Moretti) who reinvented *commedia dell'arte* and mask work after World War II in Italy. "Carlo taught us to look back on the roots of theatre, always in an historic context," Zaslove recalls. "Carlo emphasized how the great clowns, the Marx Brothers, Keaton, and Laurel and Hardy, whom we took for granted, were direct descendants of *commedia.* Those of us who did the classics were able to revitalize them for contemporary actors and audiences by using the spirit. Nothing is really new!"[5]

Zaslove remembers that in 1962 Mazzone-Clementi was the movement coach for Giovanni Poli, who was more of an academic-style director from an Italian university. Mazzone-Clementi and Poli clashed in their approach to *commedia.* Zaslove was in the cast and it was his debut in New York after his studies with Mazzoni-Clementi at Carnegie Mellon University (which at that time was called Carnegie Institute of Technology). "We used Amleto's masks. I vividly recall the Sartori masks which Amleto had lent to the Italian Cultural Institute in New York for a traveling mask exhibition. The catalogue for this mask exhibit lists eighty masks by Amleto and seven by Donato. They were made out of wood, silver papier-mâché, glazed ceramics, bronze, and leather. Carlo and I laid them out on the beautiful floor in a large ballroom type of space and catalogued them. I still have the catalogue in my collection that Carlo's first wife, Vivian Leone, put on paper. She was a writer and a great help to him. In this catalogue Carlo mentions that the masks were exhibited in the lobby of the Odeon Theatre (Barrault's theatre) in February of 1962. The exhibit at the Italian Cultural Institute in New York could have been sometime between 1962 and 1964. Carlo describes Amleto "fitting by hand the wet leather skin onto his sculptured wooden creation. He would actually carry on a conversation in pure sixteenth-century Paduan vernacular.... 'For you see ... I have a fire and a bubbling up inside me like that of a vat of new wine...,' he [Amleto] would say with words and accents from his beloved Ruzante, whose works he knew by heart. Carlo also pays homage to Donato for carrying on the fine mask traditions of his father."[6]

Zaslove goes on to describe the sun streaming in from the large floor-to-ceiling windows as the masks were laid out. "I had an 8mm camera with me," he said. "I'm going to find that film soon and have it transferred to a disc. I'm not sure now if the masks actually toured, or were on display only. Donato had packed them and sent them and was the connection to the Embassy, so he might know how they were used at that time, or how they were intended to be used."[7]

A more detailed look at the lives and work of Amleto and Donato Sartori can be found in chapter 2 but note that Donato's father died very young, at age forty-six, in 1962 when Donato was only twenty years old. Even as a teenager, Donato had learned sculpture techniques in his father's workshop while continuing his own studies in art. For this reason he was able to continue Amleto's work both as a sculptor and in the theater, collaborating with such renowned artists as Lecoq, Barrault, Peter Oskarson, and Peter Brook. He became a close friend and collaborator with Dario Fo, a relationship that continues today. He has focused particularly on experimentation involving new types of masks that combine the disciplines of visual art with theatre and gesture. In addition to his professional work described earlier, he has been invited several times to the Biennale in Venice and has conducted seminar workshops in Italy for a quarter of a century. He and Paola Piizzi regularly lecture at the University of Padua.

Several mask makers I've interviewed received training and inspiration from Donato Sartori. A significant number of Donato's students have also trained with Dell'Arte International's masters.

Cultural Context of Northern California

We tend to think that Europe, Africa, and Asia accept and encourage traditional masked performance with more familiarity and enthusiasm than does the United States. Certainly northern Italy found itself central to the flowering of Europe's *commedia dell'arte* masked performance style from the fourteenth century onward; however, the Northwest United States and Canada also have a long-standing record of masked performance dating back to ancient times when indigenous tribal communities' making masks for their festivals and rites thrived along its shores. Consequently, the mask has much historic relevance to this area.

Indeed, mask makers have found particular inspiration in the culturally diverse history of northern California. Its residents have patronized progressive arts and top-quality education for over a century. But long before its urban development, Pacific Northwest First Peoples (whose masks are still very familiar and appreciated by northern Californians) created beautifully detailed masks, often involving a shaman figure "functioning as a mediator, healer, visionary, guide and counselor ... and capable of transforming into beings, both natural and supernatural."[8] The ancient traditions of spiritualism continue to synchronize with the contemporary artistic communities in this region, no doubt making it a fertile area for more mask makers than any other in the United States.

San Francisco, of course, has significantly influenced the cultural values of California's northern cities and towns. Glenna Matthew's *Forging a Cosmopolitan Civic Culture: The Regional Identity of San Francisco and Northern California* traces San Francisco's cultural influence harkening back to the great Gold Rush of 1848. Supporting the arts symbolized affluence for its *nouveau riche* citizens. She notes that Chinese, Japanese, Chilean, Mexican, Irish, Italian, Caribbean, and African-American immigrants flooded into the area, establishing diverse multi-cultural communities with a range of religious constituencies, including Catholic, Protestant, Jewish, and Buddhist.[9] A progressive social structure and liberal urban attitude steadily evolved. Descendants of these early immigrants gradually settled beyond San Francisco and into the northern region of California.

In part due to the influx of more culturally diverse immigrants coming from San Francisco, northern California continued to challenge America's more conservative values well into the 1960s. San Francisco Mime Troupe used elements of *commedia dell'arte* and mime as a political form of popular entertainment and toured north of San Francisco in streets and parks. A group of jugglers who had worked with San Francisco Mime Troupe, Peggy Snider, Larry Pisoni, and Cecil MacKinnon, established the innovative Pickle Family Circus which many patrons believe influenced the internationally acclaimed *Cirque du Soleil*. Financial support in 1976 from the National Endowment for the Arts also allowed Pickle Family Circus to tour northern cities in California. Famed clowns Larry Pisoni, Geoff Hoyle and Bill Irwin established their careers with this company. Amidst this prolific performance activity Carlo Mazzone-Clementi and his second wife and administrative partner Jane Hill founded Dell'Arte School of Mime and Comedy in 1971 (eventually to be known as Dell'Arte International School of Physical Theatre) north of San Francisco in Blue Lake near Arcata, California. Joan Schirle notes that without Jane Hill there would have been no vehicle for Carlo's vision. Hill wrote all the grant proposals and managed the school. She also convinced the city of Eureka to sponsor a festival and co-authored Mazzone-Clementi's article, "Commedia and the Actor."[10]

San Francisco continues its progressive entertainment experimentation today and in addition to the arrival of large numbers of various culturally diverse immigrant groups, one can see other reasons why this city and the area north of it have become such a center for physical theatre and masked performance. For instance Margaret Crawford states in *Alternative Shelter: Counterculture Architecture in Northern California*, "Even before 1967, when the heavily advertised Summer of Love signaled the commercialization of the Haight Ashbury counterculture, hippies began to leave San Francisco. Searching for cheap land in remote locales, they sought more fertile ground to create radical alternatives to the middle-class American way of life. By the mid 1970s, the rural fringes of northern California were dotted with communes and experimental households of various types."[11]

Consequently, northern California residents, like San Franciscans, had long supported the sort of progressive entertainment not so readily embraced by most other areas of the United States. These residents appreciated, however, progressive entertainment that more specifically related to the rural issues that directly affected them. *Commedia* performance style, based on the concept of improvising humorous responses to local issues, easily connected with northern Californians and highlighted the approaches of touring companies. The most famous ones, San Francisco Mime Troupe, Pickle Family Circus, and Dell'Arte Company (the professional theatre company aligned with its School and established by 1976 by Mazzone-Clementi, Joan Schirle, and Jon'Paul Cook) thrived in this region. (Interestingly, in 1968 the actors of the San Francisco Mime Troupe went to Italy, to Donato Sartori's workshop, where they created masks for the performance *L'Amante Militare*, performed by Kent Minault, R.G. Davis, and Jason Marc-Alexander.[12])

Those living in Arcata/Eureka (minutes from Blue Lake where Dell'Arte was instituted) have long appreciated the handcrafted aspects of masks, particularly masks created from wild life and natural materials such as leather, bark, and feathers, as well as wood products from the great redwood forests such as paper and latex. Historically they have sought carefully handcrafted furniture and decorative arts as well. Crawford portrays northern California residents as traditionally rugged, independent individuals who built innovative homes that evolved "backward to pre-industrial times, hoping to return to a more natural and more authentic life based on handwork." She notes that pervading wild life continues to co-exist with people living close to Arcata/Eureka, where nature vividly displays her power in all seasons with natural settings along their ocean inlets and majestic redwood forests.[13] This pervasive attention to nature, and decorative arts produced with local natural products, encouraged these communities to savor the fine technical prowess required in making traditional masks.

For almost three decades, a local arts group called The Ink People in the Arcata/Eureka area of northern California has sponsored a unique and very popular annual exhibition called *Maskibition*, featuring masks from abroad as well as masks by local artists. Dell'Arte faculty members Schirle, Marrs, Foreman, Fields, and others have served as judges who award prizes for the best masks in two categories: Performance Masks and Art Masks. Some mask makers teach workshops during the event. Audiences annually look forward to *Maskibition*, and mask makers learn a great deal from each other. Its influence over the years has helped local audiences develop a particular admiration for the complex challenges of mask making and mask performance.

The northern Californian rural communities still regularly celebrate and even take for granted the frequent family weekend arts, crafts, and theatre festivals (usually comprised of local performers and artists), as well as down-home, commercially sponsored events such as wine and oyster festivals.

While traditional handcrafted masks have not held the appeal for American audiences as much as those in Europe, one must remember that the United States lacks the traditions of masked theatre found in Europe and major areas of Asia and Africa. Yet citizens in northern California seem more inclined than most Americans to appreciate the aesthetic and communicative resonance of masks in part because of the area's rich influence of the arts, crafts, and theatre festivals as well as the influence of nearby native Pacific Northwest groups and their mask-making traditions. This local familiarity with masks made it much easier for the physical theatre companies of the '60s and '70s to incorporate them in their performance work. Masks work especially well for performance work emphasizing gesture.

Mask maker Donvieve, with assistance from Bruce Marrs along with Joyce Radtke (all introduced in chapter 2), has provided significant leadership and they have well represented this community-conscious cultural Mecca for the arts. For several years Lauren Raine (also introduced in chapter 2) has likewise helped plan and has participated in the annual Spiral Dance Ritual in San Francisco. This ritual event, now in its third decade, incorporates masked performance and pays homage to the ancestors and the inevitable spiral of rebirth. Underscoring the progressive atmosphere of northern California, three of these mask makers are women, reversing the predominant global trend of male mask makers. Not surprisingly, Dell'Arte has flourished within this accommodating environment since 1971.

Dell'Arte International's Global Legacy

Dell'Arte International has an educational and entertainment mission that focuses on topics relevant to local, social, or environmental issues, partly because the community strongly supports this emphasis. They seem especially appreciative of its performance style, rooted in European popular traditions. And despite the organization's rural location, its professional theatre company tours worldwide, and students often come from Europe and Asia. The School currently offers a one-year certificate program in physical theatre (the PTP or Professional Training Program) as well as a three-year Master of Fine Arts degree in ensemble-based physical theatre, plus summer workshops and residencies in Bali and Denmark. Its professional touring ensemble, the Dell'Arte Company; its annually produced Mad River Festival; its Dell'Arte Youth Academy; and study abroad programs have all enjoyed support in terms of progressively increasing local and national arts grants as well as increased public attendance.

The history of Dell'Arte has not yet been formally written. But Joan Schirle briefly summarizes the institution's development as "a center for the exploration, development, training, and performance of the actor-creator. Its mission is to employ and revitalize the traditional physical theatre forms to explore contemporary concerns." Schirle says that while Dell'Arte occasionally uses masks in its presentations, it particularly focuses on the power of physical movement and gesture, influenced by, though not limited to, *commedia dell'arte*. This emphasis on physical movement and gesture allows its audiences to experience a broader level of sophisticated presentational skill required by masked performances, relying more on impeccable timing and specific characterization, dance, movement, and visual detail than on dialogue. Schirle describes the distinctive character of Dell'Arte as one of a handful of rural professional ensemble theatres in the United States, internationally recognized for its unique contribution to American theatre via its non-urban point of view, its thirty-plus year history of ensemble practice, its work to push the boundaries of physical theatre forms in professional productions, and its actor-training programs.[14]

She explains that the initial motivations of co-founders Carlo Mazzone-Clementi and Jane Hill came from their belief that creativity bloomed best away from urban distractions. Dell'Arte's entire pedagogy became based on the observation of nature as a primary source for the actor. Mazzone-Clementi and Hill were largely influenced by Jacques Copeau, whose early-twentieth-century school and theatre company, *Le Vieux Colombier*, was located in a rural area where he believed the actor would experience more integration with natural elements.

In 1957 Mazzone-Clementi first came to the United States, where he introduced a number of masks that Amleto Sartori had given him to students at American institutions (such as Carnegie Mellon University) as he guest lectured and conducted demonstrations. In the fall of 1966 (the inaugural year of the New York University's program in theatre), Mazzone-Clementi started to work with a young partner, Hovey Burgess, known as a circus reformer. Together their collaboration developed into "New Circus" which still influences circus entertainment.

As mentioned earlier, Lecoq's meeting with Amleto Sartori in Italy had led to the creation of the now famous "neutral mask" as well as Lecoq's development of a pedagogy which explored the idea of "neutrality" through practice with the neutral mask. When Mazzone-Clementi commenced his own workshops in the United States, he commissioned his old friend Amleto Sartori to develop another kind of neutral mask, which Mazzone-Clementi called the metaphysical mask. While the neutral mask resembles a human face in an expression of calm wonder, the metaphysical mask is based on geometric forms of the two elementals: the line and the curve. Its eyes are a circle and a triangle and its shape more resembles a fencing mask than a human face.[15]

"The metaphysical mask, which is still in use at Dell'Arte today," says Schirle, "requires a very strong projection from the actor. The severity of the form throws the body into even stronger relief than the neutral mask." Dell'Arte has for many years used copies of the original in class work, and the original male plaster model and the original leather female mask are on display at the School. In 2007 a Dell'Arte alumna, Dee King, created a new set of neoprene metaphysical masks for Schirle.[16] Eldredge and Huston describe the metaphysical mask of Mazzone-Clementi as "the extreme of abstraction and one that has a distinctive centerline, a browline" and assert that such an abstract mask "leads the actor beyond psychology to the intrinsic qualities of movements and body shapes."[17]

According to Schirle, Mazzone-Clementi, like Joseph Campbell, believed that there are interconnections throughout world mythology and religions that can be found in their spirit figures. For example, he believed the local Native American spirit figures of Coyote, Loon, and Raven had their parallels in the stock characters of *commedia dell'arte.* "The first original work of the company we founded in 1976 was based on this connection. It was called *The Loon's Rage* and toured in 1977," she said. "Many of the subsequent plays of Dell'Arte Company have been based on our concept of 'theatre of place' which uses local themes, issues, and characters to create plays that nonetheless are universally accessible. On the other hand, it is also 'international' in the sense that it has involved international artists from its inception; it has toured widely to world festivals and it attracts an international student body. Additionally, it has created many plays which have a more 'urban' sensibility in both formal approach and content. Some pieces blend both," said Schirle. "For instance, my solo *Second Skin* draws from world mask traditions and universal themes, yet some of the characters are drawn directly from people at the local bar. Dell'Arte's 'non-urban' point of view includes an appreciation of the interface where nature and civilized life meet and which has become a battleground (and will continue to be) over water, trees, oil, wildlife, and urban development."[18]

Mazzone-Clementi wanted to bring the European physical training tradition to the United States by developing actor-creators through training in mime, mask, movement, and ensemble creation. But the initial years were not tranquil for the theatre company. Its members experienced dissenting philosophical and artistic viewpoints on how the company should evolve. It had very little financial support, making the situation even more difficult.

Originally called Dell'Arte School of Mime and Comedy, the School's name was changed to Dell'Arte International School of Physical Theatre in the late 1980s as a result of the narrowing definition of "mime" and a desire to investigate a broader vision of theatre and the work of the contemporary actor. When asked why Dell'Arte adapted the term "Physical Theatre" in its title rather than "Mime," Schirle responded, "Essentially the name 'mime' had become synonymous with whiteface mimes and Marcel Marceau, becoming the butt of jokes. It became necessary to find other words that meant the same thing, such as physical theatre, movement theatre, and theatre of gesture. Even so, Schirle admits that none of these terms are as deeply meaningful or ancient as 'mime' which comes from 'mimesis.'"[19]

Arne Zaslove agrees with Schirle about the problem of using the term "mime" even though this term is ironically more concise and descriptive for the type of theatre Dell'Arte emphasizes. "For years I kept a cartoon from *The New Yorker* pinned to my bulletin board," he said. "The cartoon shows an earnest court jester cavorting and sweating in front of his king, seated on his throne. In the foreground one spear-carrying guard whispers to the other, 'Mimes stink!' I also recall the scene in *Tootsie* when a street mime is nonchalantly pushed on the street. And then there's Antonioni's *Blowup* that includes a series of bad scenes of mimes playing tennis without a ball. I suspect that the world has seen too many clichéd, trite, sentimental street mimes (usually amateurs) who think they can do a few tricks."[20] Dell'Arte needed to get beyond that perception in order to be taken seriously as an actor-training center.

Furthermore, Producing Artistic Director Michael Fields describes the school's ambitious objectives in teaching as they relate to the School's use of masks in order to better utilize appropriate gesture for physical theatre. "Many students arrive 'blind.' Because they can't see, they can't perform. We use the mask in our work to open the students. The mask immediately reveals all that is unessential; the mask reveals what is real and what is not. If the body is closed, you cannot react truthfully. You must therefore work with the mask and with the body's readiness. It must be trained and opened."[21]

Joan Schirle identifies an impressive number of mask makers and masked performers who have been either alumni or teachers at Dell'Arte and she offers a rationale for why mask work is such a basic component of a school that emphasizes physical theatre: "The roles of mask makers and mask performance research have been part of Dell'Arte's pedagogical approach as well as its formal theatrical explorations. Copeau's and Lecoq's mask studies, as well as research into the traditional masks of Bali and other traditional cultures have influenced the work of our performance company as well as the School," she says. "The Dell'Arte pedagogy approaches the mask as an embracing metaphor for the work of the actor, not just as the object worn on the face. The physical actor commands the space of the stage. The idea that one assumes the mask of character is aided by the energy, presence, and projection required by working with a mask on your face. Some mask makers have come to study the performing arts at the School in order to expand their own relationship to the art, and a number of artists who began as students of acting, or as faculty members in the School, found their true passion in the work of crafting masks and are now part of the considerable number of professional mask makers who are part of Dell'Arte's legacy."[22]

Notable Dell'Arte alumni working as professional mask makers include Torbjörn Alström (Sweden), Stefan Vernier (Denmark), Dean Bareham (Canada), Doug Berky and Donvieve (United States), Xstine Cook (Canada), Gina Bastone (Canada), Joe and Minna Dieffenbacher (Netherlands), as well as other international figures such as Mimi Doyka, Todd Espeland, Newman, Alyssa Ravenwood, Kirby Soderberg, Wendy Gough, Tony Fuemmler, Kate Braidwood, Dee King, and current faculty member, Bruce Marrs.

In the early years some of the instructors for mask making at the School were Jon'Paul Cook, Alain Schons, Tony Pellegrino, and Robert Ernsthal. Cook teaches at the Danish National Theatre School in Odense; Schons, a theatre designer/director credited with designing the masks for Dell'Arte Company's first production, *The Loon's Rage*, and currently living in France, recently directed a production at Dell'Arte and was director of the Dell'Arte School in the early '80s; Pellegrino is still active primarily as a sculptor; Ernsthal died in the late '90s.

A number of instructors have taught masked performance at Dell'Arte over the years. Primary mask performance instructors (half of whom also made masks) have been Mazzone-Clementi, Joan Schirle, Jon'Paul Cook, Bruce Marrs, Joe Dieffenbacher, Avner Eisenberg, Stephen Buescher, Alicia Martínez Álvarez, Arne Zaslove, and Ronlin Foreman. All of these artists possess the sort of international stature in physical theatre that merit books describing their own individual, impressive achievements. Shorter workshops have been offered by Leonard Pitt, a student of Decroux and highly influenced by Carlo Mazzone-

Clementi. (Pitt also studied with Dell'Arte's commissioned mask maker I. B. Anom in Bali.) Arne Zaslove seriously collects masks; Ole Brekke serves as director of the *Commedia* School in Denmark; Michael Fields serves as Producing Artistic Director of Dell'Arte Company and Dell'Arte Mad River Festival; Julie Goell is a master clown, director, and master teacher of masked performance; Kaf Warman is mask and movement specialist at Carnegie Mellon University, Balinese dancer Nyoman Catra and Swede Torbjörn Alström are mask makers and masked performers.

Dell'Arte alumna and Canadian mask maker/director/performer/producer Xstine Cook (introduced in chapter 4), who served as one of its many guest artists, declares that she loves meeting people and experiencing different cultures and getting "that feeling of strangeness and otherness while moving through it to a smile and friendship." At a young age, she realized she would make masks for a lifetime, but quickly recognized that the performer, not the mask maker, tours. Consequently, her love of traveling encouraged her to study performance techniques at Dell'Arte. She described the school as a special environment due in part to the natural beauty of the surrounding area, including the ocean, the redwoods, and the craggy cliffs. "Spending time in nature is life changing, and Dell'Arte's program is equally intense. Students find themselves locked in a small town with one bar, fellow classmates, and twenty-four-hour access to the School, with its glorious old Odd Fellows Hall and redwood floors." She concluded, "The ten of us were deliriously committed to the program, to creating new work, discovering, trying, failing, and flying. Dell'Arte is the foundation of my practice."[23]

Students have traditionally reflected the international scope of Dell'Arte, representing England, Hungary, Korea, Mexico, Belize, Guatemala, Chile, Holland, Germany, Austria, Denmark, Norway, Finland, Sweden, Canada, Australia, New Zealand, Spain, Japan, India, Bosnia, Bulgaria, France, Italy, Puerto Rico, Costa Rica, Iran, the Philippines, Czech Republic, Croatia, and Latvia.[24]

Dell'Arte's Study Abroad Program in Bali has provided enriched tutelage for generations of students. The six-week course of study has been offered every other winter since 1996 and is now offered annually as a one-month course. Ron Naversen, who teaches at Southern Illinois University Carbondale, learned mask carving in Bali with I. Ketut Molog during Dell'Arte's 2003 workshops (described in chapter 3). He explained that Molog met British expatriate and mask maker Newman (well-known particularly for his fine leather-crafted *commedia* masks but also a master at mask wood carving) in Bali and became friends. Newman began to use Molog's studio to work on his own. In 1996 Dell'Arte International began a study abroad program in the traditional Balinese performing arts of mask carving (*Topeng*); dance (*Legong*) and shadow puppetry (*Wayang Kulit*). Newman, who was a student and later a faculty member at Dell'Arte, recognized that Molog would be the right master teacher for the carving program.

"I had a magnificent experience in Bali," Naversen recalls.

> The Dell'Arte Study Abroad coordinators are experienced Balinese travelers and began their program with several days of orientation to the language, customs, transportation, ceremonies, and arts of Bali. The Dell'Arte instructors then facilitated the formal instruction with the master Balinese artists. Most of the instruction took place in the villages and family compounds of the Balinese teachers, providing a wonderful opportunity for the students to thoroughly immerse themselves into the native life and culture. Each student selects one of the three courses of study on which they concentrate, but many opportunities are provided to experience the other subjects as well. Dell'Arte also provides a series of

> yoga and Alexander-based technique sessions during the program to help the students deal with the physical stresses their bodies encounter during their instruction. Throughout the program, Dell'Arte continues to provide excursions to Balinese festivals, performances, offer vocal workshops in Balinese singing and symposiums on the links between Balinese and Western mask performance traditions. Food, clothing, massage, motorbike rental and arts and crafts are available at low prices and the Dell'Arte instructors helpfully provide sessions on the best places to shop and how to haggle for bargains.[25]

Many students opt to stay in Bali after the course of instruction is over and the Dell'Arte instructors are very helpful in facilitating this extension. "I felt that Dell'Arte truly fed my mind, my body, and my spirit making for an incredibly fulfilling experience," Naversen concludes. "I believe the experience in learning to carve masks in the Balinese style will affect me for the rest of my life."[26]

No other physical theatre company or school in the world has perpetuated the mask and masked performance work on the level that Dell'Arte has. Its international reputation and unique emphasis has had a major wide-ranging influence on masked performance. Rooted in *commedia dell'arte,* it often combines that style with other physical theatre techniques and masked performance styles from the United States, Asia, Africa, and Europe. It regularly commissions international faculty and artists who collaborate at the School in significant performance settings and educational forums. It continues to maintain and support major masked performance traditions while initiating innovative contemporary directions for the mask in theatre settings.

Carlo Mazzone-Clementi's Influence

Dell'Arte's influence on mask makers worldwide as well as its international success and outreach from the small town of Blue Lake, California, harkens back, fittingly enough, to its founder, Italian performer Carlo Mazzone-Clementi. Summarizing his involvement with Dell'Arte, one should note that above all, his impressive skills and charismatic power over young artists made him a dramatically inspirational personality during the formative years of the School. He had a great knowledge of and love for the European classical theatre heritage as well as a strong belief in the power of rural settings to reveal essential truths found in nature. (Joan Schirle has perpetuated this philosophy over the years by offering workshops abroad entitled *Believe, Behave, Become: The Carlo Legacy.*) His philosophy regarding the significance of physical movement in theatre came from his extensive personal involvement with *commedia dell'arte.* This foundation serendipitously happened to intersect with the convergence of the seminal group of mid-century artists mentioned earlier in northern Italy and France who re-explored *commedia* and mask work with renewed fervor after World War II.[27]

Zaslove maintains that Mazzone-Clementi, already an experienced performer, acquired major acclaim when he played Brighella in Strehler's initial version of *The Servant of Two Masters* at *Piccolo Teatro* in Milan in 1947. Amleto Sartori did not make masks for that production (according to Donato Sartori, the first leather masks by Amleto appeared in the '50s[28]); the actors painted their faces. Lecoq had conducted the research on classical movement of *commedia* characters, which inspired his work as movement coach for this production. Zaslove believes that "this production and work with Lecoq may have been Amleto's initial motivation for experimentation in reviving the ancient art of performing in the leather masks." He goes on to say, "Perhaps it is only legend, but I remember either Lecoq or Carlo telling me that Amleto went into an Italian museum that held original *commedia* leather masks and bribed a guard to look the other way while he cut a tiny piece of the leather from the inside of the mask to have it analyzed." (Donato Sartori insists that this story is pure fabrication.[29]) In any event, Zaslove observes that Amleto "eventually enjoyed tremendous success in molding leather masks, and his carved wooden molds are unrivaled. His son Donato still has them and uses them."[30]

"I was nineteen when I met Carlo in 1957," continues Zaslove. "He and his first wife, Viviene Leone, had a studio in New York City. It was a vibrant time and the studio attracted talented performers from Europe and the States. Carlo was a wild and crazy guy—in another zone. He was one of Shakespeare's 'poets, lovers, and madmen.' [Dell'Arte's Michael Fields called him 'an original.'[31]] I have to admit he was not a great teacher. He was frequently incoherent, but somehow right away I understood what he meant. He inspired me greatly. We Jews have a saying, 'Sit at the foot of the rabbi and catch the crumbs from his beard.' I treasured Carlo's crumbs. Once you understood Carlo's lesson, you never forgot it—it became so vivid."[32]

Zaslove compares Carlo's teaching methods with Jacques Lecoq's, with whom he studied in Paris from 1964 to 1966. "Lecoq was French; organized, coherent, methodical. Carlo was Italian and much more flamboyant; larger than life. Lecoq was reluctant to stroke or flatter his students. Carlo validated everyone's talent, at least those who possessed talent. Carlo was full of compliments and enabled you to try. He would rescue you if you were sinking; he never let you drown. He had no subtext; he thought out loud. He never stopped talking and he could cross reference aspects of literature, philosophy, and poetry. He remembered everything he ever read or did."

It was well-known among Carlo's friends that he could antagonize relationships. "Admittedly there were periods when relationships between him and other Dell'Arte performers were strained," Zaslove said. "Carlo could be quite egotistical and oblivious to the havoc he caused around him. I think I served as a bridge (as his artistic son) to re-connect Carlo with Dell'Arte activity once or twice just by gently encouraging both parties to move closer together." Zaslove recalls one such time in Padua when he had "bridged a brief confrontational misunderstanding between Carlo and Donato Sartori in Padua, though consequently I had to escape from Carlo, but that's another story."[33]

Zaslove directed a theatre/vaudeville/circus piece for Pickle Family Circus entitled *Café Des Artists*. "Eventually I became serious and rather successful at directing in Seattle," adds Zaslove. "An important moment for me in this new effort came when Carlo came to see one of my productions and exclaimed that I was a 'great director!' This encouraged me considerably because at that point I realized that I had incorporated his teachings of classical theatre and physical theatre while maintaining my own distinctive and unique vision as a director. This is the legacy I took from Carlo. Even now, almost forty years after its inception, Dell'Arte is the only North American institution that has fully embraced the artistic foundation of physical theatre which was initiated by Carlo."[34]

As recently as 1989 there was a gathering of some of the masked performance giants of the past century. Zaslove recalls it as "a highly significant symposium in Padua" and it was organized by Donato Sartori and Paola Piizzi in collaboration with the Padua Town Council, entitled *Oriente-Occidente a confronto* (Confrontation of East and West).[35] For the first time, everyone was assembled together: Carlo Mazzone-Clementi, Lecoq, Dario Fo, his wife Franca Rame, and Swiss Erhard Stiefel, the official artist for masks and puppets for world-renown French stage director Ariane Mnouchkine, and whom I consider to be the greatest mask maker and sculptor in the world. [Erhard Stiefel learned his mask making technique from Amleto Sartori[36] and early in his career studied at Jacques Lecoq's School in Paris.[37]] Maas Sogen, a great actor from Bali, some American students, and I were there plus an Italian company or two." Donato Sartori says that Hideo Kanze (the most important actor of the Japanese *Noh* Theatre); Namura, director of the old company and actor of *Kyogen* Theatre, and many other representatives of the masked theatre, such as the Peking Opera, also attended this unique, historical event. Donato Sartori also notes that Zaslove was on vacation in Padua at that time and the Sartori family invited him to attend the symposium.[38]

While there has been no formal connection between Dell'Arte and the famous Italian mask maker Amleto Sartori and his equally renowned son, Donato, a number of mask makers who have worked at Dell'Arte over the years have had training and/or collaborations with the Sartoris. Joan Schirle acknowledges that all of Carlo Mazzone-Clementi's masks were made by Amleto Sartori and she recalls that all of them were stolen in Berkeley during a Dell'Arte Company tour in the early '80s. Quite a few years later, to help make up that loss, Donato sent him seven masks from his father's molds, which Schirle now has and exhibits. Dell'Arte served as the United States' distributor of the Sartoris' book, *The Commedia dell'arte and the Masks of Amleto and Donato Sartori: Centro maschere e Strutture Gestuali,* (Casa Usher, publisher) in the early '80s. Several of Dell'Arte's graduates who make masks have studied with Donato, including Newman, Torbjörn Alström, Xstine Cook, and Mimi Doyka. Schirle also participated as a performer in *Second Skin* at the same symposium where Donato lectured in Italy in 2003.[39]

The complicated (some would add, tormented) clown artist who bridged this remarkable span of masked performance activity from the end of World War II to the present was clearly Carlo Mazzone-Clementi, who died in 2000 at the age of seventy-nine. No doubt he failed to realize the important part he played in the flowering of this art form and its development in the northern regions of two countries: the cradle of *commedia* in Padua, Italy, onward to the most significant formal site for the study of masked physical theatre in the United States. No doubt he underestimated his dream of a school that would eventually hold such extensive global impact on contemporary masked performance and mask makers.

Dell'Arte officially notes on its website that "his teaching helped ignite a rethinking of the very purpose of theatre that led to the creation of the new vaudeville and a theatrical circus renaissance." Schirle adds, "Carlo burned with a primal fire; the light he spread can be seen round the world in the hundreds of people who have been influenced, inspired, and touched by his vision. He was not an easy man to understand, but he always said that what he taught wasn't in the books. He called it 'learning by the heart.'"[40]

Carlo Mazzone-Clementi's innovative clown spirit allowed him to embrace the mask in his performances. Influenced by such European artistic giants as Copeau, Lecoq, Fo, and mask makers Amleto and Donato Sartori (particularly Amleto), Mazzone-Clementi provided the spark needed to carry on masked performance traditions in the United States. Northern Californians readily responded to the nuanced sophistication of this masked clown spirit, sparked not only by Mazzone-Clementi but also the superb artistic and technical skills of Dell'Arte Company co-founders Joan Schirle and Jon'Paul Cook, along with its early mask makers Alain Schons, Tony Pellegrino, and Robert Ernsthal. These Dell'Arte pioneers as well as current master mask maker and teacher Bruce Marrs have encouraged generations of international mask makers who have reinvented the mask to function as it gloriously functioned in earlier centuries. Ronlin Foreman, perhaps Dell'Arte's quintessential darker foil to Carlo Mazzone-Clementi's zany characters, still finds a wellspring of potential in his use of the red nose. Carlo must be smiling somewhere.

For information on Donato Sartori's International Mask Museum and annual summer workshops in creating traditional *commedia* masks, visit http://www.sartorimaskmuseum.it/.

For information on Dell'Arte International School of Physical Theatre and their programs, contact them through their website http://www.dellarte.com/.

6

Commercial Mask Makers and Traditional Mythic Concepts

Traditional Mask Iconography

Traditional mask iconography continues in contemporary fantasy film productions and in fantasy Broadway productions. Contemporary adaptations of classic fantasy narratives in popular film draw on four classic mask categories: protector-heroic, demonic, Everyman, and transcendent characters. The last century's mechanical masks (android, robot, cyborg, and avatar masks) in science fiction films continue to use Romantic mask iconography but reflect contemporary anxieties regarding technology.

Traditional characteristics of protector-heroic and demonic masks still represent a range of periods and cultural styles in contemporary popular works. The most effective masks are found in fantasy stage and screen because this genre makes use of universal mythic themes and dramatic heroic journeys with such clarity. Victoria Nelson in her book *The Secret Life of Puppets* defines the "fantastic" as "incorporating elements by turns supernatural, antirepresentational, and grotesque ... born in the Renaissance and revived during the Romantic era as an aesthetic revolt against the eighteenth century's rising Aristotelianism. The Romantic storytelling mode, whose model was set by the stories of Hoffmann, flowered in America in the work of Edgar Allan Poe.... Over the course of the eighteenth and nineteenth centuries a second variant of fantastic literature, the Gothic novel, together with its stepchild the Victorian ghost story, became perhaps the first fictional literary form to penetrate popular culture."[1]

Romantic style especially favors the exotic. What could be more exotic than ethereal, Gothic, cybernetic, and extraterrestrial worlds found in fantasy—and most notably in science fiction? Nelson believes that, "for now, we still enter the realm of ... transcendental self-knowledge ... mostly [by way of] popular modes of horror and science fiction" and she identifies contemporary popular entertainment as "our main subterranean entry." She notes that we inherited the Western concept of Romantic expression "via the German Romantics, who got it from the Renaissance natural philosophers, who found it by foraging in newly discovered classical texts as well as Roman ruins."[2] But of course the Romantic tale began much further back in time. Some of the earliest Paleolithic stories told around the fire at night must have been exotic, horrifying, and full of characters and forces from the supernatural realm.

Susan Mackey-Kallis in *The Hero and the Perennial Journey Home in American Film* states that George Lucas is especially drawn to "adventures in far off lands" and to the value of "modern fairy tales" that he creates in *Star Wars*.[3] But just as other exotic fantasy narratives and the modern fairy tale have morphed into film versions, fantasy film genres have morphed into film animation genres. If we perceive fantasy animation characters as wearing masks (they obviously function artistically as masked characters), we see the traditional mask maker evolving into the role of commercial film animator, possessing strong illustration skills rather than sculpting or molding skills. Film animation projects masks in movement in the same way that medieval audiences perceived puppets projecting masks in movement. Nelson writes, "In England puppets were known as 'motions' and puppeteers as 'motion-men' or 'motion-masters.'"[4] These terms are not so different from terms such as "film animators" or "claymation artists." The "fantastic" mask inspired (and essentially exists in) all other versions of puppets, Trinidadian walking mobiles, parade characters, robots, film animation characters, and digital avatars.

Mackey-Kallis describes fantasy and fairy tale film genres, but especially the science fiction film genre, as most effective in rendering the spiritual qualities of humanity and she adds "that science and technology can also reveal such elemental aspects of the human condition." Mackey-Kallis warns, however, that "science and technology paradoxically obscure those same spiritual truths." She identifies our contemporary fascination with the struggle to reconcile technological issues (or the "logical/rational ways of knowing") with spiritual issues (or "nonrational ways of knowing") as the ultimate anxiety of our time and concludes that the historic tendency to favor one path over the other has failed to resolve this anxiety.[5]

This contemporary anxiety reflected so pervasively in fantasy stage and screen productions becomes a significant motivation for masks that often accompany them. Traditional fantasy myth conventions likewise affect their mask styles. As traditional mask iconography morphs into high-tech animated and motion-capture versions of androids, robots, cyborgs, and avatars in the new millennium, the fundamental characteristics of protector-heroic and demonic imagery continue to dominate.

The contemporary fairy tale, like the science fiction story, still conveys a sense of wonder even as it allows violence and brutality to lurk just beyond the next breath. At times the sinister ambience remains palpable, propelling threatening characters into a sublime evocation of eerie tones in voices, music, and dark shadows. That indescribable atmosphere, which threatens order and security, is "precisely what appeals to children," according to Alec Worley in *Empires of the Imagination*: "[F]airy tales are not so much about fairies as the perilous realm they inhabit."[6] Masks have traditionally indicated such perilous realms more vividly. For example the Beast mask in Cocteau's *La Belle et la Bête* (1946) underscores the mysterious, threatening wildness of the elegant beast just as effectively as the mask in Disney's *Beauty and the Beast*, still being performed on Broadway in the early twenty-first century, but of course the archetypal seductive beast image harkens back to ancient times.

Frequently heroes, particularly masked heroes, appear in fairy tale, fantasy, and science fiction films precisely because they resolve conscious and unconscious threatening possibilities. Hero and protector masks take on human facial characteristics, functioning in similar ways, and together they are a major category of fantasy masks. Heroes (or anti-heroes) such as Superman and Batman often protect the vulnerable in warrior-like ways. Heroes such as Wonder Woman can also return with good fortune, renewed vitality, and insight. Protectors can easily appear as heroic warriors. Even an animated burlap puppet such as 7 fights valiantly—complete with warrior bird mask helmet over her "puppet mask" in Shane Ackers' 2009 post-apocalyptic film, entitled *9*.

Protector-hero and Demon Masks

Broadway designer, director, and mask maker Julie Taymor describes the grand protector lion king Mufasa in *The Lion King* as:

> powerful, terrifying, compassionate, all of which I had to build in his face [mask]. The essence of Mufasa is symmetry: he is an extremely balanced and straightforward personality. I designed Mufasa's mane to form a circle around his head. He is like a Sun God, the center of the universe. There, in father/hero, the mane symbolizes the circle of life that *The Lion King* celebrates. In the first conceptualization, Mufasa's mask was designed to operate like a shield, which the performer held on the front of him with both hands. When not in use, the mask lived in a kind of backpack behind the actor.[7] Scar's characteristics are more misshapen psychologically, with one eyebrow up and the one down; a completely twisted face with spiky porcupine-like hair.[8]

A significant number of contemporary, Romantically based adventure fantasy stage and film productions utilize protector-hero and demon masks following the aesthetic parameters of traditional Western (and frequently Eastern) mask iconography. The protectors, whose goals have to do with balancing disharmonies, strive to establish a stable and symmetrical world for those they guard and defend.

Consequently Romantic protector-heroes typically appear with balanced proportions in hairstyle, attire, and symmetrical facial features to signal their quest for order and security. Even when protector masks have demonic iconography they intentionally have heroic characteristics of balanced harmony in order to signal their power over worse demons. Yet unlike "authentic" demon masks, warrior-type protector-heroic masks maintain an essentially symmetrical quality. Batman, for example, wears a symmetrical, non-distorting mask even as it projects the demonic, threatening qualities of a bat. Conversely, Scar's visually misshapen image implies that he can never serve as a demon spirit who ultimately protects. In postmodern fashion, *The Matrix* deconstructs traditional protector/demonic signals in order to deceive the viewer (for a while) by generating the guise of seemingly "neutral, symmetrical faces with sunglasses" to project seemingly beneficial protector characters that are similar to FBI agents. Audiences eventually realize their sinister qualities. These evil forces disguised as protectors in business suits cause havoc while handsome anti-hero hacker Cypher wears no mask but instead "hides" symmetrical artificial sockets at the base of his neck and back that support his superhuman efforts to save humanity.

Don LoCicero writes that nowhere in mythology is there "a scoundrel more cleverly conceived than the perpetually smiling Joker," Batman's arch-rival. LoCicero cites Bridwell's description of the Joker as "the perfect blend of clownish humor and malevolent evil."[9] The bizarre and distorted clown makeup of Heath Ledger's Joker in *The Dark Knight* (2008) becomes increasingly distorted as he triumphs in evil deeds. The Joker frightens people with what should be benign makeup that is actually his "war paint." We see his constant frown juxtaposed with his bizarrely painted, smiling face. "Does it distress you just how alone you are?" he sneers at Batman. "They need you but they will cast you out. These civilized people will eat each other." The Joker obviously speaks from experience. "I'm not a monster, just ahead of my time."

Contrast the Joker's painted mask (and intentions) with that of Rafiki in *The Lion King*. Both masks are clown-like and distort facial features. But although Rafiki's mask distorts the face to look more exotic and animalistic, it maintains symmetry and always has clearly defined lines and features. Joker's distorted, exaggerated smile and lurid colors transform his character in a disturbing, frenzied, and chaotic way. The purely geometric abstract make-up mask of Rafiki's shaman figure (though just as colorful if not more intense than Joker's) underscores her stable and powerful nature. Rafiki can conjure, quicken, and blend the animal spirits with humanity's spiritual/divine realms and vice versa. She is a prime mover in the musical: a primal earth mother who encourages the life force within all the others. Taymor describes her character and mask as "a shaman baboon who stands apart from the rest as a benign presence and who views the action as an outsider while serving as the musical's spiritual center. The mask (three-dimensional) is absent — using only colored red, yellow and blue make-up — creating an abstract emphasis on the eyes while also suggesting the contours of a baboon's face.... The idea was to link the animal spirit with humanity wearing totemic trinkets and amulets.... Rafiki in the form of a shaman brings the jungle community together as both a character and as a sort of force of nature."[10]

Not coincidentally, Rafiki guides Simba in resolving his fears of assuming the heavy responsibilities of his father's kingdom despite his self-doubts. She reminds him that he is not alone. The critical evocative moment occurs at "the sweet caress of twilight" (the crucial moment of Time's gateway to darkness) when Simba's yearning for integration with the sublime (defined in this case as the supreme unity with nature and mankind) is heightened in a Romantic ambience invoking total harmony and balance within the spirit of the protective ancestors. Note also that Rafiki admonishes Simba to "have faith" (that is, to avoid contemplating forbidden knowledge outside the realm of the protective spiritual world). She reminds Simba that the power to remain connected to the protective spiritual world resides within and around him.

Contemporary commercial masked performances typically project hero, anti-hero, and protector characters that most resemble human beings, even when masked, as a way of underscoring our human ability to protect ourselves and forge ahead. Wonder Woman wears only makeup. Batman's mask, which defines his own facial features rather than those of a bat, fits closely to his face. (Catwoman, Batman's love interest, has similar human facial features under her potentially sinister black cat mask. She looks more human than cat because Batman perceives her as redeemable rather than purely evil like some of his archenemies.) Spider-Man wears a tight, contour-fitting red and black spider mask. Even the animated heroic burlap puppet, 7, has large human-looking eyes and an expressive human mouth. In Cameron's *Avatar* (2009) both the hunter and the prey (indicated by the masks of Marine Jake Sully's humanoid avatar on the extraterrestrial moon and his extraterrestrial Neytiri) have similar heroic looks (human blended with bright blue cat-esque features) and indeed they experience role reversals. Nevertheless they ultimately project protector-warriors as they and their cohorts attempt to save their races while striving to live in harmony with nature (the moon's natural environment.) The theatrical Angel who crashes into Prior Walter's New York apartment in Tony Kushner's *Angels in America*, although perhaps androgynous, looks undoubtedly human. Most contemporary commercial stage and screen productions use this concept of maintaining realistically proportioned human features when projecting heroic or protector masks.

While predominantly human-looking, animal imagery also inspires iconic templates for hero and protector masks, as the examples above demonstrate. The animal imagery of Rafiki's mask suggests a shaman baboon, an example of animal totems and tutelary spirits also frequently signifying protector masks. Animal protectors function in many cases as the ancestors of humans. When contemporary stage and screen productions present animal protector imagery, the masks tend to realistically or abstractly resemble the specific animal, bird, or fish that each represents in real life, such as Hawkman's mask or *Avatar*'s cat-esque humanoid mask, mentioned earlier. While Western protector masks might simultaneously incorporate references to human elements as well as specific animal (or bird or fish) elements, the imagery rarely incorporates image references of "non-worldly" creatures. (This gets complicated when extraterrestrial characters are introduced — though the visual template stays consistent.) Admittedly, Hopi and Eskimo masks have traditionally bucked this trend with fantastic, chimerical abstract versions of protective forces and spirits. Also the Balinese *Barong*, the Indian Ganesh, and the Greek mythical firebird Phoenix are all fabulous protectors. (Eastern mask iconography generally assumes simultaneous elements of good and evil in all natural and fantastic forces/personas — making them less visually predictable.) But popular Western performance venues today tend to ignore fabulous protector images in favor of images — or exaggerated images — of actual living creatures found in nature.

Contemporary Western heroic human-like masked characters contrast with demonic characters which appear in various stages of facial and body distortion. Likewise, demonic, fierce, or wild non-human forces in the mask often appear as distorted or unbalanced versions of animals, birds, or fish. The imaginary combinations of animals, birds, and fish frequently evolve into imaginary forms of non-worldly griffins, dragons, and gargoyles.

Why have we tended to create fabulous masked versions of demons but rarely such distorted, juxtaposed anti-human imagery to indicate protector-heroic figures? Mary K. Patterson Thornburg in *The Monster in the Mirror* makes a convincing case that our contemporary Western aesthetic formula which focuses on fantastic demons (rather than fantastic heroes) hearkens back only to the seventeenth century.

Thurnburg notes that as the Protestant Reformation swept through Europe, more people were less inclined to accept the Catholic emphasis on religious authority and instead embraced secular beliefs that "exalted the moral and societal virtues associated primarily with the Protestant middle class." She suggests that the burgeoning Protestant sentimental myth championed domesticity and the family and conversely feared dark, exaggerated, sinister, Gothic forces of isolation and suffering in the absence of this myth. This shift in religious values reflected and reinforced the cultural climate of its time.[11] While the sentimental component of this myth was conscious, its counterpart, the Gothic aspect, was virtually unconscious (except for the occasional rants by such zealots as Cotton Mather.) Puritanical propensities for suffering as a way of seeking redemption from sin supplanted the Catholic worldview emphasizing forgiveness in the face of guilt. This new religious emphasis encouraged grotesque imaginings. Furthermore Nelson cites Carlo Ginzburg's theory, acknowledging "the widespread Eurasian folk belief that anything modifying the image of the whole human body is a way of expressing an experience that exceeds the limits of what is human.... Anyone who goes to or returns from the nether world ... is marked by asymmetry."[12]

Since the Age of Enlightenment, reason has usurped spirituality. From the eighteenth century onward, ideal theatrical characters became less angelic, more heroic, and infinitely more down to earth. For the past three hundred years, until rather recently, hidden demonic forces tend not to show themselves in the light of science and rationality. Consequently, heroic figures have resembled strong, powerful, military figures while demons reside unacknowledged in the "dark" unconscious, where the imagination takes over to conjure much more distorted images that society (and religion) collectively and outwardly ignores. Bram Stoker's Count Dracula, introduced in his 1897 novel, for instance, never shows his fangs except in the vague shadows at night and just immediately before his consort becomes his victim.

Masked characters in contemporary film fairy tales or film fantasies, like Shrek, exemplify occasional dissonance between expected images of good and evil. *Shrek!* began as a children's picture book by William Steig that came out in 1990. Dream Works' 2001 *Shrek* eventually inspired Broadway's *Shrek The Musical* in 2008. In all of *Shrek!*'s fantasy venues (book, film, and stage) the ogre character Shrek lacks the foreboding qualities seen in typical fairy tale characters. Worley states that the mask in "*Shrek* is more about its mocking swagger than its review of fairy tale stereotypes."[13] His observation reverses the notion that the most significant characters (masked or otherwise) are most effective in fairy tales when they underscore the basic malevolent nature of the tale. Conversely, Shrek threatens no one and has more comic coloring and form than malignant features.

Other fantasy masked performance productions intentionally scramble traditional forms of heroic and demonic imagery when projected on stage and screen. Ludo in *Labyrinth*, who, at first glance, looks overbearing and bestial, is actually as gentle in spirit (though equally threatening in appearance) as Wookiee Chewbacca in *Star Wars*. Occasionally we also see anti-heroes on stage and screen, such as misunderstood and henpecked but brave and lovable Hellboy. Regardless, these situations still maintain the iconic visual vocabulary by posing as contradictory foil imagery.

Has our fast-paced world encouraged more exaggerated versions of violent mask imagery in fantasy and fairy tale films and on stage? Generally not, although our fascination with horror films has led to more versions of bloody, mutilated mask imagery and minions of vacantly staring zombies. Perhaps today's fast-paced lifestyles have encouraged this genre, precisely because it conveniently simplifies it into a starker, more easily produced — though clichéd — fantasy form.

Critics like Megan Stoner worry that fantasy films such as *The Chronicles of Narnia: The Lion, the Witch, and the Wardrobe* (2005) emphasize action-oriented adaptations at the expense of traditional fantasy narrative. She identifies the melting river scene as the most obviously action-enhanced sequence of this film. Here the children and their protectors, the Beavers (arguably animated masked creatures possessing human gestures and voices) "face a perilous crossing over shattering ice while having to fend off an attack by the White Witch's wolves." She notes that Lewis' classic story contains nothing similar to this. The scene on the screen lasts for a full four minutes while providing almost nothing new to the narrative. Stoner also states that the children, presented from the perspective of more contemporary movie-going tastes, are reinvented as "slightly more central and heroic than their book counterparts."[14] The "heroic" children, following traditional heroic/demonic mask iconography, remain unmasked to project an ultra-human look. Their protectors project the form of animal tutelaries (or wise, beneficent animal ancestors) while their evil antagonists project traditional sinister forces in the exaggerated form of Maugrim the snarling wolf, as well as various non-worldly ghouls, ogres, specters, and bats. Oreius the Centaur (with human head and torso) leads the good Aslan's army while Otmin the Minotaur (with the head of a horned bull) leads the evil White Witch's army. The evil White Witch "bewitches" her enemies with her deceptive, icy, heroic human features.

Everyman Masks

A third mask category, Everyman masks, looks more human (albeit less refined and ideal) than distorted. Consider films with animated Everyman characters such as the Gelflings in *The Dark Crystal* (1982) or Gollum in *The Lord of the Rings* (2002). These characters haunt audience members in unusual though compelling ways with their weirdly human qualities that exaggerate humanity's internal forces of good and evil. Versions of Everyman characters such as the Gelflings (questing to find the shard of the dark crystal), while obviously projecting distorted versions of humanity, contrast in appearance with the much more distorted versions of sinister characters such as Gollum. Thus the degree of human mask distortion reflects basic iconic impulses of protective, heroic, and demonic forces by using these impulses as inspiration for image exploration between these realms of good and evil. The good Gelflings are diminutive and rounded with wide-open eyes—rather child-like in appearance—while evil Gollum has beady eyes, a hunched back, and enlarged gargoyle-esque ears. The Na'vi in *Avatar* first appear as Everyman figures with their somewhat cat-like features, but their human features gradually emerge more clearly as audiences perceive their protector-heroic qualities. *Commedia dell'arte* masks are Everyman masks as well.

Everyman masked figures project a range of human and less human (or non-human) images precisely because both heroic and demonic inclinations reside within the human condition. Everyman masked figures dominate our popular culture. Recall the animated character masks with voiceovers by top stars such as George Clooney and Meryl Streep in the film *Fantastic Mr. Fox* (2009). *The New York Times* reviewer A.O. Scott contrasts these very human-looking and human-acting fox masks (among other animal figures in the film) with other more fantastic-looking "three-dimensional, computer-generated creatures that swoop and soar off the screen these days." He writes that the *Fantastic Mr. Fox* "stiff figurines" could actually be "animated and ventriloquized on a classroom or bedroom floor by precocious children." The masked effect "suggests puppetry and [director Wes Anderson] shows a stubborn reluctance to let story take precedence over style." The *Fantastic Mr. Fox* characters are "furry talking animals on display ... with their matted pelts, jerky movements and porcelain eyes [looking] a little quaint, like old-fashioned wind-up toys uneasily sharing the shelf with the latest video game platforms."[15]

Sesame Street puppets functioning as masked characters and *The Lion King*'s Timon and Pumbaa also belong in the Everyman category, representing both human and animal (or bird) looks. Many clown masks fall into this category, though often more abstractly. But clown makeup can project such abstract, exaggerated human features (eyes, noses, hair, smiles, and tears) that, while the makeup mask intends to indicate natural features (and a friendly persona), the clown's appearance actually borders on distortion, even when the features are symmetrical. Consequently, clown masks can unintentionally project demon features, provoking many audience members to fear clowns more than they laugh at them.

We cannot fully express humanity as "eternal" or "ideal" abstract images of good or evil. The Everyman masked figures such as Hellboy (an anti-hero but ultimately more Everyman in spirit), Gollum, Harlequino, *Kyogen* comic characters, the Tin Man, or R2-D2 provoke a blurred mixture of animal, angelic, robotic, and child-like imagery that can shift toward facets of good or evil and evoke varying states of happiness or sadness, greed or generosity, and other complex human emotions. The iconic imagery of Everyman masks is less predictable than protector-hero and demonic iconography precisely because the masks' visual signals respond to such a range of nuanced positive and negative emotional states inherent in the human condition.

The symmetrical, geometric effects of Pixar's animated *WALL-E* mask presents intriguing considerations and other plausible exceptions to traditional mask iconic signals. WALL-E the trash compactor robot starts out simply as a janitor of sorts, cleaning up centuries of

Earth's trash, long after Earth has become uninhabitable to humans. But as the film gets going, WALL-E becomes a protector figure as he collects and saves memorabilia such as a scene from the film musical of *Hello, Dolly!*, the planet's last expression of humanity. His familiarity with this collection prepares him for establishing a human-esque bond and eventual love connection with fellow robot Eve. But WALL-E is no typical protector figure. His large, hapless, drooping-angled eye lenses with no eyebrows or mouth, though robot-looking, have a whimsical, human infantile quality, especially when synchronized with his plaintive machine squeals. He bungles his way into creating a new life with Eve, and one hopes that together they will bring back a semblance of humanity to Earth, if not humans themselves. The mask has the grotesque, exaggeratedly popping eye features seen commonly in traditional demons, and yet WALL-E's less frenzied and rather confused expression is much more lovable. His large "camera lens" eyes are constantly observing and memorizing, reminiscent of a baby's innocence as he explores the world. His childish gestures make him doubly charming. Certainly no demon, but not quite a protector, he seems like a transcendent character (a category discussed next), or at least an Everyman figure.

Another version of Everyman masks which explores the idea of "scrambled mask iconic implication" appears in the form of masked monster playmates (created in a child protagonist's mind in *Where the Wild Things Are*) that simultaneously project both friendly and sinister personalities. Inspired by the classic children's book (1963) written and illustrated by Maurice Sendak, Spike Jonze and Sendak present these book characters in the 2009 film version and illustrate how the monster playmates seem simultaneously threatening and harmless. In a 1986 interview with Terry Gross for National Public Radio's *Fresh Air*, Sendak describes the inspiration behind his monsters: "Well, ... I didn't want them to be traditional monsters, like griffins and gorillas. Just like, I wanted them to be very, very personal, and they had to come out of my own particular life.... I realized they were all my Jewish relatives. They were all the adults who treated us in such silly fashions when we were kids, and they were the real monsters of my childhood. So the only entertainment was watching how— watching their bloodshot eyes and how bad their teeth were. You know, children are monstrously cruel about physical defects. So my entertainment was to examine them closely ... and they became the wild things."

When Terry Gross responded that they seemed "really goofy ... not really frightening," Sendak countered:

> That's true, but at the same time they are threatening. I mean, if Max were not in control of them, they could indeed be in control of him, and when they say oh, please don't go, we'll eat you up, we love you so, they mean just that, and he knows that, and I think children know that too, that the fun of that book is a perilous tightrope between him being a little boy and very vulnerable to these huge creatures and the absurdity of his having control over them by staring into their yellow eyes. It's what every child would like, to have control over such things. Kids are not afraid of them because Max is not afraid of them, and see, the kids clue in onto Max right away, and they follow him, and if he's okay, they're okay.[16]

Many parents felt that *Where the Wild Things Are* was more frightening on screen than the images in the book. Regardless, while these monsters project facets of demonic or at least frightening personalities, the monsters seem more like humans than evil forces.

Admittedly, with the mixed signals of anti-hero characters such as Shrek and Hellboy, as well as the complicated Everyman characters like Gollum, WALL-E, and Sendak's wild beasts, we cannot simply divide fantasy and fairy tale film masked characters into protector-heroic, demonic, or even Everyman stereotypes. But the contrasting iconic imagery suggesting good and evil generally seen in the protectors versus the demons clearly underscores a standard traditional visual vocabulary with which to compare and contrast personalities and forces in commercial masked performance. This traditional Romantically based protector/demonic iconography pervades current fairy tale, fantasy, and science fiction productions. Everyman figures appear as masked forms in fantasy stage productions as frequently as on screen.

Transcendent Masks

A fourth category of contemporary stage and screen masks increasingly includes (especially in science fiction film) somewhat "superhuman" or "extrahuman" characters who project as transcendent messengers rather than protector/demon/Everyman personalities. This fourth, entirely different iconic facial fantasy category includes both unmasked performers and masked performers (or frequent animated cartoon versions of masked characters) that consistently draw on exaggerated juvenile imagery. Transcendent characters usually appear without masks, precisely to emphasize their human characteristics. But unlike protector-heroes, these characters, when masked, invariably emphasize the innocent qualities of young children.

Movie audiences especially enjoy these transcendental characters. Characters in this category again reflect our anxiety regarding the rise of technology and its influence on contemporary spirituality. Transcendent characters intentionally — or not — assist in guiding humanity toward an enlightened reconciliation of the technological and rational realms with the spiritual and non-rational realms. Makey-Kallis points out, "Usually the relationship [between these realms] is resolved by offering a third or transcendent way of knowing that combines the best impulses of both" or by introducing a non-biased character frequently seen as a Jungian child archetype who can "symbolize not only innocence but also receptivity to creative potential, the nonrational possibilities of alien life, and the transcendent."[17] The transcendent character maintains quest and search agendas rather than seeking to destroy alien influences or foreign ideas, and motivates others accordingly.

Makey-Kallis recalls the child-like countenance of transcendent characters such as Spielberg's E.T. and the *Close Encounters of the Third Kind* aliens. She notes that Lucas' Jedi-master Yoda looks simultaneously childlike, old, and diminutive. (His power resides with his wisdom, in spite of his fragile appearance.) Wizard-in-training Harry Potter (with his enlarged glasses) almost falls into this category of transcendent masked characters as he navigates between imaginary and natural world situations. On the other hand, film versions of Alice sans mask in *Alice in Wonderland* or Peter Pan in *Peter Pan* or five-year-old Carol Anne Freeling in *Poltergeist* present ultimate transcendent child archetypes precisely because they look like "real" children.

Finally, Mackey-Kallis suggests that the round, child-like qualities observed in such masked transcendent characters as E.T. and the aliens in *Close Encounters* lie in the imagery associated with the ancient mandala process of harnessing our unconscious realizations. I mentioned aspects of her traditional theory in chapter 2 when mask maker Donvieve elaborated on the use of the mandala to assist in her mask making inspiration. The circular mandala captures and "frames" our inner imaginings, allowing them to transcend reality. Mandalas function as windows (or eyes) to the soul. The exceptionally large, blank but all-knowing, luminous eyes of a small child can appear as versions of traditional mandalas, suggesting earlier realms before worldly birth. Hence, the mandala provides a traditional rationale for very young-looking transcendent characters. (Mackey-Kallis even suggests that the frequent round "camera eyes" indicate monolithic computer Hal in *2001: Space Odyssey,* who "appears" as such a transcendent albeit perversely as both a naïve and simultaneously a frightening character.) She describes the mandala-like images in these transcendent characters as "symbols of the unconscious ... similar to [Jung's] child archetype, representing transcendence, unity, or centeredness of being," and mentions Jung's theory that "they express the idea of a safe refuge, of inner reconciliation and wholeness."[18] The child transcendent can function as a non-threatening vehicle for change, open to new ways of understanding and unhampered by useless worn-out perspectives. On the other hand, the new perceptions (eternal youth or computers replacing spacemen) are not necessarily ideal for humanity, as Peter Pan and Hal the computer eventually demonstrate.

Contemporary Mechanical Masks Inspired by *Frankenstein*

Another mask category that projects android, robot, cyborg, and avatar characters found in so many science fiction films and occasionally in apocalyptic films has been around for the past two centuries. Or have we seen masked versions of artificial humans much earlier? J. P. Telotte in his book *Replications* traces robot-like creations back to Homer's *Iliad* when "Hephaestos, the blacksmith (or technician) god devises mobile tripods to serve his divine fellows at their banqueting." He goes on to mention Daedalus's bronze man designed to serve King Minos of Crete, and the production of "various statues to amuse him [Minos], including one of Venus." Telotte then reminds us that Pygmalion the sculptor created a statue that Aphrodite proceeded to bring to life. He recounts "later historical creations" such as "clock-tower figures popular in Europe during the Middle Ages and later, to the *theatrum mundi* of the eighteenth and nineteenth centuries, Vaucanson's celebrated mechanical duck and musicians, and even Edison's talking doll of 1894" as non-mythical examples of technological explorations designed to imitate humans.[19]

But Telotte (and others) consider Mary Shelley's *Frankenstein* to be most significant in introducing artificial life as a reflection of the major anxiety of the past two centuries regarding technology and its influence on humanity. This novel was the first work of science fiction. Mary K. Patterson Thornburg notes that Shelley "explores the relationship between humanity and its scientific or technological creations—including its own changing nature...." She describes the Monster as "more than a psychological and philosophical construct" but also notes the "equal reality of creator and creature" and that the "Monster's actions are separate from Frankenstein's, beyond his control though in a sense determined by him by virtue of his having designed the Monster, and they have real consequences in a real world." *Frankenstein* (whose protagonist can be seen as the ultimate fictional mask maker) reflects in Thornburg's words, "humanity's scientific achievement but also its moral inadequacies and its guilt."[20] Shelley's bold tale at the onset of the Industrial Revolution foresees the promise as well as the horrors of machines and scientific technological advancement. Frankenstein unwittingly loses control of his newly developed scientific and technological triumph. Indeed, the Monster illustrates both Frankenstein's God-like creative triumph and his hubristic inability to imagine the fatal consequences of his creation. The novel upset Industrial Age society's moral compass by disrupting the sentimental bourgeois myth of striving for idyllic domesticity, supposedly achieved by enlightened earnestness and "simple" hard work. The great "new modern myth" advocating science and technology as the answer to the limitations of the human condition — along with universal anxiety regarding questions of technology's constructive interlacement with humanity — arrived with *Frankenstein* and continues to pervade our psyches today. This dominant contemporary myth justifies and even sanctions our popular fascination with science fiction and its accompanying new masked forms of extraterrestrial, artificial, and humanoid versions of humanity.

Continuing Romantic Emphasis on Forbidden Knowledge

Telotte writes that our desire to craft artificial images/beings like ourselves "carries a price, as we are also warned against overstepping the limits of our nature, at being *too* crafty — too technological."[21] He adds that the early twentieth century's machine age quite naturally ushered in the golden age of science fiction with Fritz Lang's seductive and "classic dystopian vision *Metropolis*" in 1927.[22] While robots in the form of androids and cyborgs have regularly appeared in novels throughout the past two centuries, we now see them dominating the multiplex. Movie audiences enjoy films like *The Terminator* series, *The Matrix* series, *RoboCop* series, *Star Wars* series, *Blade Runner* series, *Transformers* series, *9*, and *Avatar*, in theatres and on DVDs in their homes.

Ultimately, the relatively recent introduction of android, cyborg, and digital avatar masks marks a distinct diversion from the traditional Romantic motivations for masks even as the Romantics with Mary Shelley introduced our concept of mechanical masks. Nelson reminds us that we have had androids for only the past one hundred years, robots for the past seventy-five years, cyborgs for the past thirty years, and "the virtual-reality constructs or 'avatars' for a mere decade."[23] While these mechanistic creations continue to reflect our yearnings to maintain and conjure higher forces to help protect us from lower, baser, and evil forces (or to accept, celebrate, or abhor our human condition with Everyman masks), the android/robot/cyborg mask maker's quest has transitioned into a more anxious existential realm. What if no higher forces exist? Victoria Nelson suggests that "the new cosmogonic myths" found in science fiction with their "extraterrestrial 'aliens' have supplanted the old deities." She argues that the concept of the machine can also be considered a sort of Platonic ideation of God: "It is the machine, not humans, that dissolves the boundaries of time and space, creates life and new species, duplicates or mutates old species, violates and transcends the laws of nature. This unconscious belief in the divinity of machines has carried over into the popular language used to describe real scientific inventions, everything from giant computers that 'conquer space and time' to robots that 'reproduce.'"[24]

Fantasy films signal a new perspective in science fiction with its introduction of "replications of our own imagined humanity." Telotte concludes that the mythos of the robot "reflects the human, but in a 'more than superficial' way. It sketches the technologized being in depth, a depth that might help us realize what the technological can offer and yet keep us sovereign over it, save us from our own craftiness."[25] If we accept the premise that we are all versions of monsters — at least at an unconscious level — might mechanical versions of humanity at least be more controllable? Conversely, should our human monsters attempt to control more humane — though "mechanized mask" versions — of humanity? *Metropolis* introduced this dilemma in 1927, and while *2001: A Space Odyssey* dramatically continued the debate, we still see other forms of this issue in recent science fiction films such as *Avatar*.

Resurgence of Romantic Masks

Thornburg states that "traditional science fiction seems to be moving into mainstream literature or into a subcategory of its own, while increasingly popular audiences favor heroic fantasy, a self-consciously mythic representation of sentimental, Gothic, and realistic themes in deliberately nonrealistic, Romantic terms." She also identifies the contemporary horror novel or film which resembles the "traditional Gothic novel in its realistic presentation and tale of terror atmosphere."[26] Popular films with masked characters follow these science fiction and horror trends as well — often presenting versions of their literary predecessors, such as *Blade Runner, The Puppet Masters, Bicentennial Man, Alien,* and plenty of masked horror/monster personalities seen in *Dracula, Dr. Jekyll and Mr. Hyde, Frankenstein* sequels and in more ludicrous versions of *Godzilla, Brotherhood of the Wolf,* and *The Fly.*

Traditional Romantic masks for both stage and screen show no signs of disappearing. But according to Nelson, "the first real signs of decline in the three-hundred-year-old tradition of the grotesque as preeminent definer of the supernatural" is at hand. She cites such examples of this trend as *Terminator 2,* with the protagonist "as noble" as the protagonist in *Terminator 1* was "implacably evil."[27]

Wicked's Elphaba (the younger version of the Wicked Witch of the West in *The Wizard of Oz*) is one more contemporary Romantic masked protector. *Wicked,* which premiered on Broadway in 2003 (songs and lyrics by Stephen Schwartz and book by Winnie Holzman), is based on Gregory Maguire's novel *Wicked: The Life and Times of the Wicked Witch of the West* (1995), inspired by L. Frank Baum's novel *The Wonderful Wizard of Oz* (1900) and MGM's film *The Wizard of Oz* (1939). Elphaba's evolution from her 1900 bad witch masked version to the 2003 good witch masked version emphasizes ancient Romantic yearnings for spiritual union and social interconnectedness and engages with our technological anxieties.

As with so many Romantic tales that pose critical moments at night — the time when men and women yearn most intensely for safety and security against the reality of mortality — the Oz community members turn against the misunderstood anti-heroine Elphaba at night and she "defies gravity" by losing her "self" and flying off into the darkness of her self-doubts. Willing to trust her instincts, she returns to her internal sources of divine protective powers. Her green persona (not disfigured as in *The Wizard of Oz* but symmetrically and beautifully proportioned in *Wicked*) becomes the demonic protector of the animals (derived from the Latin *anima* or soul) who have been rejected by the grand "unfeeling" (and highly technological) wizard.

Elphaba not only learns to fly on her own, but also she is accepted into the community that misunderstood and feared her. Increasingly, however, contemporary Romantic masked characters, like Elphaba, realize that the essential demand of the life force requires not only technical mastery but also self-acceptance and accountability to oneself.

Our society at large understands this premise, at least unconsciously. And yet accountability to oneself can only go so far in relieving the tensions we confront in an overpopulated world and an over-stimulated and unpredictable global climate. We still need protectors — the sort that protect in Romantic ways. Yet Nelson distinguishes between heavenly protectors and fantastic protectors, pointing out that since the Renaissance, we have doubted divine inspiration and "Western popular films of the supernatural before the year 1990 featured no real deities, good or bad. (With its benign 'superhuman' daemons and their malign counterparts, the American comic book cosmology has always been, like the Hindu pantheon, inherently more balanced.) Not until the ascendance of the new/old virtual worldview do we begin to see, along with a smattering of angels, a mini-trend of, for example, benevolent female demigoddesses."[28]

At the beginning of the new millennium, we frequently hear pronouncements from Talking Heads about the need for "sustainability," for which we have numerous definitions. We need a sustainable earth, sustainable economy, and sustainable corporate mission statements. Sustainability has become our new (old) solution for protecting our earth and protecting our lifestyles. Columnist Rod Dreher of the *Dallas Morning News* expressed this cultural commonplace in 2008 when he wrote that he hoped that this world crisis would "generate a revival in localism, personal asceticism, and traditionalism." A change in the culture toward sustainability might "produce a new, more responsible politics, one that keeps the excesses of a culture in material and social crisis from damaging the common good and public order."[29] But, of course, this perspective is actually an ancient one.

Today's science fiction film audiences recognize and support this ancient beckoning already, and masked characters abound in this "back to the future" realm. This ancient emphasis on a Platonic rather than Aristotelian "scientific" sensibility encourages more focus on spiritual (Romantically inspired) solutions combined with (rather than dominating over) the advanced state of our technological progress. Nelson argues that the virtual reality of the web, "divorced from time and space is ... has singlehandedly moved the dormant Platonic sensibility in Western culture." It has "powerfully resurrected the old premodern construct of a unified hierarchical cosmos with a transcendent level that rules the material plane we lesser mortals inhabit, a level we now view as accessed in a quasi-magical way by high technology rather than by meditation, prayer, or incantation."[30]

Traditional masked performance, transformed but still vital on today's commercial stage (*The Lion King, The Phantom of the Opera, Wicked, Beauty and the Beast, Shrek,* and *Cirque du Soleil*) still draw on ancient tribal community sensibilities by incorporating masked performances in relatively intimate theatre spaces (rather than coliseums). The mask has always required its audience to be at a relatively close distance. But film has allowed the smallest detail to be magnified on screen, perpetuating the mask's effectiveness for much larger audiences. While fantasy and popular science fiction film audiences regularly continue to experience masked performance as a local community (at the urban movie house), they collectively experience these films as a worldwide phenomenon. Consequently the medium of film has managed to perpetuate the magic of the mask, its ancient and traditional Romantic mask realms that highlight archetypal protector figures — and their counterparts — suitable for a global universal sphere.

In her essay "Hollywood Enters the Dragon," Véronique Flambard-Weisbart cites French philosopher Paul Virilio, who predicts "the failure of Babel and a return to myth." She goes on to express his suggestion that some sort of universal world myth will encourage a more global sense of community and discourage our current emphasis on regional and national economic competition.[31] With our dramatic world economic fluctuations and threats of global warming, his audacious prediction seems more apparent with each daily virtual newspaper. And where there is myth, there will always be mask makers. But how are traditional myths evolving on the global stage and screen? I take a closer look at this issue in the next chapter. The Romantic quest for new global myths — or a return to the ancient local myths — becomes an essential challenge for the contemporary mask makers, both traditional and commercial.

West Coast United States mask makers Donvieve, Lauren Raine, and Joyce Radtke

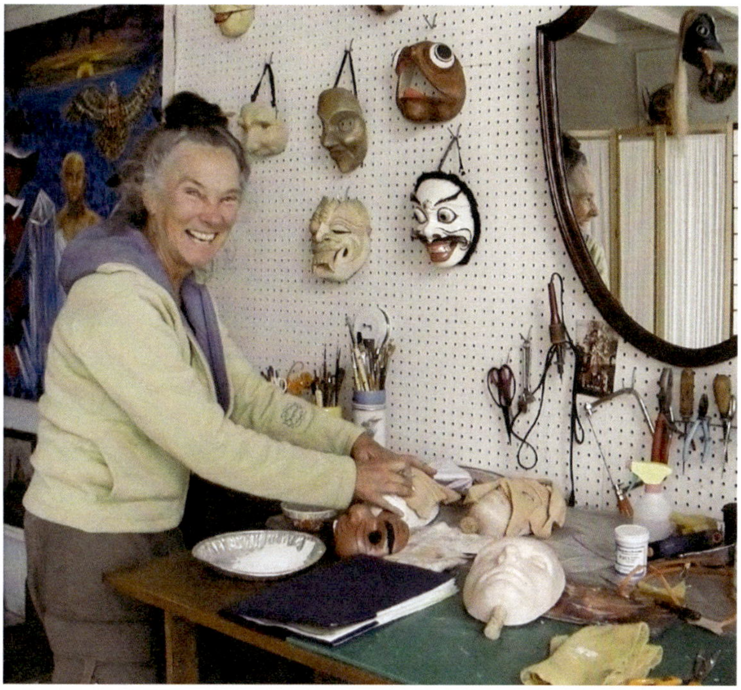

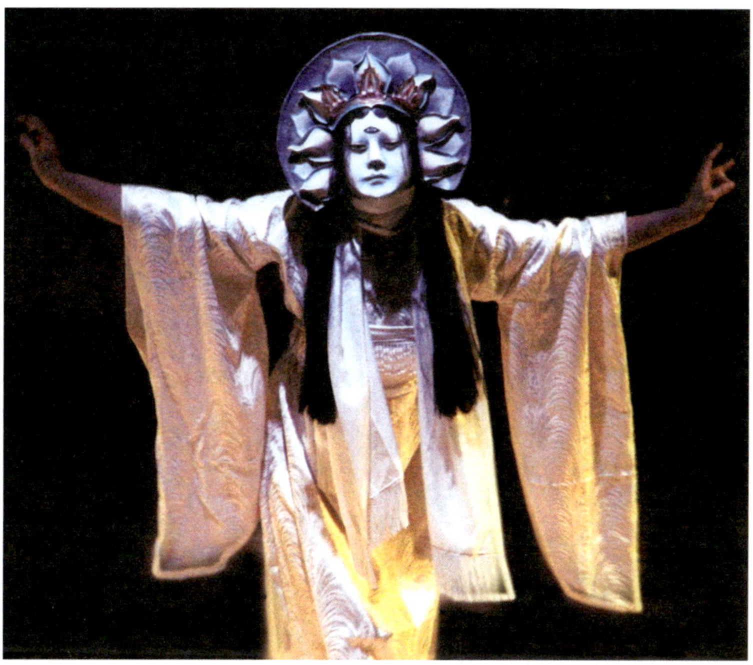

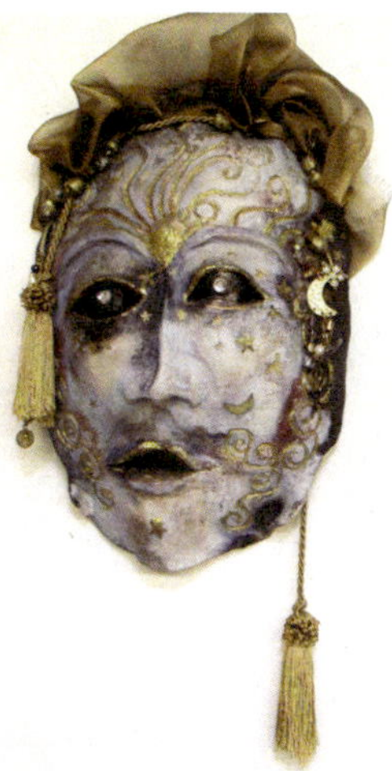

Top—Mask maker Donvieve at her studio in Arcata, California. She believes that the act of making masks has the potential to establish community. ***Bottom left***—Lauren Raine's rendering of White Tara, the revered female Bodhisattva of Tibetan Buddhism. According to Raine, Tara is "She Who Hears the Cries of the World," the embodiment of unconditional love. Performer: Mana Youngbear. Photographer: Ileya Stewart, courtesy of Lauren Raine. ***Right***—Joyce Radtke introduces masks as a way to promote successful relationships and empowerment. One of her Persephone Project participants created this mask. Radtke assists others in coping with catastrophic illnesses.

Italian mask maker Donato Sartori

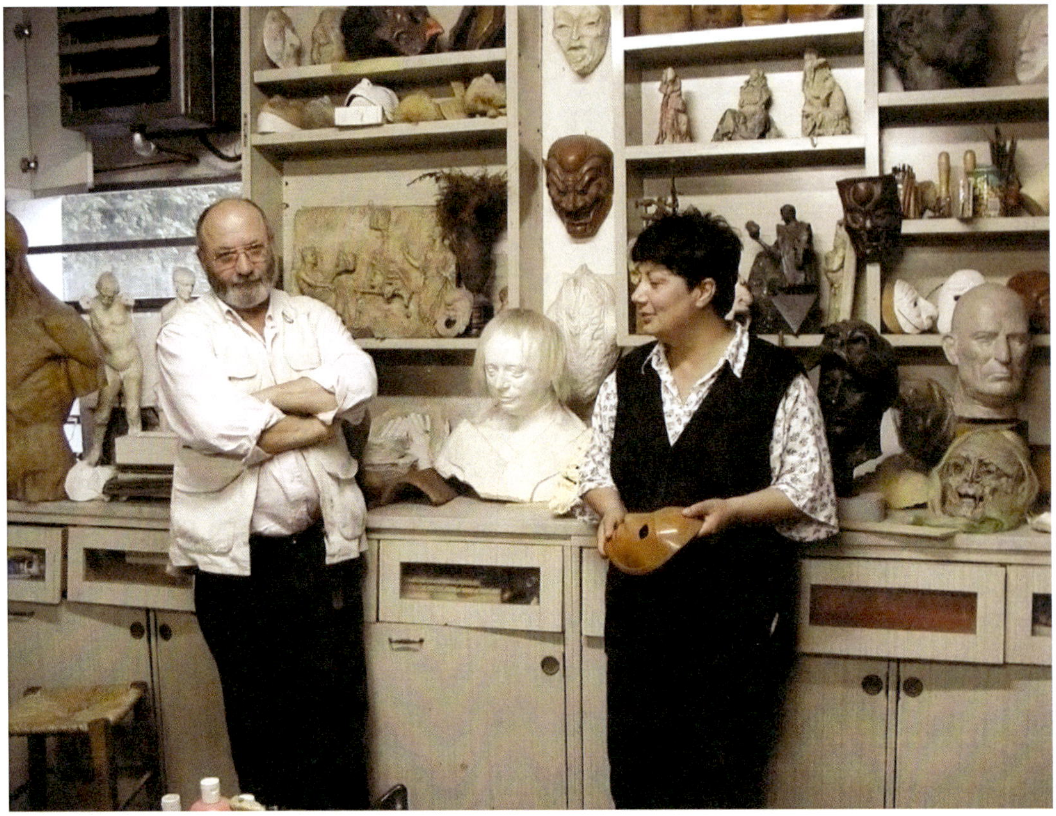

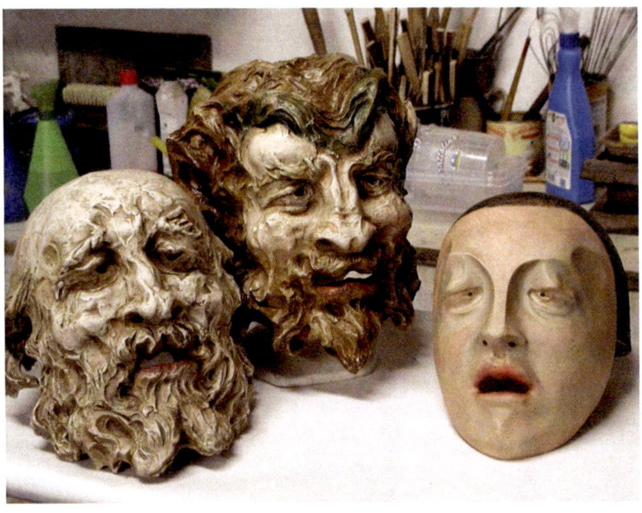

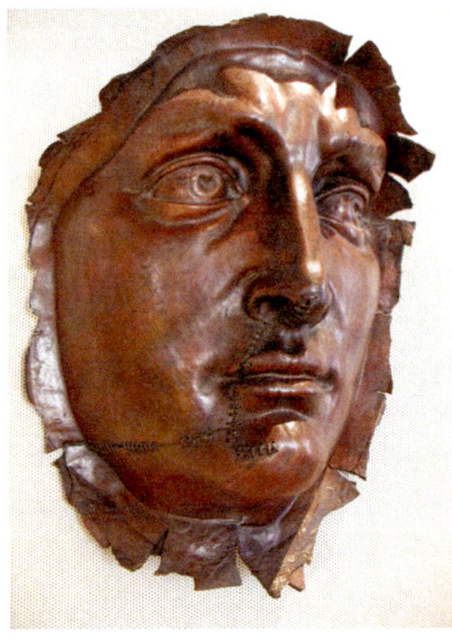

Top—Donato Sartori and Paola Piizzi in the workshop at Abano Terme, Italy. ***Bottom left***—Vibrophonic masks for the ***Oresteia*** by Aeschylus, directed by Peter Oskarson, Folkteatern, Gothenberg, Sweden, 2001. ***Right***—***Davide*** by Michelangelo—Gestural structure, dubbed leather, Art School of Porta Romana, seminar-workshop, 1981, created by Donato Sartori and sponsored by ***Centro Maschere e Strutture Gestuali.***

Swedish mask maker Torbjörn Alström

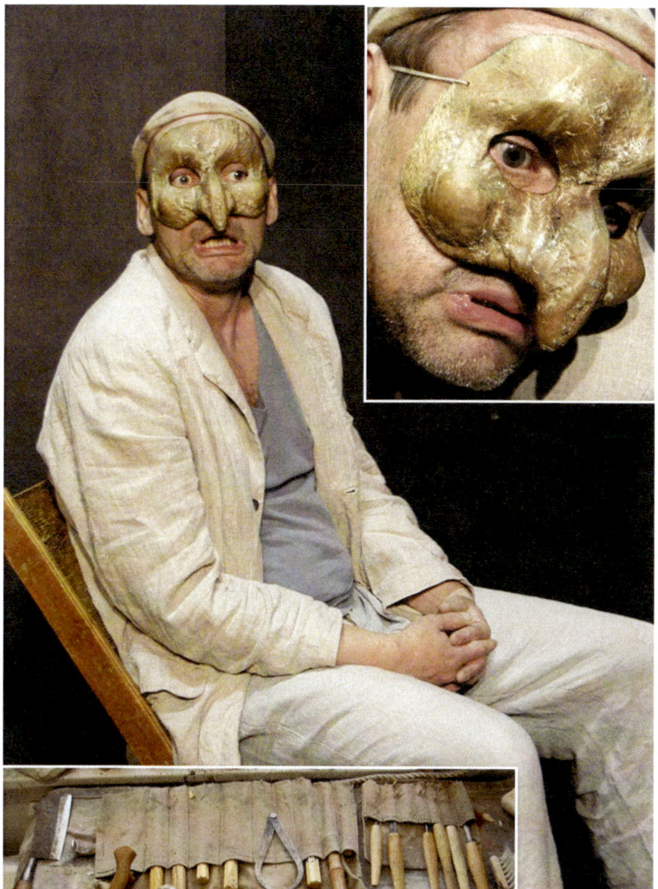

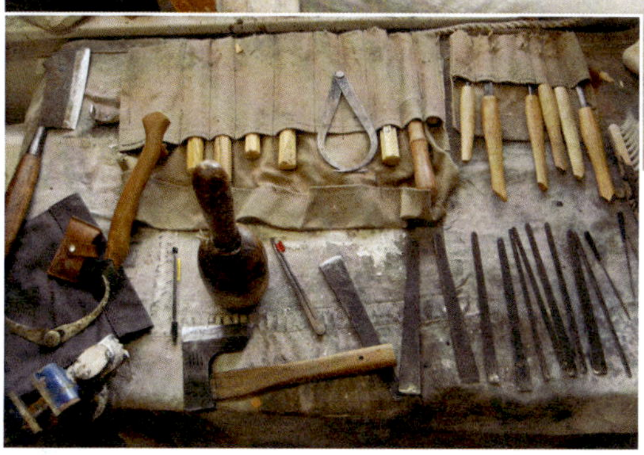

Right—Alström poignantly renders contemporary ***personae*** with ease and sensitivity. Here he performs in his Pulchinella mask, created from fish skin. ***Middle***—Alström's carving tools. ***Bottom, left to right***—(1) His artistry emerges from visceral archetypal details. (2) Alström's full mask in birchwood is for the solo dance piece ***Shadows in Water*** (2009) in collaboration with choreographer Maria Volmersson. The lips are made of black oak (oak that has been lying on the bottom of a river or lake for more than fifty years, darkening and starting to turn to stone) and the mask's forehead features silver wire fixed into the wood. Photograph courtesy of Torbjörn Alström. (3) He works in wood, leather, resins, and even fish skins. He created this fish mask from sea cat and salmon skin. Alström achieved this haunting effect while experimenting with various materials his ancestors in Sweden might have used to make masks. Photograph courtesy of Torbjörn Alström. (4) Alström's disturbing gas mask characters are as timeless as his versions of Pulchinella. This gas mask is from the dance performance ***Inaff*** (2007), created in collaboration with the dance company Raande Voo and choreographer Lena Josefsson. Photograph courtesy of Torbjörn Alström.

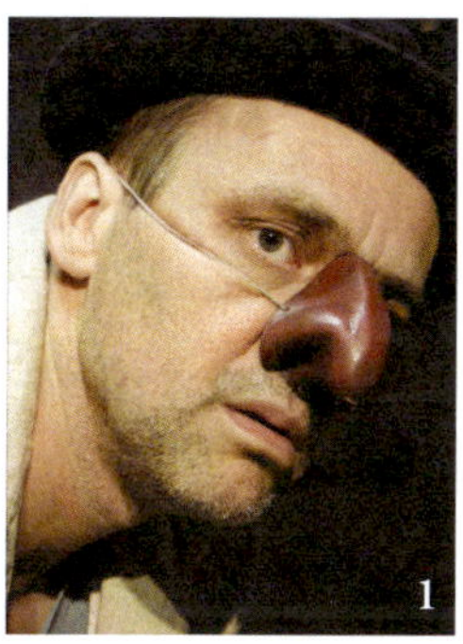

1

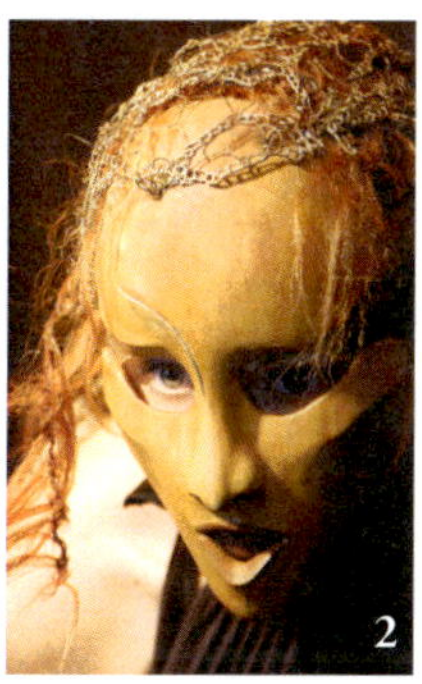

2

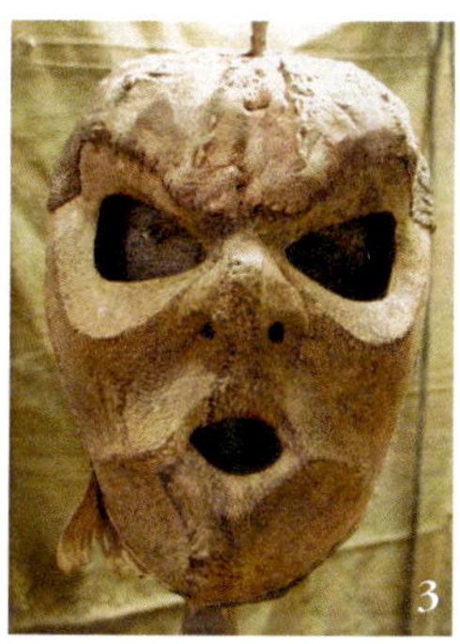

3

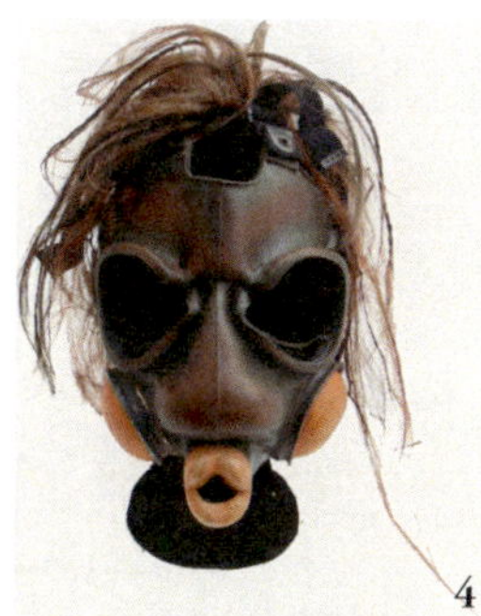

4

Japanese mask maker Iwasaki Kyoun

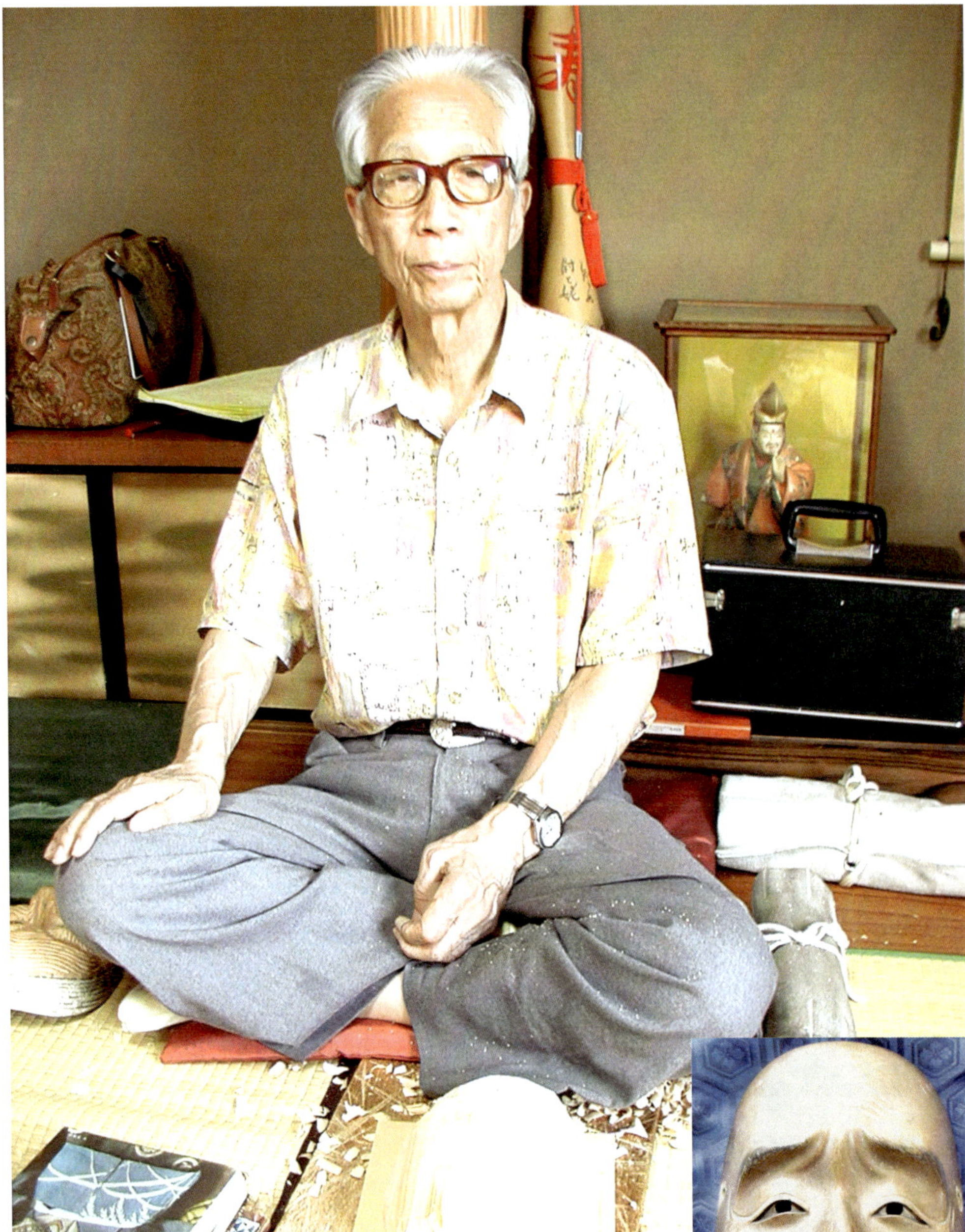

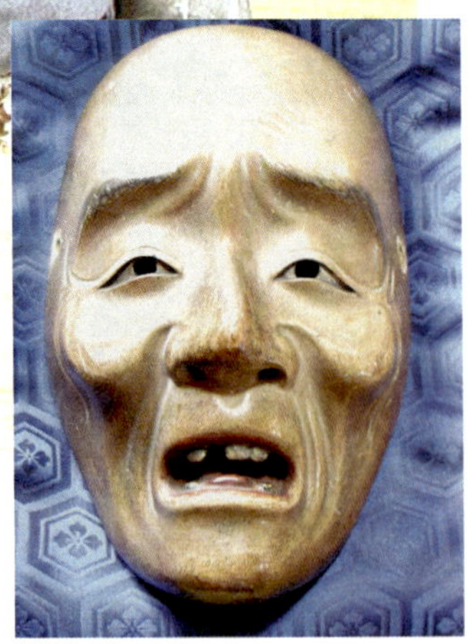

Above— Iwasaki Kyoun, now deceased, in his studio. He regularly performed in his masks well into his 80s, specializing in *Noh* masks. *Right*— Kyoun considered his carved wood "Despairing Woman" mask to be one of his triumphs in complexity.

Japanese mask maker Noboru Yoshikawa

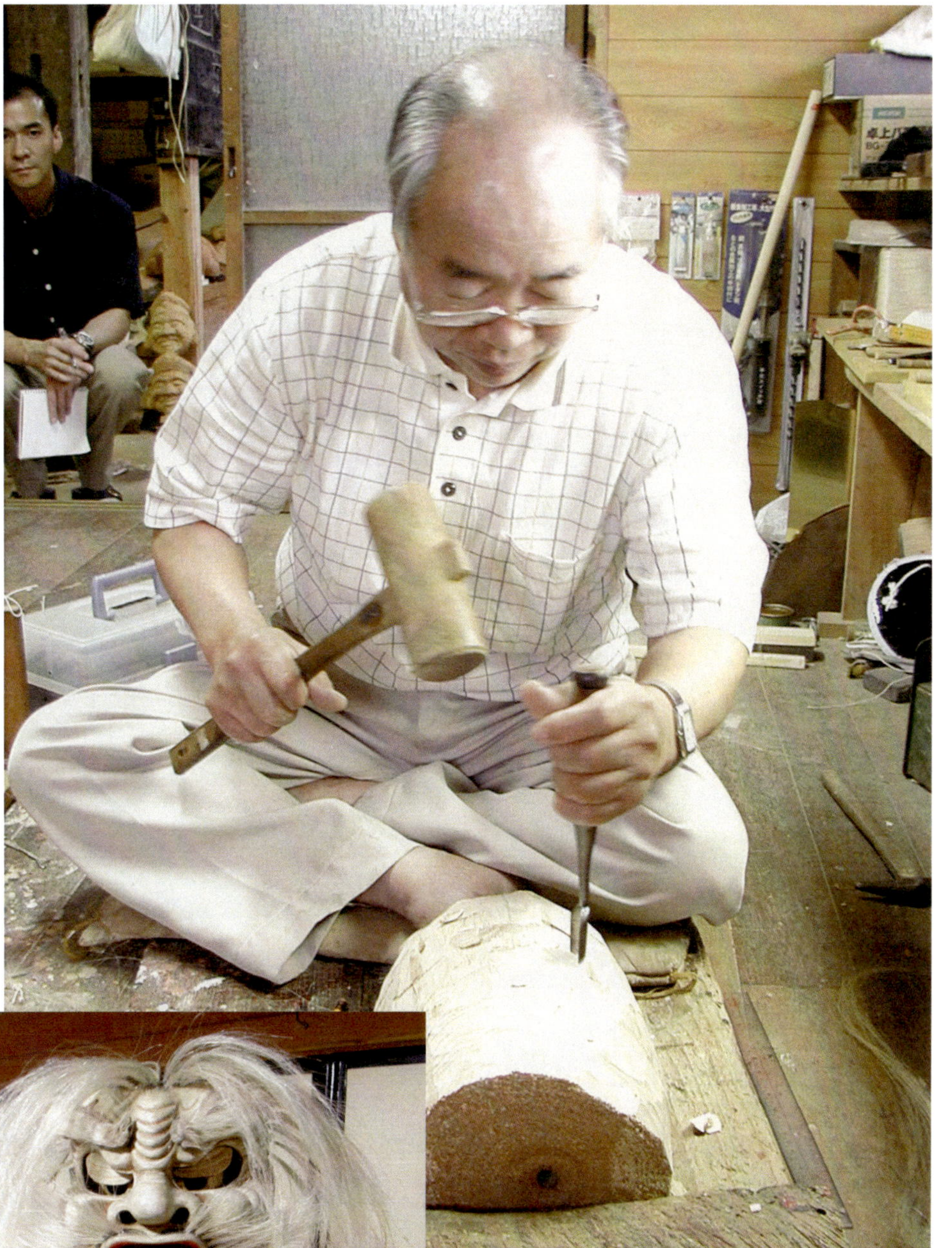

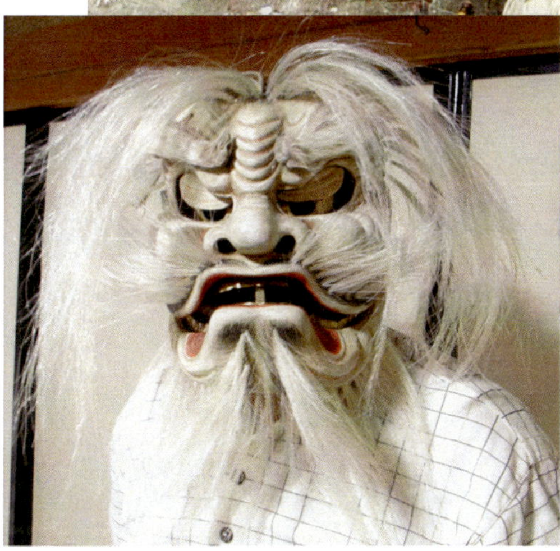

Above—A former mayor of his hometown, Noboru Yoshikawa delights in creating masks that represent his region's dragon spirit of the mountains. He also makes *Noh* masks. *Left*—Yoshikawa's elaborately carved wood dragon mask (representing the spirit of his nearby mountains) with movable mouth.

Mexican mask makers Juan Horta Castillo and Dalio Angel Perusquia

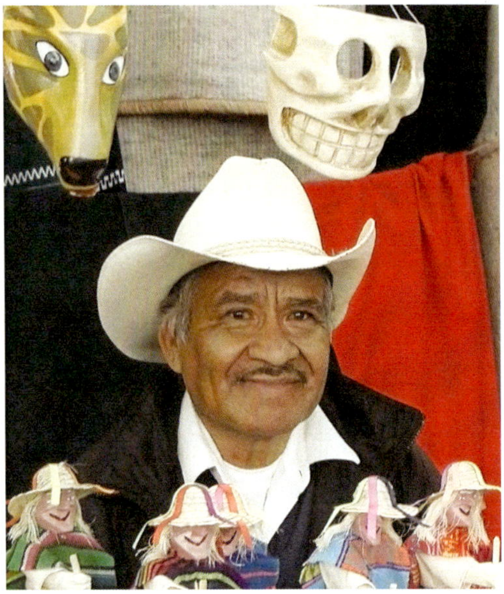

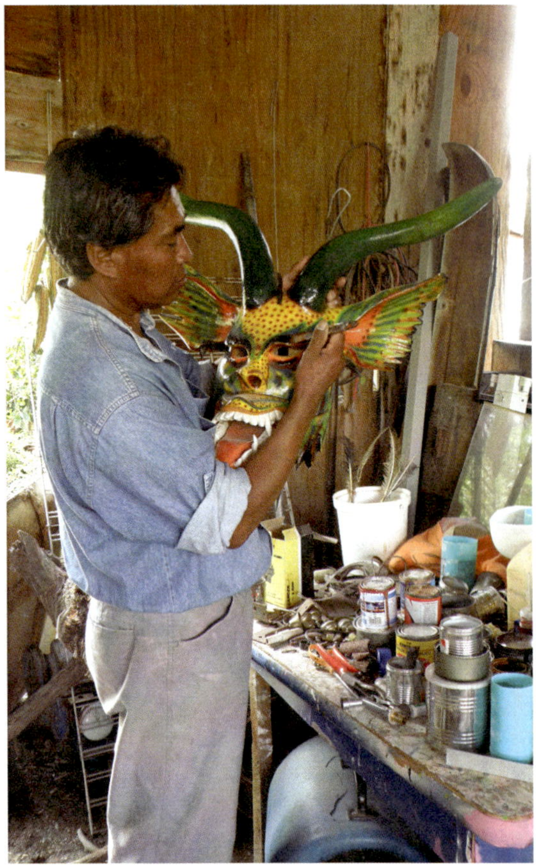

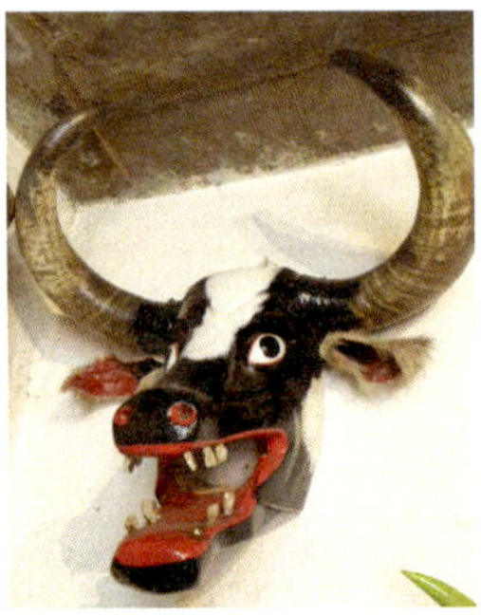

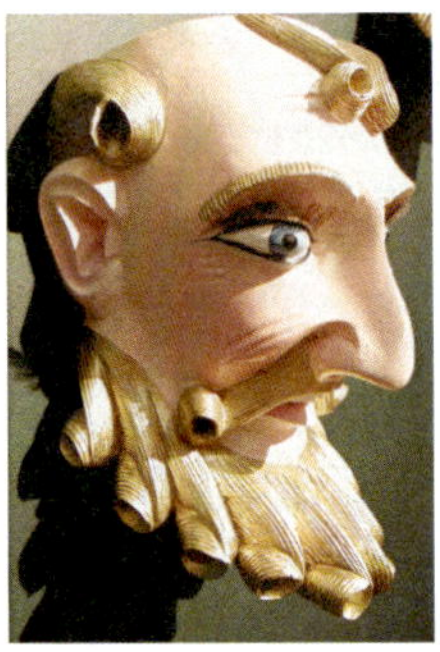

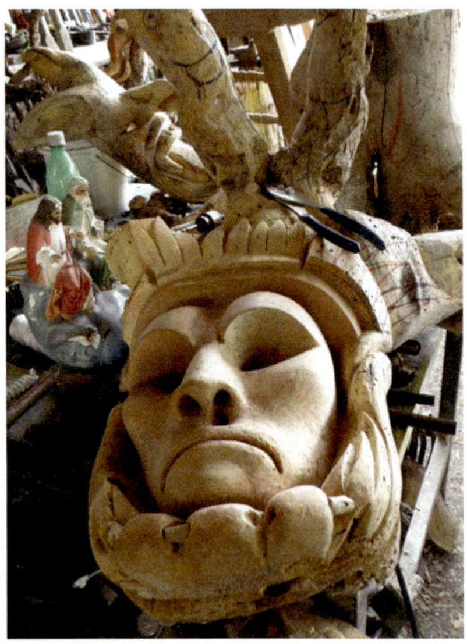

Top left—The late Mexican mask maker Juan Horta Castillo selling tourist masks in Pátzcuaro. Horta won many prizes over the years for his devil masks. His son, Manuel Abeiro Horta carries on his artistry. *Two masks above*—Carved wood devil mask by Juan Horta Castillo; and Castillo's hermit mask with gold hair and pink skin, which typically indicates a European complexion that easily burns in the Mexican sun. Many masks depicting Europeans/Spanish are derogatory, but the hermit is a gentle, kind, reclusive character and shows up in *Pastorela* celebrations along with Mary, Joseph, Jesus, and the shepherds. *Top right*—Dalio Angel Perusquia at his studio in San Bortolomé de Agua Caliente, painting finishing touches on an elaborate, brightly colored devil mask in carved wood. Devil masks are his speciality. *Right*—Perusquia's Pharisee mask for the Easter Holy Week celebrations in his hometown.

Mexican mask maker Antonio Cervantes Delgado

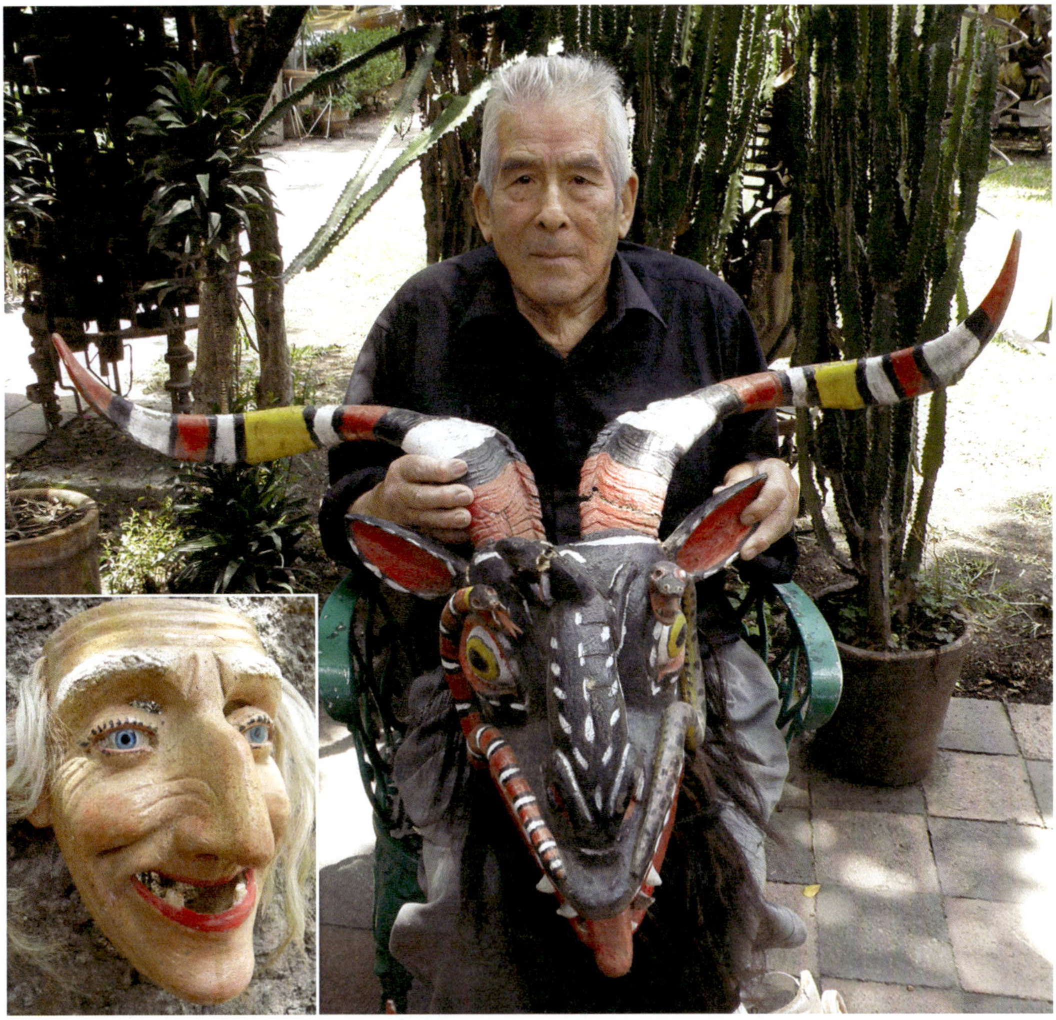

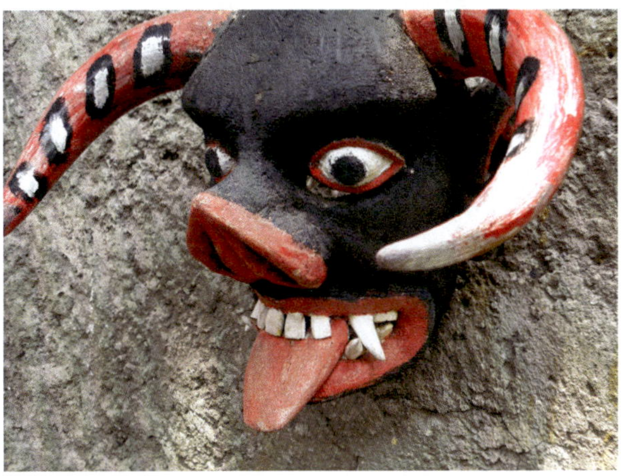

Top—Antonio Cervantes Delgado with carved wood devil mask. Several varieties of lizards indicate its facial features. Delgado has lived in Mexico City for most of his life. *Insert*—Delgado's carved wood hermit mask projects more vitality than the typical teenager. Slightly larger than head size, he has meticulously knotted and glued strands of human hair around the mask's perimeter. *Bottom left*—His devil bull mask created from *colorin* (a lightweight balsa wood). This increasingly rare wood still grows near Delgado's hometown in Michoacán.

Mexican mask makers Alicia Martínez Álvarez and Manuel Valencia Chavez

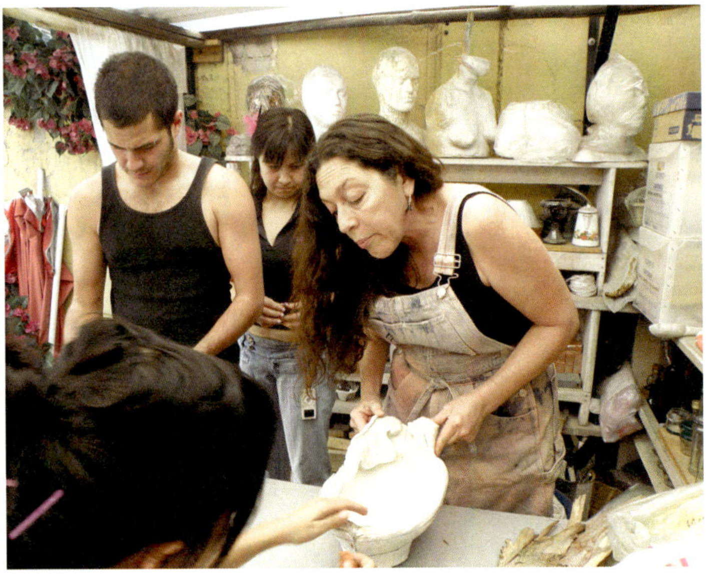

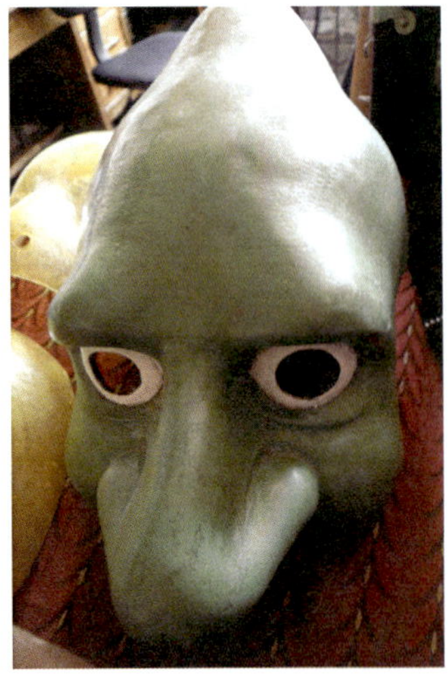

Top—Alicia Martínez Álvarez and performers from ***Laboratorio de la Máscara*** discuss ways to make the plaster negative mold for her Flute Mask (Chapter 3, page 127) at her studio in Mexico City. Her resin mask for Ubu in ***Ubu Roi*** (2006)—performed by members of her theatre company. ***Bottom left***—Manuel Valencia Chavez begins to carve the inside section of this mask. He uses an ax to make broad gouges. It takes as much exertion—perhaps more—to remove wood from mask cavity as it does to carve the mask's surface. ***Right***—His unique version of the carved wood "Little Mary" mask (***Maringuilla***) shines with an outer glaze coating and regularly appears in ***Pastorela*** celebrations.

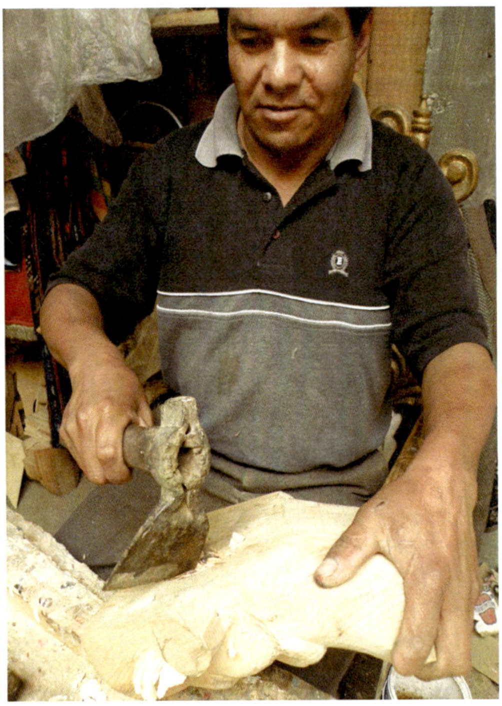

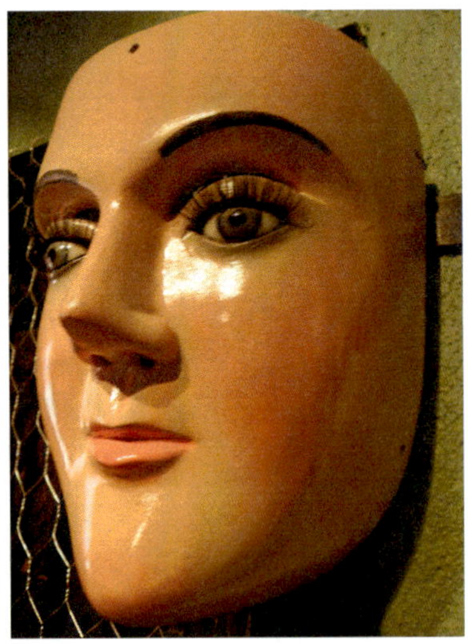

7

New Global Directions for Mask Makers

Artistic Considerations in Adapting Traditional Myths and Their Masks

In her book, *The Implied Spider*, myth theorist Wendy Doniger defines myth as a true sacred story believed by a group of people. Myth is deeply relevant to their existence. The myth is assumed to have been "written in the past, or more rarely, in the future." Myths and masks use metaphoric imagery to express meanings beyond the literal imagery. Earlier I quoted Victoria Nelson's explanation for the Greek and Latin artistic significance of the terms *metamorphosis* and *transformation* as descriptions of undergoing deep, unspoken, and often unconscious change. Doniger adds that "translation" and "metaphor" are English derivatives for Latin and Greek words that mean "bringing across." Just as a translation from a foreign language translates only so much, likewise a metaphor suggests a level of reality but not quite the full extent of that reality.[1] We use metaphor just as we use foreign phrases such as *joie de vivre* because they communicate a level of reality not easily expressed in the language at hand. Ultimately, a successful metaphor articulates a reality that is more truthful than actual reality.

Both myth and masks function artfully by using varying degrees of exaggerations found in metaphorical imagery and magically become more descriptive at a sublime level. For example, the mythic story of Adam and Eve in a garden "translates" as a garden of blissful union with God; the mask worn by a Balinese *Topeng* dancer "translates" into a supernatural character such as the heroic monkey king Sugriwa, found in the Hindu epic *The Ramayana*. The exaggerated image of the garden as blissful and non-violent or the exaggeration of both human and monkey features found in the Balinese *Topeng* mask are examples of metaphoric images that project realities beyond the immediate appearances.

While myths and masks function by using metaphorical imagery, William Bascom in his book *The Forms of Folklore: Prose Narratives* agrees with Doniger (and a number of other contemporary myth theorists) that the myth is indeed regarded as a sacred truth, at least within its own sphere of influence.[2] Conversely, the mask by itself is not generally considered to be a sacred truth, even when used in ritual or performance. We recognize the mask more often as an artifice that conjures up a more essential aspect of the supernatural force or character represented by the mask. Exceptions can be found in some archaic masks such as those used in African *Egungun* ritual, some Balinese sacred masked performances, or Eskimo shamanic rituals where the performer literally becomes the ghost, divinity, or spirit. But for most masked performances and masked rituals, the magic lies in a metaphorical image readily accessible within its audience's cultural, aesthetic, and historical boundaries.

This basic premise is worth repeating in order to underscore the mask's intent. That is, the traditional masked performance (and much of Western theatre throughout history) rarely denies its intention to project metaphorical illusion in order to present a deeper level of reality whereas the traditional myth suggests a literal level of truth inherent within its metaphorical illusion. For example, the raven mask in a Tsimshian performance or a *commedia dell'arte* mask are accepted at poetic levels, not as literal facts, while the majority of Christians believe that Jesus was literally resurrected on the third day after his death and ritualistically celebrate this event at Easter. Likewise, contemporary Balinese believe that witches and demons, along with manifestations of God, literally influence daily life and set artful sacrifices of food and flowers outside their homes and shops each day to appease the bad spirits and encourage the good.

Theodor H. Gaster in *Myth and Story* agrees with Raffaele Pettazzoni in acknowledging the myth as true story precisely because it is "sacred and explains creation from a religious point of view." He astutely compares memory and hope with myth by saying that what memory is to the past and what hope is to the future, likewise myth is to the present.[3] Robert Brockway in his book *Myth from the Ice Age to Mickey Mouse* further describes mythic thinking as "imaginative and also imaginal" but notes that mythic thinking is also "connected, structured, and linear." He considers myths ultimately as stories having a "beginning, middle, and end."[4]

Traditional masks tend to reflect the context of the myth by projecting specific characters or forces that also proceed sequentially in a narrated performance. Brockway makes a strong case in favor of defining Disneyland as a contemporary myth with a sequential order in its development as a cosmos. He does this, in part, by identifying (the masked) Mickey Mouse as an example of a contemporary archetypal figure who serves as the "prime mover" of this cosmos, projecting the Disneyland myth as a realization of the American Dream. Although the mask of Mickey never changes, Brockway recognizes that the plot lines of Mickey's various stories underscore various stages of development as they relate to the quintessential American pursuing the American Dream in various stages: as a young idealistic boy or man, and then as the corporate executive or wizard-artist in middle age.[5] Of course Mickey Mouse, like all divine forces, is eternal; he never grows old nor will he ever die.

Contemporary Viewpoints

No one has an absolute definition of masks. Trinidadians create huge motorized walking structures that theatrically function as masks. *Bunraku* puppeteers wear mask-like coverings while operating puppets with mask-like features. Nigerian festivals include masks worn on top of the head rather than on the face. Some consider the fashion show, with the model strutting down the runway to pulsating music, as a theatrical event and view her makeup and exaggerated expression as a mask used in performance. Peking Opera singers, some rock stars, and Japanese *Kabuki* performers wear white makeup with colorful accents as masks, indicating specific characters or states of being. Designers will occasionally refer to the embellishment around the mask (such as the headdress or stylized hair or collar) as the "frame" of the mask while others refer to a highly stylized costume in its entirety as a mask or masquerade.

Still, purists will claim that only a three-dimensional covering of the face can be called a mask. Others will only consider masks to be masks when they function in performance rather than hanging on a wall. We seem to recognize traditional masks most clearly as masks (in a variety of forms) when used in ritual and in legendary, folkloric, and mythic performances.

While masks might suggest a range of blurred definitions and assumptions according to the viewer, the task of defining myths also provokes a range of opinions among theorists. Most myth theorists agree with Doniger and Bascom regarding their premise that the traditional myth is sacred for the audience it serves, though they concurrently acknowledge the irony that recent popular sentiment more often assumes any myth to be a "lie" or at best "fiction."

The problem of defining myth increases in complexity when we attempt to compare and contrast myth with other types of narrative. Bronislaw Malinowski categorizes the idea of myth within the context of "clearly distinguishable types of story" such as "the fairy tale, the legend, and the saga," though he consistently refers to myth as "the sacred tale" and at least according to archaic viewpoints a myth suggests a "living reality."[6] Bascom explores a range of opinion regarding basic characteristics of myth and how these characteristics blur in comparison and contrast with other narrative prose. At one point, he cites Hultkrantz's description of one particular example of myth as the "true narrative of gods and divine kings whose actions take place at the beginning of the world." Bascom then describes Hultkrantz's related example of legend which is comprised of humans, heroes, and supernatural forces (like myth) but pronounces legendary stories (like myth) also true. Later, Bascom quotes the great cultural anthropologist Sir James Frazer, who distinguishes myth as having its source in reason (science) while the legend has its source in memory (history) and the folktale has its source in imagination (Romance.)[7]

Robert Brockway cites a number of scholars of popular literature when he asserts that since the beginning of the nineteenth century, the definition of myth has broadened to include sacred history, literary epics, and popular genre literature such as Westerns, Gothics, science fiction, fantasy tales, and romances. He states that "even if not all these categories are considered forms of myths, they have mythic overtones and implications." This broader, more contemporary definition allows him to propose that the cosmos of Disneyland be considered a current global myth with Mickey Mouse as a current mythic [masked] character.[8] Apparently, just as an audience defines a mask, a myth is ultimately defined according to the myth's interpreter.

Contemporary Mythology as Psychology

Not coincidentally, according to a number of myth theorists and psychologists, the realms of mythology and psychology intersect because both address the great dramatic tensions of living: emotional states of fear and desire. In her book, *The Absence of Myth*, Heller identifies a number of myth theorists over the years who have stated in various ways that mythology is, indeed, psychology.[9]

Perhaps the concept of personal myth simply implies a synthesis of imaginative personal narration and the articulation of personal artistic and spiritual values. Brockway declares that myth has descended to the underworld "like a river that plunges underground. Myths are consciously rejected and persist sub-consciously and unconsciously."[10] He agrees with Campbell's theory that "the modern and post-modern mythogenetic zone is actually the psyche of the creative artist, poet, novelist, playwright, and short story writer. Since the artist is in touch with the inner depths from which fantasies and dreams emerge, he plays a role in modern and post-modern society akin to that of the shaman in archaic societies. He [the artist] is the medium of the psychic underworld. In a figurative sense, he communes with spirits."[11]

Heller recalls Joseph Campbell's assertion that "myth is the public dream and the individual's dream is the private myth."[12] Furthermore, she cites Campbell's Romantic belief that mythology can be considered both "a social as well as spiritual necessity."[13] Some theorists reject the notion that myths have potential to be universally recognized (that is, springing from the deep wells of a collective unconscious). Others suggest that myth has relevance at most for the local collective unconscious of the audience it serves and springs from a personal interpretation. Heller summarizes this dilemma by noting that myth has not only been "split between the archaic and modern it is now further divided between the collective and the individual."[14]

Yet Heller remains skeptical about the "problem of gods and goddesses within us" and is convinced that "personal mythology is far more concerned with the personal than it is with myth, citing Joseph Campbell biographer Stephen Larsen's position that, 'Personal myth is born out of humankind's unwillingness to endorse the loss of myth.'" She doubts the concept of accessing the god or goddess from within and persuasively questions the validity of a collective unconscious, suspecting that a problem ensues when people assign more significance to personal narrative than can be measured. She wonders, for example, why "motherhood must take on the sacred qualities of earth and mother goddesses and cannot just be plain motherhood. Never mind that any appropriation of the goddess is only partial and abstract, unable to incorporate the full range and power of what she represented when actively, obediently, reverently, communally, and fearfully, if need be, worshipped."[15]

Another vagary regarding myths' influences on either personal or collective unconscious states rests with the artistic agendas of the myth maker and mask maker. While the popular artist or folk artist, according to Brockway, "caters to popular moods," the innovative artist "articulates a personal vision, draws upon his or her own imagination, and expresses his or her own soul. Brockway goes on to compare the innovative artist to a "mystic in religion," whereas the popular artist is like the "shaman or popular preacher."[16] He summarizes the polarities of these two artistic strategies:

> While the serious novelist or artist plunges deep into his own psyche and produces a work of individual self-expression, the popular writer paradoxically draws from deeper wells, those of the collective unconscious. The commercial writer does not reveal his soul. He is a craftsman who uses his technical skills to perform a pragmatic function. The aim is to entertain [or, one could add — to heal]. The process is impersonal and does not draw on his life experience, affects, yearnings, hopes, and fears. Yet precisely because the professional writer works from formulas, he reveals the archetypes of the collective unconscious. His stories are mythic. To be sure, the novelist plunges far deeper than his own psyche, but since all he says emerges through the medium of his consciousness, the archetypes are camouflaged.[17]

However one views the relevance of these correlations between mythology and psychology, the range of perspectives provides clues to the unique creative response of a specific traditional mask maker toward his or her mask.

Global Issues Concerning the Balance Between Universal and Local Knowledge

Another issue when analyzing the creative challenges of traditional mask makers on a global scale lies with the dilemma of comparing quite divergent artistic and spiritual agendas. Additionally, how does one describe archetypal, subliminal forces found in masked performance? Some (especially Jungian proponents) will classify archetypal forces as part of the vast universal collective unconscious of humanity while contemporary anthropologists will contest local artistic expression as having little if any universal impact spanning time, place, and cultures.

Indeed, while Brockway introduces the concept of universal mythic influences by describing Frazer's literary work *The Golden Bough* as "a vast, encyclopedic study of magic, totemism, and myth" and tracing the universalism held by later myth theorists such as Freud, Jung, Eliade, and Campbell back to Frazer's early-twentieth-century influence,[18] cultural anthropologist Clifford Geertz explores this topic from a substantially different viewpoint in his book *Local Knowledge*. He initially introduces the issue by stating that "the question is not whether art (or anything else) is universal; it is whether one can talk about West African carving, New Guinea palm-leaf painting, quattrocento picture making, and Moroccan versifying in such a way as to cause them to shed some sort of light on one another."[19] Later he insists, "we can never apprehend another people's or another period's imagination neatly, as though it were our own,"[20] concluding that "the giving to art objects [such as masks and masked performances] a cultural significance, is always a local matter ... no matter how universal the intrinsic qualities that actualize its emotional power may be."[21]

Eventually, however, Geertz admits that "the hallmark of modern consciousness is its enormous multiplicity,"[22] which essentially subscribes to Doniger's theory that "the mind itself, the basis of language and myth is part of what could truly be called a World Wide Web."[23] While she suggests that "globalization and diversification have come to power simultaneously and continue to egg each other on,"[24] she and Geertz apparently believe that ultimately universality lies within the multiplicity of local detail.

Bascom adds to this perspective by suggesting that native myths are not "universally recognized but can be meaningfully applied cross-culturally."[25]

Recognizing the wide range of opinion between the relevance of universalism versus local knowledge, some artistic forms of expression still invariably take on profound significance across cultures, or at least collective cultures. Most people from any locale can viscerally relate to the scene in *The Gold Rush* in which Charlie Chaplin (arguably wearing a mask of moustache and eyebrows) cheerfully cooks, eats, and savors a shoe because he is starving. Likewise, masked performances easily span cultures and historical periods, partly because human facial expression itself (if not the localized myth associated with the specific facial expression and style) universally occurs across continents and time. And as the Internet makes our global village increasingly smaller, the issue of local knowledge's impact becomes perhaps less significant regardless.

New Myths or New Perspectives

If the Internet is making our global village smaller as we assimilate various local myths, traditions, and styles into a global consciousness of Doniger's "multiplicity of local detail," do we need new, more universally recognized myths to help unify an Internet-driven global society that could conceivably assist us in withstanding threats of terrorism, overpopulation, global warming, and nuclear destruction? Or have we moved beyond mythic solutions for social and psychological harmony?

Susan Mackey-Kallis cites the conclusion of Janice Rushing and Thomas Frentz when they assert that "the new myth for humankind needs to be a *quest,* not a *conquest*; its purpose, to *search* rather than to *search and destroy.*"[26] Since traditional masks tend to reflect local myths, legends, or folklore (not new myths or "a" new myth for our time) perhaps this lack of a new myth is one reason why many contemporary traditional mask makers have reached a critical creative juncture. They tend to find themselves either creating masks for increasingly obscure local myths or struggling to respond to vague (or as yet unidentified) global myths that are perhaps still evolving into coherent forms. Even more problematic for non-traditional mask makers, Heller states that "the postmodern myth maker or myth-seeker [or postmodern mask maker] does not choose fabrication as a means toward self-satisfaction or blissful anesthetization. Rather, the postmodern myth-seeker has no choice but to follow where the gods may lead, even if into an abyss."[27]

One could speculate that traditional mask makers seem to be disappearing because they are clinging to the old forms of traditional myths in spite of increasing global recognition that local cultural values are giving way to more universal (some would argue, diluted) cultural and spiritual trends. One point of commonality that might lead toward a resolution of local versus universal tensions between (local) mythic time and postmodern time is Heller's suggestion that "both are [ultimately] outside of history." She adds that "for a new myth of consciousness, the 'meaning' is apprehended neither through ritual or a collective center but through absence, through disengagement and nonattachment. The nothingness or emptiness that is not an existential, personalized crisis but rather a gateway into the formless engendering all life, the space between the two breaths, or the logical negativity of the soul — this negative opening understands the questions of meaning and meaninglessness to be irrelevant."[28]

Several contemporary traditional mask makers I've interviewed increasingly wonder why their masks are not revered or appreciated as they once were. As Heller's global postmodern consciousness takes on more universal appeal, the sacred local traditions of the mask maker begin to appear as distant, blurred memories. The masked performance religious rituals receive less attention in the communities they were meant to serve. The folkloric mask presents local characters and forces no longer relevant to its community.

Brockway, drawing on eighteenth-century philosopher and historian Gianbattista Vico's theory of universal cyclical patterns in history, suggests similar cyclical patterns found in the evolution of myths. Each historic cycle, according to Vico, commences with an "Age of Gods," then progresses to an "Age of Heroes," and culminates with an "Age of Men," only to repeat the pattern throughout history. Likewise, Brockway perceives a similar cyclic pattern in myth development.[29] Based on this premise, one could also assume that contemporary myths have evolved to an "Age of Men" phase, with an emphasis on the power of the individual to influence existence and creation.

If this is true, those traditional mask makers who pursue the creation of self-expressive masks over traditional mythic or folkloric masks have potential to forge a creative connection between the traditional local myths and today's universal myths in various stages of development. Ironically, universal concepts of the human condition seem more vividly evident within the most personal experiences of the individual, regardless of one's views on the collective unconscious or lack thereof. Doniger considers this circumstance a valid perspective as she cites soprano Jessye Norman's observation that "art brings us together as a family because it is an individual expression of a universal sentiment."[30]

Furthermore, Brockway maintains that myth currently flourishes "in the popular arts where it is purest," that is, where myth is most effectively and unconsciously experienced.[31] Using Brockway's more contemporary definition of myth, one could entertain the notion that Mickey Mouse's Disneyland is a universally recognized (or at least internationally recognized) global cosmology for our time by mass audiences who do not think of Disneyland in terms of traditional myth. Nevertheless the average family assumes Disneyland to be a highly valued point of destination reflecting a true reality that aspires to an ideal lifestyle in a mythic manner of thinking.[32]

Meanwhile Brockway notes additional "human-generated" examples of significant mythic themes, such as those found in children's fantasy literature.[33] Heller offers a similar viewpoint, identifying the clearest expressions of myth as found in "fantasy fiction or films such as ... *The Lord of the Rings, Harry Potter, The Matrix*" yet acknowledges, "No matter how deeply these creations may engross and inspire us, we still look for the ordinary human being behind the curtain pulling all the strings."[34]

Bruce Butterfield, adhering to a different version of cyclical pattern of myth, suggests, "In the end of course, ancient myths are also our new-age myths — a body, labyrinthine, within, moving outward into the universe, weaving new stories from old, telling the universal story, always becoming."[35] Joseph Campbell voiced a similar consideration when he suggested that *Star Wars* might be just such an ancient myth, forever becoming new by incorporating "new," though essentially archaic, archetypal heroes and demons into a "new" plot.[36] One can argue that the *Star Wars* myth was at least new (within the context of the history of mythology) in its cinematic form and indeed offered new mythic heroes along with protective and demonic forces. It has captured a wide range of international audiences (conceivably defining it as a global myth). Still others will insist that even this international screen story simply projects yet another American Western cowboy myth using Caucasian characters and robots.

As discussed in chapter 6, if we accept current popular fantasy films and children's literature as fertile ground for either new myths or recycled old myths, we can more readily understand why traditional masks which so often accompanied the ancient myths and legends still linger to portray elemental divine, heroic, demonic, and protective forces in our current popular forms of entertainment. We frequently see examples of exaggerated "masked" characters not only in versions of children's literature such as *Alice in Wonderland* and *Winnie the Pooh* but also see many masked characters on the Broadway stage in musicals and dramatic works (*The Lion King, Avenue Q, Wicked, Beauty and the Beast, Phantom of the Opera, Gem of the Ocean, Blue Man Group*) or in fantasy or animated films (*The Hobbit, The Lord of the Rings, The Chronicles of Narnia*, and *Toy Story*).

While Brockway's proposed Disneyland myth readily correlates to his reference to the "Age of Man" mythic period (as does Heller's and Campbell's considerations of children's fantasy literature as human mythic inventions underscoring our current ages of heroes, antiheroes, and good guys), we might conceivably expect the next cycle of an "Age of Gods" to be forthcoming, also at a global level. How better to project this new global "Age of Gods" if not by masked religious sacred rituals as well as secular performances on stage and in film? Whatever cycle comes next, the artifice of the mask in its various forms with universally recognized human facial expression holds the strongest potential to make upcoming evolutions in global values most evident.

Contemporary special-effects artists do well to observe the attitudes and creative approaches of traditional mask makers before their traditions disappear along with themselves, often representing generations of cultural, spiritual, aesthetic, and historical perspectives toward mythic masks. We need both the traditional folk artist and the innovative contemporary artist to find some balance between the world's great spiritual traditions and the tensions of life in our current precarious time. Heller reminds us that "the stories, the poesis, still seek to tell the truth of living in a particular culture in a particular time, whatever the truth may be."[37] Even if these truths hearken back to earlier times, they provide insight and perspective for our current crises. Once these mask makers disappear, contemporary special-effects mask artists lose the insights of traditional mask making forever, unless we document traditional work and creative processes.

On the other hand, by seeking inspiration in the archaic myth traditions, rather than accepting these myths as sacred truths, we all pay a price. The artists and audiences today lose the greatest potential level of vitality regarding the myths' truths. To a much greater extent, current generations must accept and seek the forbidden knowledge beyond the myth. The traditional myths become much more distant echoes of the ideal and the eternal; truth becomes (even more) relative. This is not necessarily negative. A number of contemporary traditional mask makers I've interviewed obviously already make masks with the assumption that their masks no longer relate directly or literally to the myths and legendary stories that originally inspired them. Many no longer believe in their masks' power to conjure up literal divine forces, for example, though their masks invariably possess some level of archetypal and mythic expressions.

Wendy Doniger explores this basic assumption of relative truth in *The Implied Spider*, asserting that regardless the level of truth one ascribes to a sacred myth, it can consistently function as a "tool" or "lens" to describe the various layers of relative truths behind myths. She believes that one can interpret a myth through the "broad lens" of the universalist view, the "middle view" of the naked eye, and the "theorist's microscopic view," suggesting ultimately that God is in the details, however one interprets the details.[38] Joseph Campbell makes a similar statement in his eloquent conclusion to his major work *Primitive Mythology: The Masks of God*:

> Mythology—and therefore civilization—is a poetic, supernormal image, conceived, like all poetry, in depth, but susceptible of interpretation on various levels. The shallowest minds see in it the local scenery; the deepest, the foreground of the void; and between are all the stages of the Way from the ethnic to the elementary idea, the local to the universal being, which is Everyman, as he both knows and is afraid to know. For the human mind in its polarity of the male and female modes of experience, in its passages from infancy to adulthood and old age, in its toughness and tenderness, and in its continuing dialogue with the world, is the ultimate mythogenetic zone—the creator and destroyer, the slave and yet the master, of all the gods.[39]

And yet, as Heller insists, "We cannot have it both ways. We cannot be the ones wielding myth as a tool or lens and then act as if something outside of us has all the power."[40]

For mask makers, this becomes a crucial issue. Are the divine forces that inspire the makers of the mask external rather than internal? If so, masks that reflect divinity and eternal truths are indeed sacred. If mythic divine forces exist instead within ourselves (and not within a global context), each mask maker plays God on some level. The question becomes how one mask maker's mask can be universally divine at the exclusion of another mask maker's mask.

The Absence of Traditional Myths

Heller reflects that, "far from serving as a unifying force that can restore a lost connection between humankind and the divine, myth ... becomes a great detractor." She declares that "it is one thing to ask whether there is myth today and another to ask whether we are between myths."[41] If we assume that myths no longer exist, obviously we are not in a transitional stage in which traditional local myths are evolving into new globally (as yet fully recognized) universal myths.

The belief that myths no longer exist haunts a number of today's myth theorists and seems the basis for the anxiety of a number of mask makers I've interviewed. Heller clearly articulates this perspective in *The Absence of Myth*: "Myths are gone; the gods are dead." Even the natural elements of the world are no longer "divinely personified." She observes that they have been gone for at least hundreds of years, though this premise has yet to be universally acknowledged by the world. "In many respects we are truly alone. Perhaps it is the fear of this aloneness that lies at the bottom of the yearnings for life, people, God, even ourselves, to be so much more than everything already is. And perhaps it is the notion that life must be far more than it is that leads to the expectation that we be filled with something we do not have and cannot see that we might not need."[42]

Yet humanity might be incapable, at least in the near future, of accepting the idea that existence is never eternal. All living things (and myths) eventually fade away, even if existence appears temporarily cyclical (as Brockway's description of traditional cyclical "eternal return" myths indicates) or constantly progressive (as Brockway's description of the traditional hero vs. dragon myths indicates).[43] Accordingly, Heller reflects on Joseph Campbell's musings on the necessity of myths when he asks, "What is the meaning of a flower? And having no meaning, should flowers, then, not be?" She also recalls Campbell's reference to traditional myth as "a secure circle," while recognizing that without the traditional myth today, "the circle is open and its circumference is nowhere and its center is everywhere."[44]

At the end of her exhaustive exploration of the relevance (or lack of relevance) of traditional myths at this time, she acknowledges the probability that Campbell's notion of "experiencing the act of being alive" is as good as it gets. Furthermore, "we have to be willing to release the attachment as to how life should be and be penetrated by life—and by things far less idyllic than bucolic summer walks."[45]

Heller concludes by citing Peter Homans' view that the symbolic loss of our myths is worth mourning over and observes that "cultural forms such as film and theatre [especially theatre of masked performance], for example, can function as [public] monuments."[46] But must the monuments be dreary? Perhaps performers of the Everyman masks (such as those wearing *commedia* masks) have at least unconsciously acknowledged the abyss, but mask maker and masked performer Rob Faust offers an intentional glimpse into the abyss with today's humor.

Rob Faust: Mask Messenger

Rob Faust's superb work as a mask maker and masked performer vividly blends the traditions of this ancient art form with a hip, contemporary vision. He easily adapts to modest or elaborate performance spaces while humorously integrating a range of provocative topics that explore the pathos and yearnings of our human condition. He encourages reflection at both elementary and sublime levels with seemingly effortless skill. Faust personally develops and makes all of his expressive masks and is equally comfortable working with wood, leather, Celastic (a carcinogen no longer legal to produce), and neoprene. He has also experimented with fiberglass, papier-mâché, and bronze.

As an American expatriate living in Toronto since 2001, Faust has continued to perform with Faustwork Mask Theatre, a company he created as a one-man show in 1983. He has trained over a dozen masked performers to present his acclaimed, long-running touring shows, *The Mask Messenger*, *Little Big Frog*, and *Faustwork in Concert*, taking these productions throughout the United States and Canada and beyond to countries in Asia and Europe for over two decades. He has toured theatres, festivals, universities, corporate events, and schools in England, Australia, Italy, South Africa, Hong Kong, Singapore, Israel, and Brunei. Examples of significant venues where he has appeared include the Sydney Opera House, the Metropolitan Museum of Art, the Kennedy Center, and the Maui Arts and Cultural Center. His original, provocative, and frequently humorous work has a level of sophistication that goes beyond most masked performances. He enjoys substantial commercial success, although this has never been his primary objective.

In addition to a company manager and outreach coordinator, Faust currently commissions six performers; four tour the United States and two tour Canada. He himself performs frequently and over the years has used these performances as laboratories in which to hone his craft along with the original masked personalities created for *The Mask Messenger*.

This long-standing experience in masked performance work has served as a foundation for Faust's current corporate entertainment and speaking engagements, along with workshops that focus on a variety of themes, such as leadership, non-verbal communication, and sales techniques. When communication master and celebrated speaker Nido Qubein first saw Faust's performance at a corporate event, he declared Faust not "just" an entertainer, but an innovative speaker who uses masks. Qubein encouraged him to develop more of these inspirational guest appearances for business corporations, focusing on entrepreneurial activity and leadership skills, using masked role playing and character development as workshop exercises. Rob Faust still manages to tour with *The Mask Messenger* while also offering his successful corporate presentations, which he has entitled *Behind the Mask*.

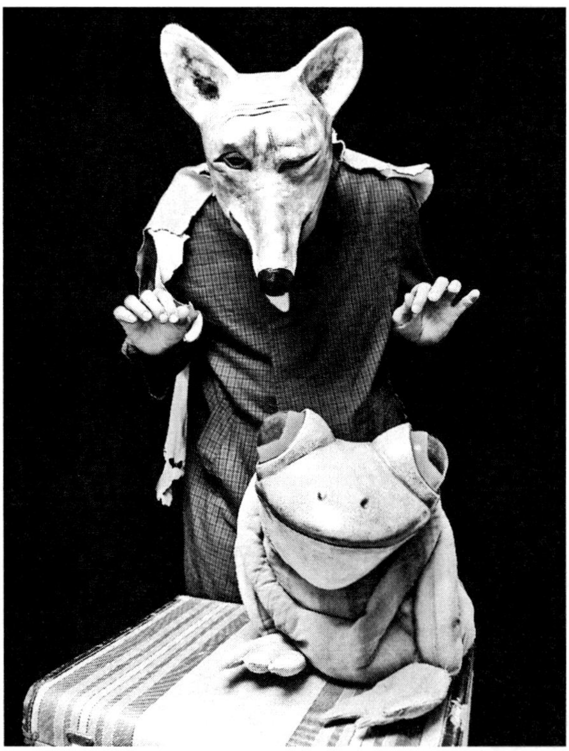

Scene from Rob Faust's *Frog Prince* skit. Photographer: Ron Naversen.

The Importance of Play in Faust's Work

Faust credits his delight in "the act of play" as well as his ability to savor the wonderment of playfulness for much of his success. "Play/fun onstage is indeed very important but linked as well to my approach toward living and developing my masks," he says. "Several clown workshops I've taken over the years with Philippe Gaulier, Avner Eisenberg (Avner the Eccentric), and Sue Morrison have strongly influenced my work. Clowns wear their hearts and feelings on their skin; reveal reveal reveal; and have fun on stage so that the audience will too. Clowns work the room and consider accidents such as ringing cell phones, subways rumbling, babies crying, and latecomers as gifts to acknowledge, use, and play with. These accidents keep us all in the present, in the room. The audience feels as if anything can happen. *The Mask Messenger* is play, not a play. I will stop performing it when it the work of it outweighs the joy of it."[47]

Although his work is hugely popular with young audiences, Rob Faust considers his public and corporate masked performances a "thinking man's form of entertainment" that builds on the premise that we are all fifth graders at heart. "Young and old audiences alike want me to mystify them, trick them, play with them," he says. His corporate presentations utilize his mask projects in order to illustrate the human face of business. He considers his workshops most successful when his corporate audience members recognize the childlike aspects within themselves when they see or wear his masks. "We all want permission to believe in magic again."[48]

"It took me a long time to define myself as an artist," he continues. "I find my mask work fun and compelling. I'm not sure why. Before making masks, I used masks as a training tool in physical theatre performance preparation. My masks evolve from my instincts and natural abilities as a dancer and actor. I can make them as art, or use them as tools, toys, and craft. They serve as my inner dialogue, 'my take' on people. I have great fascination for the fact that people are so similar, yet so completely unique. Masks and masked performance encourage a playful way to see human nature and engage the world. The motivation behind my mask work is not so much a spiritual quest or a search for the meaning of life; it expresses, in the words of Joseph Campbell, 'the experience' of being alive."[49]

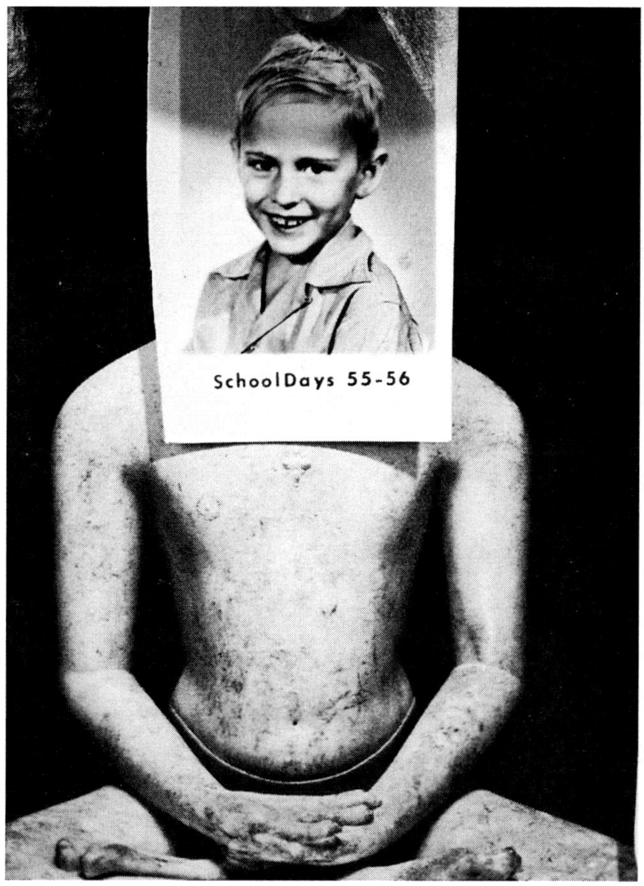

Inspirational photograph in Rob Faust's mask studio, Toronto.

Faust savors this experience of "being alive" by bringing a playful attitude not only in the final activity of formal presentation but earlier when he is actually creating the mask and developing the character for the mask. Like any artist, he has recognized this sense of wonderment as a quality in the act of play from his earliest years of artistic development. No doubt this has been historically part of the creative process for typical traditional mask makers, though I have never heard any of the mask makers I've interviewed specifically describe this activity of play as an important consideration for them.

For Faust the act of play is as simple and as crucial as the act of fishing. Indeed, he considers these acts synonymous in terms of the creative state they generate for him. He experiences the same level of curiosity and unpredictability inherent in a typical fishing excursion as he experiences in the act of play. "I'm not sure what is under the water," he says. "I must be totally in the moment and improvise at will. My imagination becomes crystallized with the moment of reality. I escape the pressures and concerns of my life." Many people describe the consciousness of fishing as similar to daydreaming. The actual experience of fishing induces a heightened level of awareness yet still allows for an awareness of the actual act of fishing. Faust describes fishing as an activity where "I must see and read the wind, the light, the currents, the surface of the water, the birds, and the other critters around me. These elements become the pressures and demands of that moment. For me fishing is serious but playful; technical but imaginative; and most of all, restorative. It allows me to empty out, and to then refill with a re-energized imagination. I re-engage with my life with a more playful spirit. This playful quality invariably surfaces in my mask work."[50]

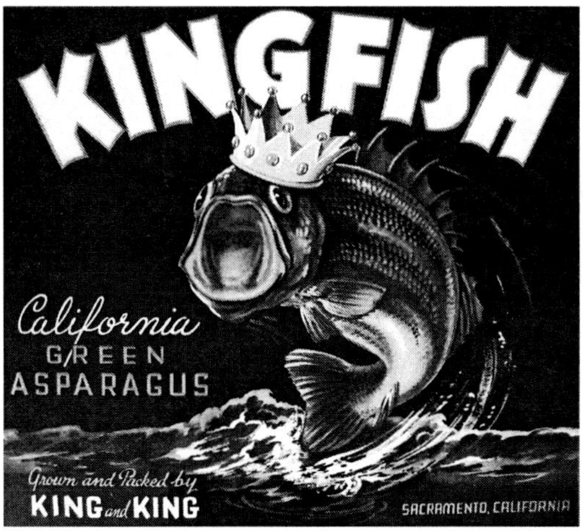

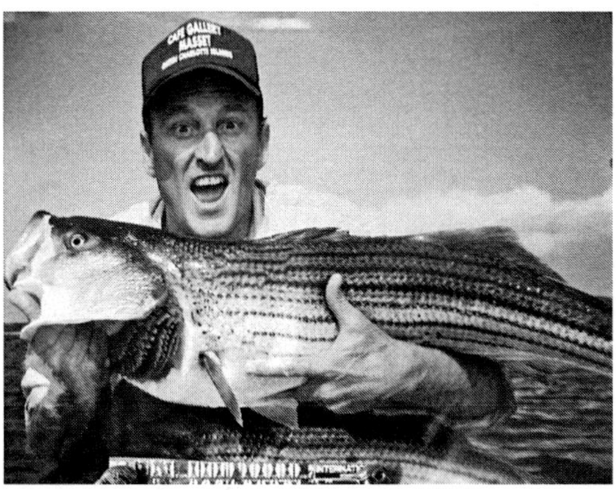

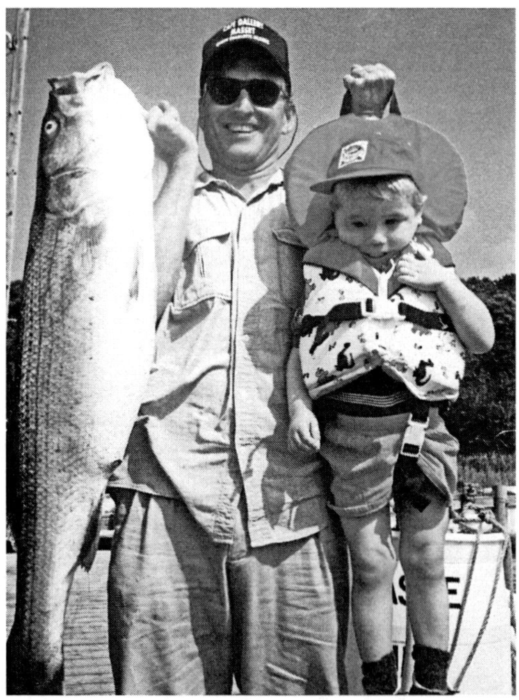

More visuals displayed in Rob Faust's mask studio. Obviously fishing is a significant component of Faust's creative process in mask making. Yet *Nyau* Secret Society mask makers in Malawi also have used fishing as a part of their transformation rituals for centuries.

At first glance, the act of fishing might serve as a rather unusual way to describe anyone's creative process. But, though seemingly far-fetched, Faust's description of the creative state that fishing encourages recalls the centuries-old rites of the *Nyau* Secret Society members in Malawi, which also require initiates to undertake fishing activity before they create their masks. These initiates also rely on day dreams and dream-like states generated by this activity as part of their creative process.

Growing up in New Orleans, Faust has vivid memories of "mask madness" while masquerading during Mardi Gras every Carnival season. The sense of play in these annual events help to conjure dream-like images of grotesque devils juxtaposed with angelic or seductive sirens on every street corner. A semblance of fishing also occurs at these events when the masquerading parade participants throw their beads out into the streets for delirious, masked, costumed characters to grab.

Rob summarizes his continuing inspiration from childhood memories of New Orleans. "I think I've tried to stay a free spirit, and the masks help me to that end ... something in my blood and hometown ... nature and nurture both conspire, as always, yes? Don't forget that New Orleans is the 'city of sin' and 'the city that care forgot.' Carnival season and Mardi Gras are as sacred as you get in the Crescent City. I was a rebel. I tuned in, turned on, and didn't quite drop out; I found dance, theatre, and masks instead. I derailed from the track that would have had me working at One Shell Square in a seersucker suit. Randy Newman sings 'nobody from dere never come to no good.' It's too easy and too hot to hustle. We make do ... set a spell in the shade ... have our ambition wilted, and settle for fun or rest or just getting by. So I guess you could say that I've put my urge for fun and play to work for me."[51]

He goes on to say that he does not dwell on spiritual issues in his work, but he tries to capture a spirit of joy, laughter, amazement, and transformation. "I'm an athlete who found dance and physical theatre and a class clown who found red noses and masks. I'm a Southerner who doesn't want to work too hard unless it's fun. Turns out I had a knack for mask making and the stage ... and a good business sense as well. The masks," he concludes, "are both an end in themselves and the tools of my theatre trade."[52]

Portrait of Another Artist as a Young Man

As a teenager, Faust wanted very much to please his father, a conservative German Catholic surgeon. This motivation led him to earn an undergraduate degree in Education from the University of New Orleans, though Faust did not have much enthusiasm for this traditional pursuit. Faust's mother, an ultra-radical feminist, divorced his father and "split for the Coast" in the mid–1960s. Soon after graduation, Faust joined her in San Francisco and fondly recalls exhilarating days watching *avant garde* physical theatre produced by such groups as San Francisco Mime Troupe; Pickle Family Circus with performers like Bill Irwin, Larry Pisoni, and Geoff Hoyle; and Dell'Arte Company.

Always athletic in high school and college, reveling in hiking, biking, climbing, swimming, and body surfing, his youthful love of movement and physical challenges eventually led him to take his first dance class at the University of Oregon at the age of twenty-five in 1975. "My innate clown then lured me, kicking and laughing, from dance into theatre," he said. He played co-ed volley ball at the local community cultural center and while there, discovered contact improvisation dance classes, a form that emphasized counter balance, natural movement, and flow without having to point toes or worry about looking pretty.

Teams and pairs of performers literally rolled around and on top of each other. Faust was attracted to the work's sense of collaborative playfulness that eventually led him to join a men's contact improv dance collective called Mangrove. This became his introduction to serious professional dance work, even though he did not have extensive formal dance training. During one of his early performances with Mangrove, his family came to watch when his very proper paternal grandmother, according to family lore, anxiously whispered to Faust's brother, "Is he going to do this the rest of his life?"

By 1978 he wanted to get more into choreography and structured performance work so he took classes with Leonard Pitt in Berkeley. Pitt, a student of Decroux (Marcel Marceau's teacher), had studied in Bali and at this period was offering workshops in masked performance with Balinese masks. While attending Pitt's workshops, he met fellow student Wendy Duke, who offered to teach him how to make Celastic masks built from clay molds over the course of two Saturday afternoons. She gave Faust all the training he needed with two directives: "Remember, a face is not flat" and "always look at the clay from different angles." Also during this time Bari Rolfe (author of several books on physical theatre performance techniques) and he experimented with making leather masks, after she learned the basic technique from mask maker Jack Schutes who sold them at art fairs. Eventually Faust learned wood-carving techniques with traditional folk carvers in Maine and, years later, with mask makers he met and studied with when he traveled to Ubud, the arts capital of Bali.

Faust has experimented with a technique for making a leather mask using a fiberglass resin positive mold (described in chapter 3). He discovered that he favors calfskin or "kip" leather best, along with Hydrocal plaster (white gypsum cement), leather dye, and acrylic paint. These preliminary sessions of experimentation with leather masks were the extent of his "formal training" in mask making and masked performance. The rest he learned by trial, error, and passion. Eventually other friends and mentors taught him how to work with neoprene.

In 1980 he joined Pilobolus Dance Theatre and moved to Connecticut, where he lived for twenty years. For two years he toured extensively throughout the United States and abroad, appearing on Broadway and once on *The Tonight Show*. He also toured many of the most beautiful opera houses in Italy. Even though he learned a great deal dancing and choreographing with Pilobolus and enjoyed the experience, he actually wanted to experiment with creating and performing more theatrical work. Consequently he started a small company with several other performers (including one former company member with Mummenschanz) in Italy for a year. That company eventually folded. He returned to the United States where he and six others, under the direction of Martha Clarke, created *The Garden of Earthly Delights*, which eventually won an OBIE Award.

Concurrently while working with Clarke, Faust initiated the preliminary scenarios for *The Mask Messenger* in 1983–84. In 1986 he showcased some of this early work at PACT (Producers and Associates of Children's Theater) in lower Manhattan, which organized the event to help promote theatre for young audiences. His seven-minute showcase performance at PACT led to 150 bookings the following year in Australia, Canada, and the United States, including Hawaii and Alaska. By 1988 he was performing *The Mask Messenger* 280 times a year. He liked the control he had as producer of his own show, and he could easily try out his ideas with the young audiences. "It was," he says, "a working lucrative laboratory with masks about masks." Schools appreciated the show's content because of its related topics in art, history, comparative religion, psychology, sociology, and cultural issues. The show was so successful, in fact, that he hired and trained his first company member, Larry Hunt, to perform in *The Mask Messenger* in 1990 so he could send the show out for more tours than Faust could do by himself.

He had also received rave reviews at the 1989 Piccolo Spoleto Festival in Charleston. The reviewer called his masks "often breathtaking, sacred objects" and remarked on Faust's transformative ability to "slither into the auditorium [with the head of a science fiction creature] to terrorize the crowd, only to entertainingly break the illusion ... blaming the mask for the incident."[53]

Soon after his initial Faustwork Mask Theatre production of *The Mask Man* (the original title of *The Mask Messenger* before he taught the show to a woman), he worked with his former wife Paula Styron (also a dancer) and developed *Faustwork in Concert* as an evening of masked dance theatre with such memorable pieces as *Burden of Paradise* (where Beauty and Beast contrast the tensions of civilization vs. nature, mind vs. body, and woman vs. man) and *Gingerella* (presenting gender-bender masked renderings of Astaire and Rodgers.) He also worked on projects with the Paul Winter Consort and with Jules Feiffer. Later he and cellist Eugene Friesen were commissioned by the Los Angeles Music Center to create and perform *Voice of the Wood,* a piece set in Venice during Carnivale, about a cellist and a *luthier*, a maker of musical instruments.

Later Mike Wallace (a friend of Faustwork Mask Theatre's New York producer, Lewis Allen) had seen the opening night performance of Faust's *Carnival Knowledge* in 2000 and agreed to help with a promo tape. Shortly thereafter, while sitting in front of his *60 Minutes* set, Wallace pronounced Faust's work "totally unique. I have never seen anything like it and neither have you. It is simply stunning."

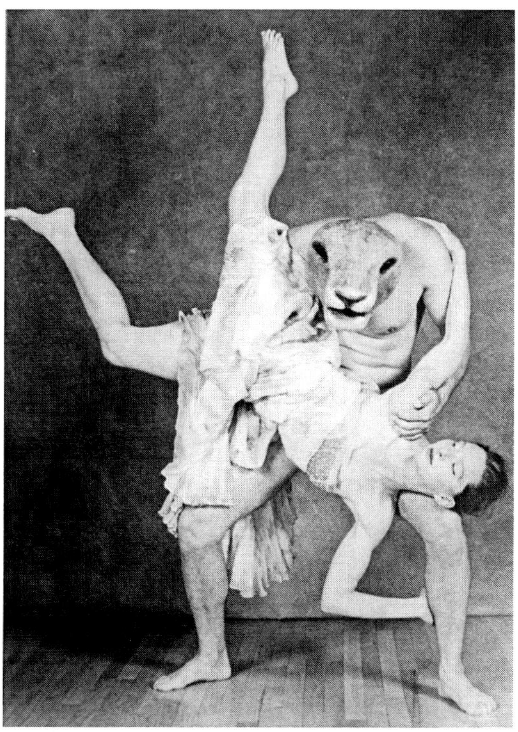

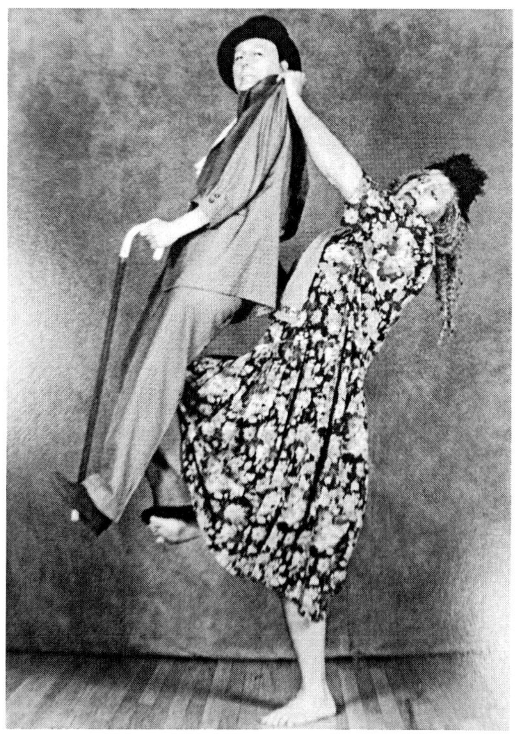

Photographs from *Burden of Paradise* and *Gingerella*, part of *Faustwork in Concert*, New York City. Photographer: Gary Gunderson.

Faust's Creative Process

Part of Rob Faust's secret for success is his willingness to try anything new. Between 2004 and 2007 he participated in several unusual masked performances with symphonies and even experimented with a physical theatre and dance rendition of Shakespeare's *A Midsummer Night's Dream* in which he played versions of Oberon and Theseus. He enjoys the element of risk in his work and continues to try out variations of the same solo show that he has performed for decades.

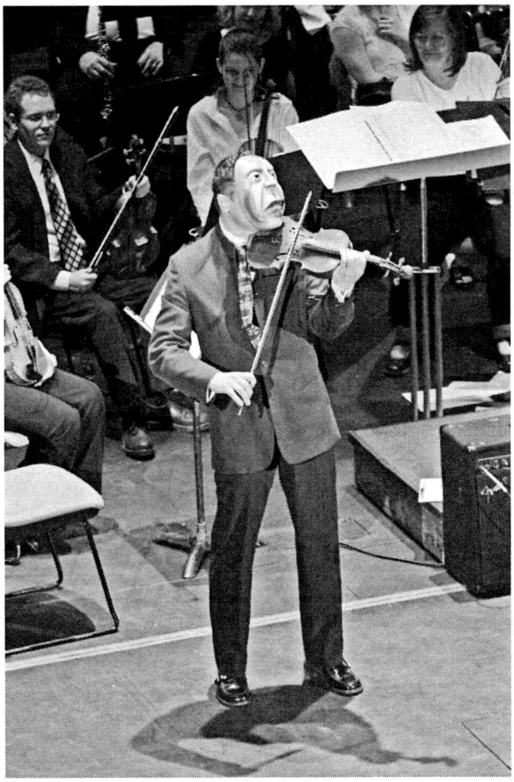

Faustwork's Halloween Symphony Show in Kansas City featured theatrical tricks and treats and classic orchestral pieces, including *The Sorcerer's Apprentice, Peer Gynt Suite: In the Hall of the Mountain King, A Night on Bald Mountain, Danse Macabre, Hedwig's Theme*, and the *Harry Potter* series.

Kansas composer/conductor Gary Gackstatter — a fan of Faustwork Mask Theatre — asked writer/director/performer Rob Faust to be a guest artist with the Winnfield Regional Symphony. Music was then composed for each of the characters. (Faust created and performed this "Sad Violinist" character.) Faust wrote the script/scenario for what has turned out to be a unique collaboration in the world of symphony performance, known as *Face the Music*. Photographer: M. Beauchamp.

He experiments within a range of performance styles and venues but a key factor in his exploration invariably requires interaction with an audience. "I work a room. I provoke a dialogue with my audience," he says. "I can't even rehearse well without an audience. Masks always involve a two-way thing with the viewer. It is the interaction for me. When I'm making a mask, I'm making something finite and immovable. I'm creating some sort of potential. Of course it is solid and finished, but everyone who wears my masks brings something different. And everyone who observes one of my masks in performance interprets it a little differently. It is the potential of the mask in performance that brings about the excitement and tension."

Faust contrasts his need for audience with his need for solitude. "On a practical level I usually need a way to be alone while scheming or planning new ideas. I like to share my explorations with others in performance, but I recognize that I need a great deal of time alone in order to generate those ideas. The actual masked performance is a paradox. It is ephemeral yet I feel strongly rooted in both the performance and the specific communication it generates. The mask becomes an artifact from the performance ritual. And finally the audience determines the success of the mask if it clearly engages, touches, and reflects the viewer."

Faust wants his masks to emphasize contrasting states. The masks' expressions need to express clusters of dualities and contrasting emotions. "I sometimes improvise with some clay by poking or slashing it to find the genesis of an expression," he says.

> Sometimes I really have no idea what sort of mask character I want to make until I've made at least twenty or thirty percent of it. For this reason, I keep a file of photos of interesting faces and a mirror on hand. But ultimately, all of my work originally comes from having enough 'alone' time while waiting in airports or gardening or watching television. Without sufficient alone time I cannot generate ideas.
>
> I tend to work backwards as a way of clarifying my performance objectives. For instance when creating a new show, I'll look at my vast collection of masks that aren't in a show yet and say to myself, "Okay, the characters and the story and the text are going to be built around, let's say, eight or nine of these fifteen masks. I don't write a story about a coyote and an ant—and then make masks for them. But I might think about a fairy frog mother character changing me, a frog, into a prince. I'll work out a rough scenario and then ask myself how these characters work for the story. My text needs to serve the masked characters rather than the reverse. It is opposite to the way a playwright usually works, where the thematic ideas generate the characters. For me, things most often revolve around the existing masks I have on hand, such as my bug mask or turtle mask."

Faust sometimes surprises himself when the end result is opposite to his original intention. "For instance consider the creep that was intended to be a happy face. This surprise effect will occasionally happen, depending on my mood or how easily distracted I am in the moment. Sometimes I recognize the opposite effect of my mask, but an audience will always let me know, even if I don't initially recognize the reverse effect myself."

Faust is not the first to believe that the human face provides the best inspiration for a theatre event. "Philippe Gaulier famously stated this premise as well as the admonition, 'You mustn't wear the theatre on your head like a big hat.'" Faust adds that, "The theatre is you and I. And it doesn't exist without simplicity. It is that simple ... good theatre requires careful attention to simplicity. What I do is pretty simple but not simplistic. I often have no plot or play—I'm just playing within a structure. The themes I choose just let me play. I do mask theatre; the masks drive it and I try to get out of the way of the masks."

Faust thinks that he is most successful when he effectively edits the information inherent in each mask.[54] Part of this editing involves a constant balance between tried and true techniques with new experimentation involving an element of risk.

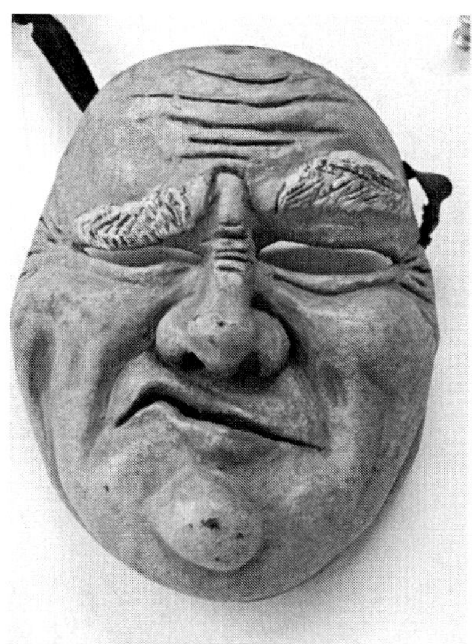

One of Rob Faust's personality masks.

> I believe most artists do versions of improvisations followed by editing. The more essentially and deeply I present aspects of myself, the more universal is my message, my connection to the audience. There is a wandering quality that is always a walk into the unknown that I've learned to embrace. Often I find myself taking on projects when I'm not sure why I'm doing them initially. Yet frequently these projects will take me into a new direction of exploration. For example, my work in Motus O Dance Theatre's version of *A Midsummer Night's Dream* later informed the poetry in Faustwork's next new piece, *Little Big Frog*. Another example involved creating a twenty-minute show with twelve masked characters for David Kirk, who wrote a children's book entitled *Miss Spider's Wedding*. He along with the book's publisher asked me to create these characters using bold shapes painted in primary colors similar to the colors used in the book. At first I thought I didn't like the project's

> parameters but as I worked on those masks, I began to like them more. The experience included making masks and directing eight performers and musicians for a toy fair event sponsored by FAO Schwarz.[55]

Regarding his use of archetypal images, Faust says he considers modern cultural archetypes such as his half-masked gruff coach/trucker character most interesting. "Coach is a character type. I had created an earlier character called Wild Man and borrowed his big eyes and buck teeth for his mask from similar masked types found in Balinese clown masks. I created a leather coach mask from the same mold used to create Wild Man, but the teeth morphed into a moustache and the bug eyes were cut out (photograph on page 114). The French artist type is showy and the colorful scarf becomes part of the framing for that mask. My nanny mask is another cultural type (photograph on page 76), as is the televangelist. I have very few specific portrait masks like Elvis, who is actually my rendition of a bad Elvis impersonator."

He added that his archetypal masks are more than specific mythic types.

> By that, I mean that most of my masked characters hearken back to Jungian themes. They are characters with dominant emotional states. They express a sense of fear and awe. We all recognize these states. I amplify them with extreme looks. They might initially be interpreted as caricatures before they get on stage, and admittedly there is a fine line

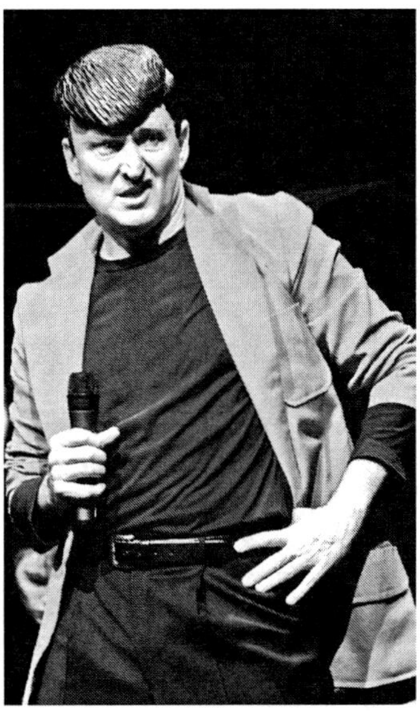

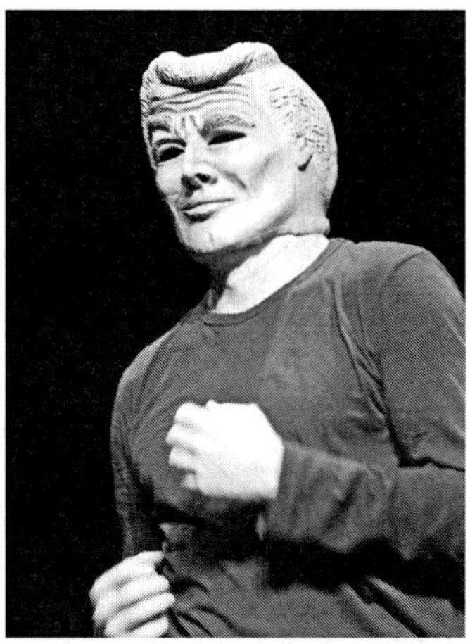

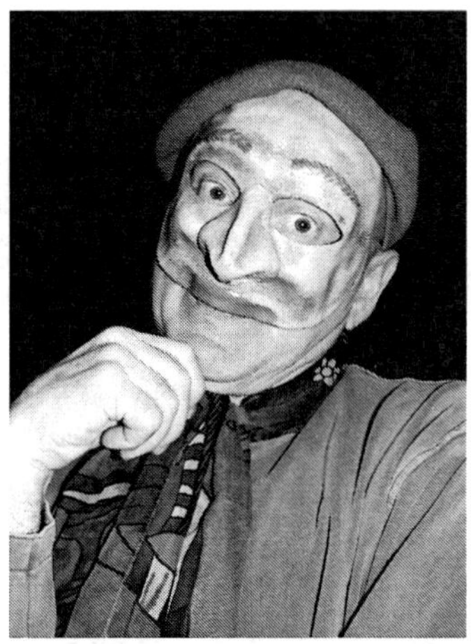

Top — left to right: **Faust's Elvis, Lifeguard, and French Artist masks in performance. Courtesy of Rob Faust.**

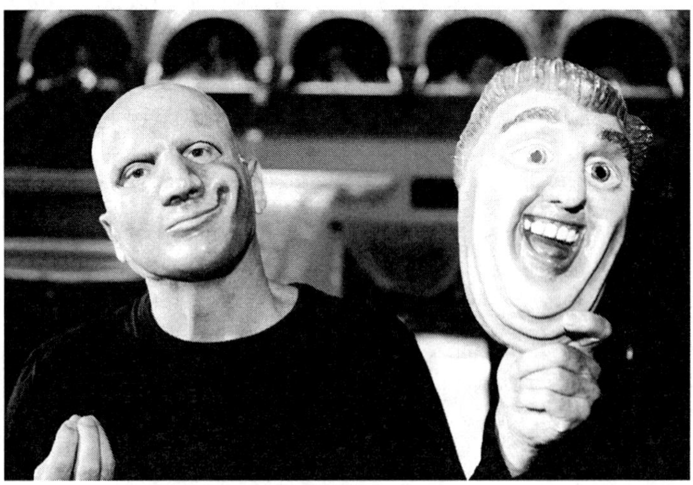

At right: **Faust holding talk show host, Toronto. Courtesy of Rob Faust.**

> between caricature and archetype. But when successful, my masks magically embody a state of mind and come to life in front of an audience with the appropriate gesture and ambience. Basically I present a tapestry of characters using masks to unify them in presentation. They are all states of mind (or heart). There is no plot in *The Mask Messenger*. The state of mind offered by one of my characters allows the audience an immediate visceral reaction. Regardless of how audiences might perceive the archetypal qualities of my masks, I certainly emphasize specificity in my masks. The closer I get to the essence of a masked character, the more each individual in the audience can identify with it.
>
> My masked performances with Faustwork Mask Theatre contain elements of hyper-realism rather than surrealism. I offer a stylized or heightened reality in which I become a kind of human puppet. Whether the intent is comic or profound, or simultaneously both, movements and intentions must be as clear and precise as those of a puppet, yet still retain an element of realism. A masked performer can live and die many times in the course of a minute or two on stage, depending on the truth and vitality with which the actor carries the mask.[56]

Faust thinks that body movement and gesture can strongly influence the search for the essence of the mask and the way the characters might emerge from behind the mask. He describes how the performer receives visual information from its shape, line, and overall design. He calls this creative process "working from the outside in." Performers can also experiment with that information by using their bodies and qualities of the movements. Consequently, a mask with exaggerated curves and heavy features will demand a curving spine and a weighty walk. A mask with a raised brow and bug eyes might require more tension in the actor's shoulder blades; a mask's pinched mouth might find expression in knees pulled together tightly.

The opposite approach, "from the inside out," requires an actor to study a mask and determine a dominant emotional state, such as sadness, and then begin to establish that sad state within. Eventually the actor will allow the shape and tension of the body to follow. He considers both approaches effective in the mask movement and physical theatre workshops that he conducts.

The inspiration for Faust's many masks (somewhere between two and three hundred now, after almost three decades of making them) comes from everywhere. For example, he was delighted when asked to create a performance piece for the Winnipeg Symphony Orchestra, based on the Eve of All Saints. "So after all these years I finally got around to making a devil mask, a task one would have thought a mask maker named Faust would have undertaken long ago. I actually made three generations of devil masks before using a half-masked

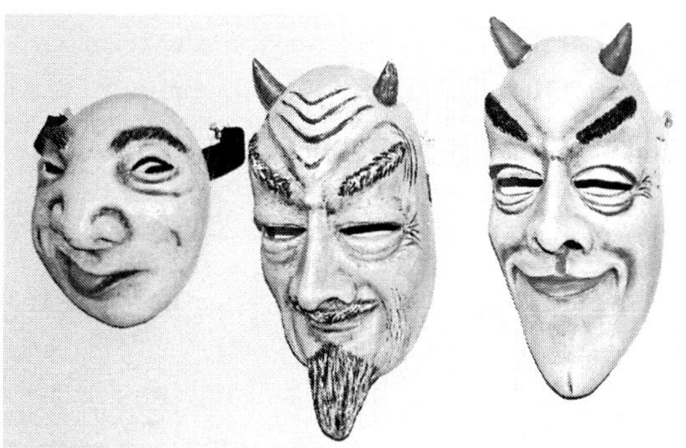

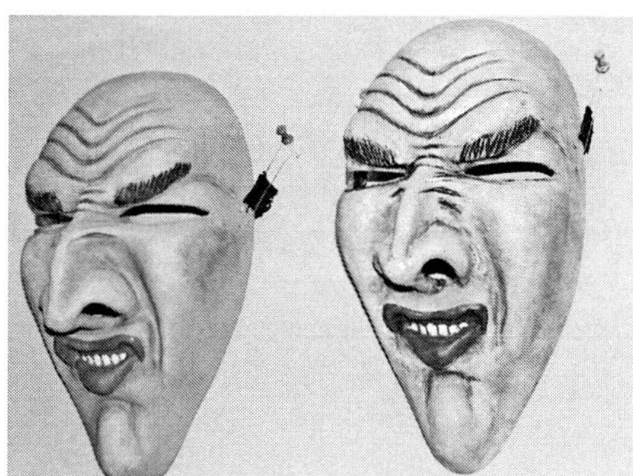

Rob Faust's devil masks and "effete" masks.

version for the *Halloween Symphony Show.* Whether the mask ultimately ends up in the performance or not, it might inspire the next mask-making impulse such as an angelic face. I'm a big believer in contrasts, the dual tensions and theatricality between seeming opposites, so the next mask-making impulse will probably be for something angelic."

He acknowledges the ultimate importance of the mirror as an important resource for mask making. "I am certainly my own most available model. After completing an angry mask, I will come away with a tremendous headache, having frowned for hours to capture the expression in the clay. Photos of masks from other cultures inspire me. The characters created from these images often get caricatured, North Americanized, and personalized. Dreams, films, books, family, friends, and people on the street: they are all fair game, fertile territory for finding the next face."[57]

Faust's Reliance on Music to Encourage a State of Heightened Awareness

When asked how he meditates or prays or focuses on a new mask creation he responds,

> I play rather than pray. I start playing with the clay. After several weeks of touring, it takes a week of being home before I can do it. I'll clean up my studio or do laundry or answer email; some sort of decompression activity has to happen. Somehow the negative quality of decompressing allows me to get to a positive quality of creating. This is a process of emptying my mind. And then something says, 'start now'; even though I don't really need more masks, I feel a deep desire to make them. I suppose I love the solitude ... and getting my hands dirty. I might start the first mask accidentally while listening to music by Randy Newman or Regina Spektor or Tom Waits. The music invariably speaks to me. Something like cool jazz works nicely late at night. It amplifies my mood and centers me. I get into an emotional mindset. I get a pulse. The trick is getting started. Once I do, I want only to continue.[58]

As with fishing, listening to music somehow induces a more relaxed, receptive state for Faust. In addition to listening to music while creating his masks, he warms up by playing music before a performance to achieve that same relaxed, receptive mental state. He particularly enjoys funky music like that of Ben Harper or Blind Boys of Alabama. "The Neville Brothers with the Mardi Gras Indians offer another favorite warm-up music experience for me," says Faust. "Music is the discipline that gives me freedom. Music helps me forget the effort I'm giving at the moment. I feel the way I do when I'm fishing. I'll have a goal at hand, yet music makes me aware of the beauty inherent in the overall process."[59]

Music seems to generate creativity beyond its own artistic agendas for many artists. Interestingly it seems to have the potential to inspire other acts of creation even as it "plays out" its own creative message. Faust and other mask makers I've interviewed recognize its power in their own work, while creating the actual masks as well as during the masked performances. Of course, music inspires the level of rhythm necessary for exaggerated gesture in masked performance but it can also aid, as Faust acknowledges, in warm-up activity to help center the performer to the project at hand. The actual act of creating music, like the actual act of creative play or fishing, seems to utilize similar conscious and unconscious states that reduce inhibition and encourage new ways of perception.

Recently, neuroscientists have conducted experiments that study the actual brain center responses of jazz musicians as they improvise simple musical phrases while inside MRI scanners. Not surprisingly, these scientists have reported that such improvisational creative activity shuts down the brain center responsible for inhibition, in much the same way as dreaming

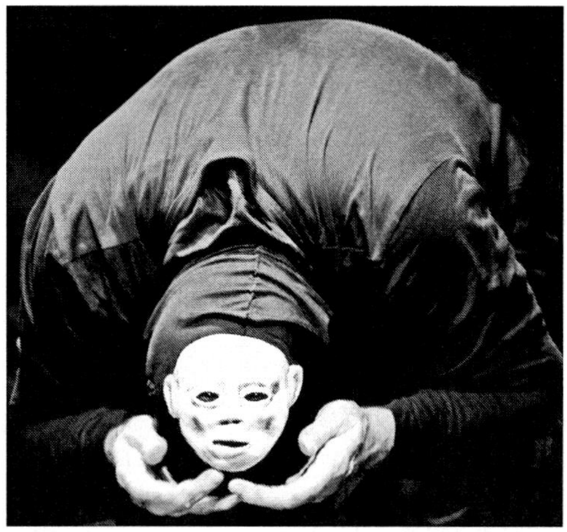

Faust's White Mask in performance, Toronto. Courtesy of Rob Faust.

triggers a drop in inhibition. Then the brain center responsible for activating self-expression (the same area linked to that activated by autobiographical storytelling) switches on. The jazz improvisation activity produces such individual styles that it's often described as telling a personal musical story. These scientists also report that the musicians demonstrate "heightened sensory awareness in the region of the brain that activates touch, hearing, and sight, even though the musicians experience none of these conditions while improvising inside the MRI machine."[60]

These preliminary experiments suggest that the process of listening to music, as well as the activity of creating music, offers similar benefits. Both processes seem to induce a heightened sense of awareness, allowing for increased creative faculties. Might these jazz musicians riffing inside MRI scanners be experiencing the same creative state found in "playful jazz improvisation" as the creative state encouraged by fishing or dreaming activity? Perhaps Rob Faust, *Nyau* Secret Society initiates, and other successful artists have long recognized this concept inherent within their creative processes without needing scientific experiments to prove it.

Bringing Traditional Mask Agendas with Contemporary Commercial Masks

Today's successful mask makers continue to find inspiration in the traditions of those who preceded them. For example, many contemporary mask makers still incorporate traditional references to plot and myth in their work. But Rob Faust breaks with traditional mask performance by presenting new work that forgoes plot and recognizable mythic personalities.

He does draw, however, on other significant traditions in mask making and masked performances. Like many traditional mask makers and masked performers, he is the "prime mover" of his masked performances by serving as the sole artist in his performances. He creates his own masks and develops his characters, using traditional materials such as leather, wood, neoprene, and Celastic. He choreographs/directs his performances. He designs his costumes and employs simple sets and lights. He designs his music cues. He performs live. He interacts spontaneously with his audience and achieves both exhilaration and dramatic tension. The human face, as in ancient times, still has two eyes, a nose, and mouth. Faust rather realistically represents facial features (or implies these features using half-masks). His mask expressions are occasionally exaggerated but often they appear exaggerated simply because they are frozen expressions. Like generations of mask makers before him, he has developed a creative process that achieves a mental state of heightened awareness during solitary activity (in his case, induced by decompressing with rest and relaxation using fishing and other forms of centering activity such as listening to music) in order to prepare himself for experimentation and improvisation.

However, Rob Faust seems especially attuned to the evolving cultural values of an increasingly global world. Unlike most mask makers a generation ago who presented their work in or near a small region beyond their hometown, a great deal of Faust's effort goes toward marketing his global touring productions beyond Toronto, where he lives. And he has experimented with less traditional materials such as neoprene and fiberglass resins. But more significantly, his approach to mask making and masked performance strikes universally relevant chords that resonate in a global society. His artistry conjures up elemental personalities (that he calls "states of being") that suggest pulses of the collective unconscious. At first glance, they seem to project specific, localized references, such as the French artist or the New Orleans nanny, but these characters live in the moment; they are defined less by locale and more by the visceral emotional states they project.

Paleolithic shamans or traditional cultures such as those of the ancient Greeks or Hindu theatrically presented mythic stories with easily recognized external protective or demonic forces. But Faust focuses on balancing the fine distinctions between archetype and caricature to present states of being rather than actual mythic figures such as the Balinese *Rhangda* (witch) or a Yoruba *Yemoja* (earth matriarch mask). Shamans and mask makers in traditional cultures want to suggest spiritual resolutions with their masked events, whereas Faust avoids formulating specific cultural or religious dogma.

Of course, Faust is not the first mask maker to project this type of universal masked personality. The tramps created by Charlie Chaplin, Red Skelton, and Samuel Beckett come to mind (depending on how one defines a mask). *Cirque du Soleil* characters often project similar universal masks. Bill Irwin's clowns have no mythic agendas associated with a specific culture. Torbjörn Alström's "gas mask personalities" possess no mythic references to specific characters or forces. Even Japanese *Noh* masks (over four centuries old) are more indicative of emotional states than actual mythic characters. But Rob Faust, more than any other traditional mask maker I've interviewed, seems rather distinctive in his ability to present (as the consummate impresario) engaging live masked performance so consistently over several decades, using a broad range of traditional mask making and masked performance techniques but in a stream-of-consciousness manner — sans plot and sans myth.

Our myths have not caught up with the ever shrinking world which the Internet has fostered. The world inherently recognizes the need for diverse communities to understand and appreciate each other, but we have no new global myths to assist with unifying our spiritual and cultural core values in ways that can be embraced by a global perspective. As mentioned earlier, according to Joseph Campbell, the myth of *Star Wars*, perhaps, came closest to projecting a new myth with the potential for global acceptance.

Communities must find ways to relate better at a global level. The village of the traditional mask maker is now much larger, with multi-cultural influences. We still struggle to balance the promotion of global understanding with tribal urges for dominance. Joseph Campbell points out that myths function in part by supporting and validating a specific social order. Campbell asserts that this function is out of date for most traditional myths. He underscores this premise with the example of Yahweh's comprehensive expectations for how to dress and behave in first millennium B.C.E.[61]

Art historians generally interpret the last five or six decades as a transitional period for the arts. Rob Faust's masked presentations function with particular success in our transitional world (bereft of globally relevant myths) by avoiding mythic characters and plots altogether. I do not suggest that Faust consciously assumes this premise. He values simplicity and editing as meritorious for a superior masked performance regardless. He also credits his audiences who let him know when he has pushed too far or not far enough, and during his successful career of almost three decades audiences clearly have not required mythic references in his performances. This conceivably indicates the transitional shift regarding the importance of traditional mythology at this point in time. However, if the past ten thousand years are any indication, we will eventually, as a global society, create and develop appropriate myths and masks that we require for our collective future.

Joseph Campbell reminds us that myths allow us to "participate in divinity ... involving the wonder and sheer beauty of existence."[62] This wonderment is at the heart of traditional masks and their myths. Ancient cultures, acutely aware of the need to survive, used heroic, demonic, or divine masks in order to ensure vitality and protection. As our world becomes increasingly precarious with global warming and a planet too densely populated to sustain itself, perhaps we are positioned to seek guidance by creating new myths (or recycling old ones) and their corresponding masks representing divine characters and forces.

Meanwhile, Faust's masked performances focus less on quintessential external mythic protective forces and more on intensely playing in the moment. His masked performances forgo the ancient mythic traditions and focus instead on emotional states that we can recognize within ourselves. We can all relate easily to his coach or his frog prince or his flamboyant Frenchman whereas Harlequin and the Balinese *Barong* are perhaps too culturally specific to be universally and fully understood.

Faust's masks still express divine wonderment with fervor equal to that achieved by traditional masks, but from the opposite perspective. That is, while traditional mythic-oriented masks typically emphasize external divine forces, Faust's masked characters emphasize internal divine forces. Faust continues to incorporate the rhythmic beat of physical gestures found in traditional masked performance in order to express most vividly the dramatic tensions of the orchestrated event. And the typical audience member attending one of Faust's performances can still appreciate the same revelation of the mask's magic unfolding on stage as did archaic audience members. The mask messenger delivers sublime reflections for us at this moment in our time.

Video Games as the New Medium for Masks

The prehistoric imaginative story told around the campfire eventually morphed into staged dramatic renderings or rites of passage on all continents, often using spectacular masks made by highly skilled mask makers who took years to develop their craft. In the last century similar stories reached global audiences via film and television. Masked characters continued to appear particularly in the special-effects realms of adventure and fantasy genres, although the development of film required audiences to view the mask as simply the interplay of light against a screen in a darkened room rather than surrounding a campfire at night.

The masked imagery in these adventure and fantasy genres demand the extraordinary skills of the special-effects film artists and production crews, who create the same exotic transformative narratives as those used by the traditional mask maker. These narratives have progressed into the area of motion capture, where a fantasy character such as Gollum in *The Lord of the Rings* can be generated by wiring an actor with sensors that, when video taped, can be reinterpreted, distorted, or exaggerated digitally with input from the camera.

Thus motion capture not only presents imaginary renderings of masking with light (and still requires performers and special-effects "mask makers") but goes further by digitally distorting the performer's and mask's shapes into more fantastical, evocative masking on screen. Even as the concept of the mask and mask making rapidly evolve, the fundamental functions still transform, disguise, or evoke as they did before. Traditional mask makers as we know them are quickly disappearing, yet their ancient Romantic agendas of valor conquering evil, love conquering hate, and life conquering death continue to beguile us. These stories continue to appear in our adventure and fantasy films as well as in Broadway musicals.

Phil May, a television producer for Disney between 1970 and 1981, created his own advertising agency that developed marketing for major film studios such as TVN, Universal, Paramount, Sony, Columbia Tri-Star, and Fox. Currently he teaches at Cuesta College in San Luis Obispo, California. May believes that the new video games are gaining momentum in power and popularity over adventure films. "From a revenue perspective, more money is currently spent on video games than on film, and this fact has the potential to change the multiplex era as we know it. These video games, such as the popular Japanese Nintendo game *Wii*, allow the 'player' to create a personal avatar that can simulate, exaggerate, or distort the player's body shape or head at will. (Other manufacturers are more aggressive about pursuing the teen demographic. Nintendo, especially in its *Wii* series, is aimed at a family audience.)"[63]

The player in these games enhances his or her storyline by generating spectacle, special-effects, sound, and music, recalling the versatility of the traditional mask maker. The player inserts his or her own image into the screen or creates a "masked persona." The television screen essentially becomes the theatrical masked event in the same way that the youngster with sunglasses posing in front of a mirror (described in chapter 2) reflects a theatrical event. The televised video game event, however, has much more power, using unlimited themes and spectacle created instantaneously by the player of the video game. There are even regularly scheduled workshops in such topics such as "Three Nights with ZBrush 3: An Introduction to 3D Creature Creation."[64]

May fears that these video games encourage an already sedentary society, particularly its youth, to withdraw from physical and social activity. Today's couch potatoes can now have the experience of playing tennis or socializing via their imagination and technology but without actual exertion. May adds that "movies now have specific scenes intended for sequential video games, ensuring additional profits. Consequently any kid can transform himself into a hero like Luke Skywalker, flying through the canyon."[65] The demand for video games has never been higher and will only increase.

The future invariably unfolds in the direction of profits generated, and this video game technology brings us to yet one more critical moment in the mask maker's historical evolution. Of course such moments can offer new vistas for both positive as well as negative paradigms. Tsimshian mask maker Victor Reece believes that with any great change comes abundant opportunity for the artists (particularly the mask makers) who can most readily respond with their imagination. May adds that video games are tremendously seductive and believes that they attract creative individuals. "Like masking, video game participation is freeing and liberating."[66] Such participation continues to draw on the mask's potential to both reveal and escape into deep psychological states.

Adolescents seem most intrigued with interactive video games. May suggests that in this stage of human development, regardless of cultural background, young people confront typical anxieties associated with self-image. "It is a time when most adolescents are least secure with their appearance. These video games give them tremendous psychological empowerment over their undeveloped skills and awkward appearances." Perhaps it is not accidental that just as the novice makers of traditional masks usually commence their training at twelve to fourteen years of age, so too the early adolescents of today initiate their quests for mastery over adulthood's anxieties via the narratives they test out on their televised Nintendo screen. Ray Bradbury's high-tech children in *The Veldt* experience all the sights and sounds of a jungle within the confines of the nursery. Today's video games describe a similar experience by setting up the quintessential "performance event," complete with both mask maker and masked performer.

Yet these young video maskers continue to tackle ancient Romantic agendas, but within the more cynical context of our twenty-first century. Today's young people lack the security and predictability which established myths offer traditional mask makers, who honor and celebrate their mythic underpinnings with their masks, and who strive to unquestioningly preserve the cosmos of their ancestors. For example, Mexican mask maker Juan Horta Castillo's son Manuel expresses deep reverence for his father's legacy of cultural values that continue to be evident in his own masks. Both Juan and Manuel have distinctive personal styles, yet they possess the cultural and iconic references of the masks created by their ancestors many generations before. This seems quite impossible for today's digitally charged youth who have access to many myths instantaneously. Our technology does not encourage specific mythic foundations, nor does the increasing intercultural atmosphere of our age.

Like traditional mask makers, current special-effects makeup and mask artists for film spend years developing their mask-making skills. But I suspect that most film artists are not as fully aware of how their work artistically and spiritually integrates with their personal aesthetic and cultural landscape. The Information Age has not as yet been harnessed, and perhaps it is naïve to believe that it will ever happen. Contemporary commercial mask makers for film have, at best, a vague sense of traditional approaches and beliefs. Surely a closer examination of those traditions and beliefs can offer insight and added richness into the work at hand. Such careful examination is certainly abundantly evident in the multicultural yet focused work of Julie Taymor. Some could argue that this is a basis for her remarkable success.

Ultimately today's youth are at critical crossroads between cultural underpinnings that embrace ancient myths (or at least synthesize them in recognizable ways) and a contemporary atmosphere much more apocalyptic in nature. In today's video games, the commercial manipulation of archetypal stories has little connection to any shared meaningful foundation. Consequently, these video games too often exemplify the spiritual emptiness of our postmodern era. The novice mask maker can potentially be anyone with a video game remote in his or her hand. Nowadays anyone has the magic wand to effortlessly conjure other realms.

Will this generation venture into the new millennium without sufficient awareness of the realms s/he is conjuring? In spite of the tremendous power that the remote wields, the traditional mask maker would admonish today's novices to take care.

Conclusion

The Mask Maker's Critical Juncture for Theatre and Film in the Twenty-first Century

Traditional masks used as a universal theatrical convention have never entirely left the stage. But they seem particularly evident today as protector-hero (or demon), Everyman, transcendent, or mechanical versions in Broadway musicals such as *The Lion King*, *Beauty and the Beast*, and *Wicked* as well as in popular fantasy films of the past few decades such as *The Lord of the Rings*, *The Golden Compass*, *Batman*, *Hellboy*, and *WALL-E*. Broadway and film have encouraged or at least accentuated the continuation of protector characters and protector mask characters (and their counterparts), in part because in spite of our post-modern lens we need the "Romance" of the protector mask perhaps now more than ever. (Even contemporary "Everyman masks" that offer humor — like Rob Faust's witty personalities or Bruce Marrs' misfits or whimsical, masked, animated film characters like WALL-E — protect our spirits.)

Why might theatre and film periodically resort to the Romantic world of traditional protector masks? Why not? The twenty-first-century global community perceives the contemporary world as the sort of overwhelming jungle or tundra that any primitive shaman experienced. Massive uncontrollable forces like Thomas Friedman's Electronic Herd in the Internet world of business have invisible powers to dramatically destroy or bless entire countries overnight in much the same way as ambivalent, capricious forces of nature could affect the shaman's world. Many of the traditional myths in world cultures that formerly promised protection have little relevance today. The fragmented attempts to replace them have yet had minimal success. Humanity has always needed protective forces, real or imaginary, to feel secure, but we currently confront precipices that perhaps demand even more increased levels of security.

Just as Gershwin's plaintive, romantic lyrics for "someone who'll watch over me" beckon the protector-lover to "put on some speed, follow my lead," the ancient primitive protector spirits evoked by the protector-hero masks likewise "followed the lead/behest" of the shaman. The protector-hero mask vividly connects with higher forces/powers/personalities by focusing on the imaginative states of consciousness in identification with the sublime. The actual reference to protection obviously implies threats of some sort. In order for the protector-hero mask to assist in overcoming threats or imbalances, the performer and the audience recognize whatever relevant adversity stands in the way of well-being. Protector-hero masks function as defenders that "work" against distinct threats in the same manner that saints or gods were invoked for specific tasks. Admittedly, they lose their power when their correlating threat is no longer relevant.

Jeff Goldblum, in the Chicago Ford Center for the Performing Arts 2005 playbill for *Wicked*, cites Joseph Campbell's belief in the inevitable violence of the world. Goldblum reflects on his character's motivations in *The Pillowman* with a quote from Campbell that "the essence of divinity is sometimes nattily sweet and lovely and ambrosial and miraculously beautiful — but sometimes it is horrifically, powerfully devastating and violent."

Humanity's protectors and heroes (divine or otherwise) provide the necessary balance in both the divine and literal worlds with their abilities to be both destroyers as well as nurturers. In order to protect against violence and disharmony, protector masks — like fathers and angels — are fierce as well as loving. Sometimes the best protector-hero masks are the demon masks or those of anti-heroes such as Batman. Our protectors (as some other force's demons) have the power and will to destroy even as they protect us. Shamans were feared more than they were loved. Shepard's archetypal "protective" (unmasked but highly exaggerated) characters in *A Lie of the Mind* all have the capacity and tendency to destroy as well as the capacity to nurture. The mobile fighter bomber "spirits" over Jake's bed represent the glories and the aggressions of warrior protectors although they haunt him because they no longer "work" for him. Kushner's Angel in *Angels in America* descends violently and threateningly in order to assist with "The Great Work." Beauty's Beast has the power to destroy her as well as nurture her, and vice versa.

All relevant "metaphorical mythic storytelling" involves a certain sense of the sacred as the participants allow themselves to be metaphorically transported from one level of physical reality to a more profound and eternal reality. This magic happens not only in masked performance but in any effective storytelling, whether experienced around the campfire; in a darkened movie house or media room at home; in the reading of a poem; or as a dance, a piece of music, or a play on stage. The image of the metaphor or event becomes more real than real in an imaginative way.

Joseph Campbell reminds us that the image of myth (as well as the image of the mask) is never a direct presentation of the total mystery of human issues and only functions as "an attitude, the reflex of a stance, a life pose, a way of playing the game. When the rules or forms of such play are abandoned, the mythology dissolves — and with mythology, life."[1] The most successful masks worn in a performance or within a community rite of passage evoke this idea of the sacred by evoking a spiritual, eternal idea of the human condition.

Efrat Tseëlon quotes a similar, albeit more profound, point made by Walter Sorrell, who states that "the mask contains the magic of illusion without which man is unable to live." However, in this case, Sorrell describes the mask (i.e., the illusionary qualities of all art) as "an imaginary shield that protects us against reality, a symbol of escape into a make-believe reality (wherein) the persona is the mask which protects us not only against the other people behind their masks, but also against our own real self." Tseëlson suggests that "the mask maker and the audience member unite in this need as the audience member bears witness to the mask maker's [artist's] message."[2]

The perspectives of Campbell, Sorrell, and Tseëlson all underscore the essential premise that the artful and protective guise (mask) of mythic illusion enables us to maintain the idea of the eternal over the temporary — that is, the spirit of life over death. Torbjörn Alström tells us that "masks eternally work because the human face is the first thing we see as babies. From then on we see faces in clouds, houses, a piece of wood. We can't be very original about mask shapes (all masks tend to have eyes, a nose, and a mouth), but we can try new surfaces and materials and techniques and expression." Indeed, those possibilities are endless — as endless as the number of characters in the world — for all time.[3]

Perhaps contemporary commercial masks do not typically claim the same appeal they still claim in Bali, where both Balinese citizens and tourists view masks daily, ensconced in forms of sacred ritual as well as in entertainment. But we still see the mask's extraordinary vitality, always with glimpses of the sacred in varied global forms of popular entertainment. The kid wearing a simple paper bag as a mask at the opening of *Titus* affirms our "hard-wired prayer" for mythic illusion in order to more deeply understand our quest for eternal truths. The mask at its most basic level metaphorically achieves this premise with each successful performance. Without the maker of the mask, and the influences of the traditional mask maker, considerable effort, indeed, crucial effort toward this universal quest is diminished.

Appendix I: Basic Functions of the Mask

- To protect (usually in ceremonies such as fertility rites and coming-of-age rites)
- To disguise (usually in pageants and theatrical presentations)
- To transform (often occurs in ceremonies and theatrical presentations)
- To establish balance between the upper ideal worlds and the lower evil realms

Mythic Qualities of Masks from Many Cultures

Protectors: angels, gods, animal totems, protective warriors
Heroes: superheroes, anti-heroes, aggressive protective warriors
Demons: witches, devils, mummers, crafty servants
Clowns: Everyman figures

Culture/ Country	*Protectors*	*Heroes, Elite Figures*	*Demons*	*Clowns, Everyman Figures*
Indonesia, Bali	***Topeng*** **masks:** Link with ancestral world	***Wayang Wong*** **masks:** Link with Hindu stories	***Calanarang*** **masks:** witches	***Topeng*** **masks:** servants: Bondresan, and other "zanies"
	Sidha Karya Putih	Hanuman (monkey)		
	Sidha Karya Salem	Jero gede Mecaling		
	Barong **masks:** protective animals			
Italy		***Commedia dell'arte:*** lovers (usually unmasked)		***Commedia dell'arte:*** servants, Capitano, Pantalone
American Indian	Sun God/Raven (Pacific Northwest) Husk faces (Iroquois) *Kachina* spirits (Hopi)		Trickster, fox Dzunukwa Bak'was	*Hactcin* clowns
	shaman masks (many cultures)			

Culture/ Country	*Protectors*	*Heroes, Elite Figures*	*Demons*	*Clowns, Everyman Figures*
Mexico	Serpent, lizard, bat, *Tigre* (wild beast), often supports fertility, rain, good harvest, and promotes strength Hermit	King and Queen Pageants: with courtiers, often Spanish rather than Indian	Pharisee devil masks, bat devils, some skeleton masks	Day of the Dead masks: begging souls, *Catrinas*, humorous Pharisee masks
Africa	Fertility Totems: *Chi-wara* masks (Mali) *Gèlèdé* masks (Nigeria) *Kasia Maliro* (Malawi) ***Dogon*** **masks**: ancestors	*Bundu* masks (Sierra Leone) Chief coronation masks (many regions) *Mfon* masks, ancestors who have reached paradise (Ibibio)	*Idiok* masks (Ibibio in Nigeria) ***Dogon*** **masks**: Dega black monkey masks (Mali)	Pedegu the orphan (Malawi)
Europe	Medieval mystery plays: saints and angels	Renaissance masque masks: beautiful/ mysterious figures	Medieval miracle plays: devil	Mummer masks
Greek	Gods: protect, but whimsically—often for self-aggrandizement	Ancestral heroes/ anti-heroes: Agamemnon, Oedipus, Jason, Achilles, Odysseus	Furies Medusa	Satyrs
India	Vishnu	Rama, Krishna human avatars (human embodiments)	Ravana	
Japan	***Noh*** **drama**: wise elder characters	***Noh*** **drama**: warriors	***Noh*** **drama**: devils, snake	***Kyogen*** **comedy**: Yamabushi and the Crab
Contemporary Britain, USA, Australia, Canada				
	The Lion King: Rafiki, Mufasa	***The Lion King:*** Simba	***The Lion King:*** Scar	***The Lion King:*** Timon, Pumbaa
		Cirque du Soleil: elegant, mysterious characters		***Cirque du Soleil***: humorous fantasy characters and clowns
			Star Wars: Darth Vader	***Star Wars***: R2-D2, C-3PO, Chewbacca
	Angels in America: angel	Superman Batman	 Joker	WALL-E

Culture/ Country	*Protectors*	*Heroes, Elite Figures*	*Demons*	*Clowns, Everyman Figures*
	***Harry Potter*:** Dumbledore	Spider-Man Hellboy ***Phantom of the Opera:*** anti-hero ***Wicked:*** Elphaba, anti-hero	Catwoman (though not as as demonic as Joker) **Carnival**: bats, devils, imps ***The Wizard of Oz:*** Wicked Witch of the West	**Rock Bands**: Kiss Slipknot, Buckethead

Appendix II: Leather Mask Materials Suppliers

Plaster

- (Most hardware supply stores)
- Alcone Company, 5-45 49th Ave., Long Island City, NY 11101; (718) 361-8373, www.alconeco.com
- Daven Ceramic Center, 5076 Peachtree Rd., Atlanta, GA 30341; (770) 451-2105, Davens@davensceramiccenter.com

Plaster bandages and alginate

- Alcone Company

Vaseline and barge/contact cement

- local craft and hardware stores

Millinery wire

- Judith M., 104 S. Detroit St, LaGrange, IN 46761; (260) 499-4407, toll free: (877) 499-4407 (US & Canada), www.judithm.com

Roma Plastilina (Plasticine) oil-based #4 white clay (for freezing) and other types of Roma Plastilina clay for basic modeling

- The Sculpture House, 38 East 30th St. NYC, 10016; (212) 645-9430, www.sculp turehouse.com

Cowhide belly leather

- (4–6 oz. vegetable tanned cowhide, preferably belly leather) Brettuns Village Leather, P.O. Box 772, Auburn, ME 04212; (207) 782-7863, www.brettuns village.com/leather/sides/
- 2/3-oz. leather. Zack White Leather Company, P.O. Box 315, 809 Moffitt Str., Ramseur, NC 27316; (336) 824-4486, www.zackwhite.com

Basic leather supplies (and natural artificial sinew or waxed nylon sinew for lacing—Osborne Round Knife, leather hole punch, rivets, leather scissors, straight knife, skiver leather tools, leather for masks including pigskin for inside edges, leather dyes)

- Oregon Leather Company, 110 N.W. 2nd, Portland, OR 97209; (503) 228-0210, www.oregonleatherco.com
- Zack White Leather Company, P.O. Box 315, 809 Moffitt Str., Ramseur, NC 27316; (336) 824-4486, www.zackwhite.com
- Daniel Smith, P.O. Box 8428, Seattle, WA 98124-5568 (rabbit skin glue)

Leather skiving tools (Swiss made chisels—#7/20, flat 05V91, curve #7, 05W91)

- Woodcraft Catalogue: PO Box 1686, Parkersburg, WV 26102; (304) 485-4050, www.woodcraft.com/stores/

Leather dyes

- The Fiebing Company: P.O. Box 694, Milwaukee, WI 53201; (414) 271-5011, www.fiebing.com

Appendix III: Contact Information for Mask Makers

Abrantes, Samuel—Brazil: samuelabrantesbr@yahoo.com.br
Adebisi, Agbede—Nigeria: C/O Adigun Ajani, adigjand@yahoo.com
Adeola, Kolawale—Nigeria: ajereagba4ever@yahoo.com
Ajani, Adigun—Nigeria: adigjand@yahoo.com
Akangbe Ogun, Kasali—Nigeria: kunlexy_olishe@yahoo.com
Alström, Torbjörn—Sweden: artmask@telia.com; torbjorn.alstrom@comhem.se
Álvarez, Alicia Martínez—Mexico: alimar@laboratoriodelamascara.org.mx
Anom, I. Bagus—Bali: C/O Newman, commediamask@yahoo.com
Castillo, Juan Horta—Mexico: deceased. C/O maskorta@hotmail.com
Chavez, Manuel Valencia—Mexico: C/O Bill LeVasseur, info@casadelacuesta.com
Clemdore, Sheldon—Trinidad: C/O Marlon Griffith, marlongriffith@gmail.com
Cook, Xstine—Canada: xpandora@go.com
Dawig, I. Wayan—Bali: made_kichen@yahoo.com phone#: +62 361 299482
Delgado, Antonio Cervantes—Mexico: C/O Karima Muyaes, Karimamuyaes@hotmail.com
Dibo, Ivete—Brazil: C/O Samuel Abrantes, samuelabrantesbr@yahoo.com.br
Donvieve—United States: maskworld@cox.net
Faust, Rob—Canada: rob@faustwork.com; info@faustwork.com; robfaust@rogers.com
Fonseca, Venicio—Brazil: C/O Samuel Abrantes, samuelabrantesbr@yahoo.com.br
Griffith, Marlon—Trinidad: marlongriffith@gmail.com
Horta, Manuel Abeiro—Mexico: maskorta@hotmail.com
Kim, Dong-Pyo—Korea: C/O Sangdae Lee, phd@inkorean.com
Iwasaki, Kyoun—Japan: deceased. C/O Akira Kiyomatsu, phone #: +81-742-44-9797
LeVasseur, Bill—Mexico: info@casadelacuesta.com
Marrs, Bruce—United States: marzilla@netzero.net, www.marzillamask.com
Meyer, Michael—United States: meyerm@uncsa.edu
Muyaes, Karima and Cana—Mexico: Karimamuyaes@hotmail.com
Ogunyemi, Agibike—Nigeria: C/O Adigun Ajani, adigjand@yahoo.com
Ojeyemi, Ojetuni—Nigeria: ojetunjiojeyemi954@hotmail.com
Orangeena—United States: C/O Deb Bell, deb_bell@uncg.edu
Perusquia, Dalio Angel—Mexico: C/O Bill LeVasseur, info@casadelacuesta.com

Radtke, Joyce — United States: radniel@humboldtl.com
Raine, Lauren — United States: www.rainewalker.com
Reece, Victor — Northwest Canada: C/O Sharon Jinkerson, Sharon@cablelan.net
Sartori, Danato — Italy: C/O Paula Pizzi, info@sartorimaskmuseum.it
Schirle, Joan — United States: www.dellarte.com
Suryasa, I. Made — Bali: C/O Judy Slattum, danu@earthlink.net
Vieira, Geraldo — Trinidad: C/O Gérard Besson, phone — 868 6244187
Vieira, Geraldo Jr. — Trinidad: C/O Gérard Besson, phone — 868 6244187
Yoshikawa, Touryu — Japan: C/O Yamamoto Yasushi Yoshikawa, yasushi@med.shimane-u.ac.jp or yasushi@shimane-med.ac.jp

Chapter Notes

Introduction

1. Jim Wren, interview with the author, June 25, 2008.
2. Eileen Blumenthal and Julie Taymor. *Julie Taymor: Playing with Fire, Theater Opera Film* (New York: Harry N. Abrams, 1995), 9, 10.
3. Sergio Martin, *Dario Fo: The Theatre of the Eye* (Florence, Ita.: S.E.S. s.r.l., 1984), 24.
4. Bill LeVasseur, interview with the author, July 2, 2009.
5. Peter T. Furst, "Foreword," in *Mexican Masks: Their Uses and Symbolism*, edited by Donald Bush Cordry (Austin: University of Texas Press, 1981), ix–xx.

Chapter 1

1. Joseph Campbell, *The Power of Myth* (1988; reprint, New York: First Anchor Books, 1991), 39, 90.
2. Joseph Campbell, *Primitive Mythology: The Masks of God* (1959; reprint, New York: Penguin, 1991), 339–344.
3. Ibid., 257, 258, 282–286.
4. Peter Brook, *The Shifting Point: Theatre, Film, Opera 1946–1987* (New York: Harper & Row, 1987), 218.
5. Xstine Cook, e-mail communication to the author, May 26, 2009.
6. Walter Sorell, *The Other Face: The Mask in the Arts* (New York: Bobbs-Merrill, 1973), 14.
7. *Webster's New Collegiate Dictionary* (Springfield: G. & C. Merriam, 1980), 1004.
8. Frank Kermode and John Hollander, *The Oxford Anthology of English Literature*, vol. II (London: Oxford University Press, 1973), 6.
9. Ted Andrews, *Animal-Speak* (St. Paul: Llewellyn Publications, 2000), 4.
10. Clare Gibson, *Sacred Symbols* (Glasgow: Chartwell Books, 2002), 28.
11. Walter Sorell, *The Other Face: The Mask in the Arts* (New York: Bobbs-Merrill, 1973), 112.
12. Victoria Nelson, *The Secret Life of Puppets* (Cambridge: Harvard University Press, 2001), 22.
13. Ibid., 22–23.
14. Peter Macnair, Robert Joseph, and Bruce Grenville, *Down from the Shimmering Sky: Masks of the Northwest Coast* (Seattle: University of Washington Press, 1998), 169.
15. Ibid., 169.
16. Sorell, *The Other Face*, 17, 18.
17. Leslie Kane, "Reflections of the Past in *True West* and *A Lie of the Mind*," in *The Cambridge Companion to Sam Shepard*, edited by Matthew Roudané (Cambridge: Cambridge University Press, 2002), 140.
18. Sorell, *The Other Face*, 112.
19. Christopher Bigsby, "Born Injured: The Theatre of Sam Shepard" in *The Cambridge Companion to Sam Shepard*, edited by Matthew Roudané (Cambridge: Cambridge University Press, 2002), 22.

Chapter 2

1. William LaVasseur, interview with the author, 6 July 2009.
2. James Laver, *Costume in the Theatre* (New York: Hill and Wang, 1964), 19.
3. Efrat Tseëlon, *Masquerade and Identities* (London: Routledge, 2001), 4, citing A. David Napier, *Masks, Transformation and Paradox* (Berkeley: University of California Press, 1987).
4. Oto Bihalji-Merin, *Great Masks* (New York: Harry N. Abrams, 1970), 179.
5. Ibid., 44–45.
6. Deborah Bell, "Masks of Transformation," *Theatre Design & Technology* 42, no. 2 (2006): 42–43.
7. Henry Pernet, "The Ritual Mask and Its Wearer," in *Ritual Masks, Deceptions and Revelations*, translated by Laura Prillo (Columbia: University of South Carolina Press, 1992), 117–135.
8. Ajani Ojeyemi and Adeola Ogunneyemi, interviews with the author, 26 July–2 August 2006.
9. Henry Pernet, "From the Dead to Cosmos," in *Ritual Masks, Deceptions and Revelations*, 64.
10. Carol Beckwith and Angela Fisher, "Yoruba Masquerade," in *African Ceremonies*, vol. II (New York: Harry N. Abrams, 1999), 119.
11. John Nunley, *Masks: Faces of Culture* (New York: Harry N. Abrams, 1999), 160.

12. Ajani Adigun, interview with the author, 26 July 2006.
13. Ibid., 4 August 2006.
14. Ojetunji Ojeyemi, interview with the author, 2 August 2006.
15. Ibid.
16. Michael Harris, "Beyond Aesthetics: Visual Activism in Ile-Ife," in *The Yoruba Artist* (Washington DC: Smithsonian Institution, 1994), 202–203.
17. Agbedi Adebisi, interview with the author, 29 July 2006.
18. Kowale Adeoloa, interview with the author, 29 July 2006.
19. Bihalji-Merin, *Great Masks*, 47.
20. Agibike Ogunyemi, interview with the author, 31 July 2006.
21. Kasali Akangbe Ogun, interview with the author, 30 July 2006.
22. Ibid.
23. Robert Pirsig, *Zen and the Art of Motorcycle Maintenance* (New York: Bantam Books, 1974), 293.
24. Ajani Adigun, interview with the author, 4 August 2006.
25. Sangodare Gbadegesin Ajala, interview with the author, 30 July 2006.
26. Ajani Adigun, interview with the author, 4 August 2006.
27. Oyabo Osunyemi, interview with the author, 4 August 2006.
28. Ajani Adigun, interview with the author, 4 August 2006.
29. Laurel Birch Aguilar, *Inscribing the Mask* (Fribourg, Switz.: University Press Fribourg, 1996), 36.
30. Martin Ott, *African Theology in Images* (Zomba, Malawi: Kachere Publications, 2000), 151–155.
31. Ibid., 181.
32. Claude Boucher, interview with the author, 24 July 2006.
33. Douglas Curran, homepage, n.d., http://www.dougcurranphotos.com/htm/nyau_04.htm.
34. Kenji Yoshida, "Masks and Secrecy among the Chewa," *African Arts* 26, no. 2 (1993): 35.
35. Ott, *African Theology in Images*, 289.
36. Claude Boucher, interview with the author, 24 July 2006.
37. Ibid.
38. Victoria Nelson, *The Secret Life of Puppets* (Cambridge: Harvard University Press, 2001), 23.
39. Aguilar, *Inscribing the Mask*, 210, 216.
40. Curran, http://www.dougcurranphotos.com/htm/nyau_04.htm.
41. Douglas Curran, e-mail communication with the author, 21 May 2009.
42. Ott, *African Theology in Images*, 201.
43. Ibid.
44. Claude Boucher, interview with the author, 24 July 2006.
45. Yoshida, "Masks and Secrecy among the Chewa," 37.
46. Curran, http://www.dougcurranphotos.com/htm/nyau_04.htm.
47. Susan Smith, *Masks in the Modern Drama* (Berkeley: University of California Press, 1984), 94, 112.
48. Aguilar, *Inscribing the Mask*, 101.
49. Joseph Campbell, *The Power of Myth with Bill Moyers* (New York: Anchor Books, 1991), 73, 81.
50. Susan Smith, *Masks in the Modern Drama* (Berkeley: University of California Press, 1984), 173.
51. Claude Boucher, *The Gospel Seed* (Mtakataka, Malawi: KuNgoni Art Craft Center, 2002), 91.
52. Ott, *African Theology in Images*, 274.
53. Claude Boucher, interview with the author, 24 July 2006.
54. Ott, *African Theology in Images*, 195–196.
55. Ibid., 479, 490.
56. Yoshida, "Masks and Secrecy among the Chewa," 39, 40.
57. Aguilar, *Inscribing the Mask*, 202.
58. Curran, http://www.dougcurranphotos.com/htm/nyau_04.htm.
59. Aguilar, *Inscribing the Mask*, 256.
60. Boucher, *The Gospel Seed*, 56.
61. Curran, http://www.dougcurranphotos.com/htm/nyau_04.htm.
62. Aguilar, *Inscribing the Mask*, 114.
63. Douglas Curran, Email communication with author, 21 May 2009.
64. Claude Boucher, interview with the author, 24 July 2006.
65. Ibid.
66. Ibid.
67. Aguilar, *Inscribing the Mask*, 207.
68. Ibid., 215.
69. Ibid., 134–136.
70. Ibid., 148–149.
71. Ibid., 151.
72. Douglas Curran, *The Elephant Has Four Hearts: Nyau Masks and Ritual* (Vancouver: Presentation House Gallery, 2004).
73. Bruce Marrs, interview with the author, 18 November 2002.
74. Ibid.
75. Ibid.
76. Ibid.
77. Ibid.
78. Ibid.
79. Ibid.
80. Ibid.
81. Ibid.
82. Barbara Mauldin, *Carnival!* (Seattle: University of Washington Press, 2004), 7–11.
83. Milla Riggio, "Play Mas — Play Me, Play We," in *Carnival: Culture in Action — the Trinidad Experience*, edited by Milla Riggio (New York: Routledge, 2004), 93–108.
84. *Webster's New Collegiate Dictionary* (Springfield, MA: G. & C. Merriam, 1980), 700.
85. Ibid., 700.
86. Riggio, "Play Mas — Play Me, Play We," 93–108.
87. Ibid., 97.
88. Milla Riggio and Richard Schechner, "Peter Minshall: A Voice to Add to the Sound of the Universe," in *Carnival: Culture in Action — the Trinidad Experience*, edited by Milla Riggio (New York: Routledge, 2004), 109–128.
89. Ibid., 120.

90. Riggio, "Play Mas — Play Me, Play We," 93–108.
91. Ibid., 102.
92. Riggio and Schechner, "Peter Minshall: A Voice to Add," 110.
93. Tracy Assing, "All in the Wash," *Caribbean Beat* 71, no. 32 (2005): 33.
94. Ann Henry, "Memories of Minshall," *The Guardian*. 10 February 2005, Ent. 1.
95. Dylan Kerrigan and Nicholas Laughlin, "Bikinis, Beads, Braids," *Caribbean Beat* 65, 2004, http://www.meppublishers.com/online/caribbean-beat/archive/article.php?issue=65&id=cb65-1-64.
96. Claire Tancons, *Lighting the Shadow, Trinidad in and out of Light*, Caribbean Contemporary Arts Exhibit, October 7–November 4, 2004, online commentary, http://www.smallaxe.net/sxspace/works_claire.html.
97. Ibid.
98. Marlon Griffith, interview with the author, 9 July 2005.
99. Ibid.
100. Milla Riggio, "Geraldo Andrew Vieira: Making Mas," *The Drama Review* 42, no. 3 (1998): 194–202.
101. Geraldo Vieira, interview with the author, 10 July 2005.
102. Annan Boodram, *Peter Minshall: Wizard of Dancing Mobile*, 2005, http://www.caribvoice.org/Profiles/minshall.html.
103. Geraldo Vieira, interview with the author, 10 July 2005.
104. Ibid.
105. Sheldon Clemdore, interview with the author, 10 July 2005.
106. Susan Makin, *A Consumer's Guide to Art Therapy* (Springfield, IL: Charles Thomas, 1994), 5.
107. Sue Jennings, *Art Therapy and Dramatherapy* (London: Jessica Kingsley, 1993), 16.
108. Ibid., 20.
109. Ibid., 23.
110. Joyce Radtke, interview with the author, 16 March 2003.
111. Megan Fulmer, "Creating a Sacred Space," in *The Palette, The Arts of Humboldt County* (Eureka: Humboldt Arts Council, 2003), 6–7.
112. Ed Duddleston, phone interview with the author, 28 August 2003.
113. Donvieve, interview with the author, 15 March 2003.
114. Susan Mackey-Kallis, *The Hero and the Perennial Journey Home in American Film* (Philadelphia: University of Pennsylvania Press, 2001), 165.
115. Ibid.
116. Sandy Phillips, phone interview with the author, 2 September 2003.
117. Lauren Raine, letter to the author, 27 June 2008.
118. Ibid.
119. Ibid.
120. Lauren Raine, "The Mask of Sedna," *Coreopsis: A Journal of Myth and Theatre* 1, no. 1 (2009), https://sites.google.com/site/mythandtheatre/Home/summer -vol-1number-2/the-mask-of-sedna html.
121. Bruce Marrs, interview with the author, 15 March 2003.
122. Donvieve, interview with the author, 16 March 2003.
123. Kate Hamm, phone interview with the author, 6 September 2003.
124. Joan Schirle, Iowa Mask Conference performance, 16, May 2001.
125. Sheldon Clemdore, interview with the author, 10 July 2005.
126. Abano Terme, *Dario Fo: Masks, Puppets, and Men Paintings*, 2005, http://translate.google.com/translate?hl=en&sl=it&u=http://www.exibart.com/profilo/eventiV2.asp%3Fidelemento%3D20856&ei=fVolSsq0ENSEtwfm6YzfBg&sa=X&oi=translate&resnum=6&ct=result&prev=/search%3Fq%3DMuseo%2BInternazionale%2BDella%2BMaschera%26hl%3Den%26sa%3DG.
127. Ibid.
128. Paola Piizzi, letter to the author, 17 September 2009.
129. Ibid.
130. Ibid.
131. Donato Sartori, interview with the author, 21 June 2006.
132. Ibid.
133. Paola Piizzi, letter to the author, 17 September 2009.
134. Ibid.
135. Donato Sartori, interview with the author, 21 June 2006.
136. Ibid.
137. Ibid.
138. Paola Piizzi, letter to the author, 17 September 2009.
139. Donato Sartori, interview with the author, 21 June 2006.
140. Ibid.
141. Ibid.
142. Ibid
143. Ibid.
144. Paola Piizzi, letter to the author, 17 September 2009.
145. Arne Zaslove, letter to the author, 21 September 2009.
146. Aguilar, *Inscribing the Mask*, 59.
147. Ott, *African Theology in Images*, 460–461.
148. Dong-Pyo Kim, interview with the author, 12 March 2003.
149. Sangdae Lee, letter to the author, 13 August 2009.
150. John Nunley, *Masks: Faces of Culture* (New York: Harry N. Abrams, 1999), 325.
151. Bill and Heidi LeVasseur, *La Casa de la Cuesta*, n.d., http://www.casadelacuesta.com.
152. Bill LeVasseur, interview with the author, 30 June 2009.
153. Ibid.
154. Ibid.
155. Dalio Angel Perusquia, interview with the author, 1 July 2009.
156. Ibid.
157. Juan Horta, interview with the author, 29 October 2004.

158. Bill LeVasseur, interview with the author, 4 July 2009.
159. Karima Muyaes, interview with the author, 5 July 2009.
160. Bill LeVasseur, letter to the author, 20 July 2009.
161. Bill LeVasseur, interview with the author, 4 July 2009.
162. Ibid.
163. Ibid.
164. Ibid.
165. Michael D. Hernandez, Jr., and Linda M. Smith, *Behind the Masks* (Carbondale, IL: Exhibit Catalogue, University Museum, Southern Illinois University Carbondale, 2005), 10, 11.

Chapter 3

1. Bruce Marrs, interview with the author, 9 July 2001.
2. Ibid.
3. Ibid.
4. Thurston James, *The Prop Builder's Mask Making Handbook* (White Hall, VA: Betterway, 1990), 136–166.
5. Torbjörn Alström, letter to the author, 27 July 2009.
6. Ron Naversen, letter to the author, 10 December 2009.
7. Manuel Abeiro Horta, interview with the author, 3 July 2009.
8. Bill LeVasseur, "Clowns (Huezquistles Dance)," in *The Other Face of Mexico*, edited by Victor Jose Moya Rubio (San Miguel, Mex.: Universidad Nacional Autonoma de Mexico, 2009).
9. Dalio Perusquia, interview with the author, 1 July 2009.
10. Dalio Perusquia, interview with the author, 1 July 2009; Manuel Chavez, interview with the author, 2 July 2009.
11. Manuel Chavez, interview with the author, 2 July 2009.
12. Manuel Abeiro Horta, interview with the author, 6 July 2009.
13. Antonio Delgado, interview with the author, 5 July 2009.
14. Ibid.
15. Manuel Chavez, interview with the author, 2 July 2009.
16. Antonio Delgado, interview with the author, 5 July 2009.
17. Manuel Abeiro Horta, interview with the author, 6 July 2009.
18. Antonio Delgado, interview with the author, 5 July 2009.
19. Michael Meyer, interview with the author, 7 August 2008.
20. Ibid.
21. Michael Meyer, interview with the author, 10 July 2009.
22. Ibid., 7 August 2008.
23. Ibid.
24. Ibid.
25. Ibid.
26. Ibid.
27. Ibid.
28. Ibid.

Chapter 5

1. Paola Piizzi, letter to the author, 17 September 2009.
2. Ralph Yarrow and Franc Chamberlain, *Jacques Lecoq and the British Theatre* (New York: Routledge, 2002), 77.
3. Paola Piizzi, letter to the author, 17 September 2009.
4. Arne Zaslove, letter to the author, 12 June 2009.
5. Ibid.
6. Ibid., 21 September 2009.
7. Arne Zaslove, letter to the author, 18 September 2009.
8. Cheryl Shearar, 2000. *Understanding Northwest Coast Art* (Toronto: Douglas & McIntyre Washington, 2000), 95–96.
9. Glenna Matthews, "Forging a Cosmopolitan Civic Culture: The Regional Identity of San Francisco and Northern California," in *Many Wests: Place, Culture, and Regional Identity*, edited by Michael C. Steiner and David M. Wrobel (Lawrence: University Press of Kansas, 1997), 211–216.
10. Joan Schirle, letters to the author, 12 July 2009.
11. Margaret Crawford, "Alternative Shelter: Counterculture Architecture in Northern California," in *Reading California—Art, Image, and Identity 1900–2000*, edited by Stephanie Barron, Sheri Bernstein, and Ilene Susan Fort (Los Angeles: Museum Associates, Los Angeles County Museum of Art and Regents of the University of California, 2000), 249.
12. Paola Piizzi, letter to the author, 17 September 2009.
13. Margaret Crawford, "Alternative Shelter: Counterculture Architecture in Northern California," in Barron, Bernstein, and Fort, *Reading California*, 260.
14. Joan Schirle, letter to the author, 21 April 2009.
15. Ibid.
16. Ibid.
17. Sears A. Eldredge and Hollis W. Huston, "Actor Training in the Neutral Mask," *The Drama Review* 22, no. 4 (1978): 19–28.
18. Joan Schirle, letter to the author, 21 April 2009.
19. Ibid.
20. Arne Zaslove, phone interview with the author, 22 June 2006.
21. Online: http://www.aasen.dk/motiv_dellarte-uk.html.
22. Joan Schirle, letter to the author, 9 June 2006.
23. Xstine Cook, letter to the author, 20 May 2006.
24. Joan Schirle, letter to the author, 9 June 2006.
25. Ron Naversen, "Learning to Carve Masks in Bali," *Theatre Design & Technology* 40, no. 1 (2004): 38–43.

26. Ibid.
27. Joan Schirle and Arne Zaslove, letter to and phone interview with the author, 22 June 2006.
28. Paola Piizzi, letter to the author, 17 September 2009.
29. Ibid.
30. Arne Zaslove, phone interview with the author, 22 June 2006.
31. Bob Doran, "Behind the Mask: Carlo Mazzone-Clementi, 1920–2000," *About Dell'Arte*, 16 November 2000, http://www.dellarte.com/dellarte.aspx?id=179.
32. Arne Zaslove, letter to the author, 12 June 2009.
33. Ibid.
34. Ibid.
35. Paola Piizzi, letter to the author, 17 September 2009.
36. Ibid.
37. Arne Zaslove, letter to the author, 21 September 2009.
38. Ibid.
39. Joan Schirle, letter to the author, 9 June 2006.
40. Doran, "Behind the Mask."

Chapter 6

1. Victoria Nelson, *The Secret Life of Puppets* (Cambridge: Harvard University Press, 2001), 75.
2. Ibid., 22–23.
3. Susan Mackey-Kallis, *The Hero and the Perennial Journey Home in American Film* (Philadelphia: University of Pennsylvania Press, 2001), 206.
4. Nelson, *The Secret Life of Puppets*, 49.
5. Mackey-Kallis, *The Hero and the Perennial Journey Home in American Film*, 162.
6. Alec Worley, *Empires of the Imagination* (Jefferson, NC: McFarland, 2005), 62, 25.
7. Julie Taymor and Alexis Green, *The Lion King: Pride Rock on Broadway* (New York: Hyperion, 1997), 41–42.
8. Taymor and Green, *The Lion King*, 42.
9. Don LoCicero, *Superheroes and Gods* (Jefferson, NC: McFarland, 2008), 223.
10. Taymor and Green, *The Lion King*, 25, 73.
11. Mary K. Patterson Thornburg, *The Monster in the Mirror: Gender and Sentimental/Gothic Myth in Frankenstein* (Ann Arbor: University of Michigan Research Press, 1987), 13.
12. Victoria Nelson, *The Secret Life of Puppets* (Cambridge: Harvard University Press, 2001), 116.
13. Taymor and Green, *The Lion King*, 82.
14. Megan Stoner, "The Lion, the Witch, and the War Scenes: How Narnia Went from Allegory to Action Flick," in *Fantasy Fiction into Film Essays*, edited by Leslie Stratyner and James R. Keller (Jefferson, NC: McFarland, 2007), 77.
15. A. O. Scott, "Fantastic Mr. Fox," *The New York Times*, 15 November 2009, http://movies.nytimes.com/2009/11/13/movies/13fantastic.html?emc=eta.
16. Maurice Sendak and Terry Gross, "Looking Back on Wild Things with Maurice Sendak," *Fresh Air with Terri Gross* (1986; interview rebroadcast October 23, 2009), interview reproduced with the permission of WHYY, Inc.
17. Mackey-Kallis, *The Hero and the Perennial Journey Home in American Film*, 197–198.
18. Ibid., 164–165.
19. J. P. Telotte, *Replications* (Urbana: University of Illinois Press, 1995), 34, 35.
20. Thornburg, *The Monster in the Mirror*, 134.
21. Telotte, *Replications*, 37.
22. Ibid., 57.
23. Nelson, *The Secret Life of Puppets*, 249.
24. Ibid., x and 250–251.
25. Telotte, *Replications*, 51.
26. Thornburg, *The Monster in the Mirror*, 142.
27. Nelson, *The Secret Life of Puppets*, 287.
28. Ibid., 284–528.
29. Rod Dreher, "Economic Crisis Is Our Own Fault," *Dallas Morning News*, 30 March 2008, http://www.dallasnews.com/sharedcontent/dws/dn/opinion/columnists/rdreher/stories/033008dnedidreher.1597db91.html.
30. Nelson, *The Secret Life of Puppets*, 278.
31. Véronique Flambard-Weisbart, "Hollywood Enters the Dragon," in *World Weavers: Globalization, Science Fiction, and the Cybernetic Revolution*, edited by Wong Kin Yuen, Gary Westfahl, and Amy Kit-sze Chan (Hong Kong: Hong Kong University Press, 2005), 242.

Chapter 7

1. Wendy Doniger, *The Implied Spider: Politics and Theology in Myth* (New York: Columbia University Press, 1998), 2–4.
2. William Bascom, "The Forms of Folklore: Prose Narratives," in *Sacred Narrative: Readings in the Theory of Myth*, edited by Alan Dundes (Los Angeles: University of California Press, 1984), 8, 9.
3. Theodor Gaster, "Myth and Story," in Dundes, *Sacred Narrative*, 132.
4. Robert Brockway, *Myth from the Ice Age to Mickey Mouse* (Albany: State University of New York Press, 1993), 7–10.
5. Ibid., 133.
6. Bronislaw Molinowski, "The Role of Myth in Life," in Dundes, *Sacred Narrative*, 196–198.
7. William Bascom, "The Forms of Folklore: Prose Narratives," in Dundes, *Sacred Narrative*, 24–26.
8. Brockway, *Myth from the Ice Age to Mickey Mouse*, 2.
9. Sophia Heller, *The Absence of Myth* (Albany: State University of New York Press, 2006), 178.
10. Ibid., 91.
11. Ibid., 108.
12. Ibid., 140, citing Joseph Campbell and Bill Moyers, *The Power of Myth with Bill Moyers* (1988; reprint, New York: First Anchor Books, 1991), 40.
13. Ibid., 176.
14. Ibid., 69.
15. Ibid., 697–703.

16. Brockway, *Myth from the Ice Age to Mickey Mouse*, 119.
17. Ibid., 124.
18. Ibid., 154.
19. Clifford Geertz, *Local Knowledge* (New York: Basic Books, 1983), 11.
20. Ibid., 44.
21. Ibid., 97.
22. Ibid., 161.
23. Doniger, *The Implied Spider*, 64.
24. Ibid., 68.
25. Bascom, "The Forms of Folklore," 10.
26. Susan Mackey-Kallis, *The Hero and the Perennial Journey Home in American Film* (Philadelphia: University of Pennsylvania Press, 2001), 238.
27. Heller, *The Absence of Myth*, 120.
28. Ibid., 190–191.
29. Brockway, *Myth from the Ice Age to Mickey Mouse*, 7–10.
30. Doniger, *The Implied Spider*, 77.
31. Brockway, *Myth from the Ice Age to Mickey Mouse*, 3.
32. Ibid., 119–145.
33. Ibid., 15.
34. Heller, *The Absence of Myth*, 1.
35. Bruce Butterfield, *Mythology from Ancient to Post-Modern* (New York: Peter Lang, 1992), xiv.
36. Campbell and Moyers, *The Power of Myth with Bill Moyers*, 177–182.
37. Heller, *The Absence of Myth*, 215.
38. Doniger, *The Implied Spider*, 10.
39. Joseph Campbell, *Primitive Mythology: The Masks of God* (New York: Penguin, 1991), 339–344.
40. Heller, *The Absence of Myth*, 217.
41. Ibid., 216.
42. Ibid., 218.
43. Brockway, *Myth from the Ice Age to Mickey Mouse*, 52.
44. Heller, *The Absence of Myth*, 55.
45. Ibid., 222.
46. Ibid., 219.
47. Rob Faust, interview with the author, 27 April 2008.
48. Ibid.
49. Ibid.
50. Rob Faust, interview with the author, 28 April 2008.
51. Rob Faust, email to the author, 27 June 2008.
52. Ibid.
53. David M. Cohen, "Mask Men May Be Cream of Piccolo Crop," *Post and Courier* (Charleston, SC), 5 June 1989.
54. Rob Faust, interview with the author, 28 April 2008.
55. Ibid.
56. Ibid.
57. Ibid.
58. Ibid.
59. Ibid.
60. "Your Brain on Jazz: Creativity Soars when Inhibition Takes 5," *News & Record* (Greensboro, NC), 11 March 2008.
61. Campbell, *Power of Myth with Bill Moyers*, 39.
62. Ibid., 258.
63. Phil May, interview with the author, 3 July 2009.
64. *Center for Design Innovation*, http://www.centerfordesigninnovation.org/ (accessed 28 July 2009).
65. Phil May, interview with the author, 3 July 2009.
66. Ibid.

Conclusion

1. Joseph Campbell, *Primitive Mythology: The Masks of God* (1959; repr. New York: Penguin, 1991), 131.
2. Efrat Tseëlon, *Masquerade and Identities* (London: Routledge, 2001), 25, citing Walter Sorrell, *The Other Face: The Mask in the Arts* (London: Thames & Hudson, 1974).
3. Torbjörn Alström, lecture, 2005 International Mask Conference, Southern Illinois University Carbondale, October 8, 2005.

Bibliography

Books and Articles

Aguilar, Laurel Birch. *Inscribing the Mask*. Fribourg, Switz.: University Press Fribourg, 1996.

Andrews, Ted. *Animal-Speak*. St. Paul: Llewellyn Publications, 2000.

Assing, Tracy. "All in the Wash." *Caribbean Beat* 71, no. 32 (2005).

Bascom, William. "The Forms of Folklore: Prose Narratives." In *Sacred Narrative: Readings in the Theory of Myth*, edited by Alan Dundes. Los Angeles: University of California Press, 1984.

Beckwith, Carol, and Angela Fisher. "Yoruba Masquerade." *African Ceremonies*, vol. II. New York: Harry N. Abrams, 1999.

Besson, Gérard A. *The Angostura Historical Digest of Trinidad and Tobago*. San Juan, Trinidad: Paria Publishing, 2001.

_____. *Folklore & Legends of Trinidad and Tobago*. San Juan, Trinidad: Paria Publishing, 2001.

Bierlein, J. F. *Parallel Myths*. New York: Ballantine Books, 1994.

Bigsby, Christopher, and Matthew Roudané. "Born Injured: The Theatre of Sam Shepard." In *The Cambridge Companion to Sam Shepard*, edited by Matthew Roudané. Cambridge: Cambridge University Press, 2002.

Bihalji-Merin, Oto. *Great Masks*. New York: Harry N. Abrams, 1970.

Blumenthal, Eileen, and Julie Taymor. *Julie Taymor: Playing with Fire, Theater Opera Film*. New York: Harry N. Abrams, 1995.

Bonds, Alexandra B. *Beijing Opera Costumes: The Visual Communication of Character and Culture*. Honolulu: University of Hawai'i Press, 2008.

Bonnefoy, Yves. *American, African, and Old European Mythologies*. Chicago: University of Chicago Press, 1991.

Boodram, Annan. *Peter Minshall: Wizard of Dancing Mobile*. 2005. http://www.caribvoice.org/Profiles/minshall.html.

Boucher, Claude. *The Gospel Seed*. Mtakataka, Malawi: KuNgoni Art Craft Center, 2002.

Brockway, Robert. *Myth from the Ice Age to Mickey Mouse*. Albany: State University of New York Press, 1993.

Brook, Peter. "The Mask: Coming Out of Our Shell." In *The Shifting Point: Theatre, Film, Opera, 1946–1987*, edited by Peter Brook. New York: Harper & Row, 1987.

Cairns, Christopher. *The Commedia dell'Arte from the Renaissance to Dario Fo: The Italian Origins of European Theatre*. Lampeter, Dyfed, Wales: Edwin Mellen Press, 1989.

Campbell, Joseph. *The Hero with a Thousand Faces*. Princeton, NJ: Princeton University Press, 1949.

_____. *The Power of Myth*. 1988. Reprint, New York: First Anchor Books, 1991.

_____. *Primitive Mythology: The Masks of God*. 1959. Reprint, New York: Penguin, 1991.

Chilton, Meredith. *Harlequin Unmasked: The Commedia dell'Arte and Porcelain Sculpture*. New Haven, CT: Yale University Press, 2001.

Cohen, David M. "Mask Men May Be Cream of Piccolo Crop." *Post and Courier* (Charleston, SC). 5 June 1989.

Collen, Jean-Paul, editor. *Bamana: The Art of Existence in Mali*. Zurich: Museum Reitberg, 2001.

Corey, Orlin. *An Odyssey of Masquers: The Everyman Players*. New Orleans: Rivendell House, 1990.

Covell, Alan Carter. *Folk Art and Magic: Shamanism in Korea*. Elizabeth, NJ: Hollym Corporation, 1986.

Crawford, Margaret. "Alternative Shelter: Counterculture Architecture in Northern California." In *Reading California—Art, Image, and Identity 1900–2000*, edited by Stephanie Barron, Sheri Bernstein, and Ilene Susan Fort. Los Angeles: Museum Associates, Los Angeles County Museum of Art and Regents of the University of California, 2000.

Curran, Douglas. *The Elephant Has Four Hearts: Nyau Masks and Ritual*. Vancouver: Presentation House Gallery, 2005.

_____. Homepage. n.d. http://www.dougcurranphotos.com/htm/nyau_04.htm.

Desilet, Gregory. *Our Faith in Evil*. Jefferson, NC: McFarland, 2005.

Doniger, Wendy. *The Implied Spider: Politics and Theology in Myth*. New York: Columbia University Press, 1998.

Dreher, Rod. "Economic Crisis Is Our Own Fault." *Dallas Morning News*, 30 March 2008. http://www.dallasnews.com/sharedcontent/dws/dn/opinion/columnists/rdreher/stories/033008dnedidreher.1597db91.html.

Ducharte, Pierre Louis. *The Italian Comedy.* New York: Dover Publications, 1966.

Duda, Heather L. *The Monster Hunter in Modern Popular Culture.* Jefferson, NC: McFarland, 2008.

Edson, Gary. *Masks and Masking: Faces of Tradition and Belief Worldwide.* Jefferson, NC: McFarland, 2005.

Eldredge, Sears A. *Mask Improvisation for Actor Training and Performance: The Compelling Image.* Evanston, IL: Northwestern University Press, 1996.

_____, and Hollis W. Huston. "Actor Training in the Neutral Mask." *The Drama Review* 22, no. 4 (1978): 19–28.

Ernst, Earle. *The Kabuki Theatre.* New York: Grove Press, 1956.

Fava, Antonio. *The Comic Mask in the Commedia dell'Arte.* Evanston, IL: Northwestern University Press, 2007.

Fischer, Eberhard. *Guro.* Zurich: Museum Rietberg, 2008.

Flambard-Weisbart, Véronique. 2005. "Hollywood Enters the Dragon." In *World Weavers: Globalization, Science Fiction, and the Cybernetic Revolution,* edited by Wong Kin Yuen, Gary Westfahl, and Amy Kit-sze Chan. Hong Kong: Hong Kong University Press, 2005.

Foreman, Jennifer. *Maskwork.* Portsmouth, NH: Heinemann, 1999.

Fulmer, Megan. "Creating a Sacred Space." In *The Palette, The Arts of Humboldt County.* Eureka: Humboldt Arts Council, 2003.

Furst, Peter T. "Foreword." In *Mexican Masks: Their Uses and Symbolism,* edited by Donald Bush Cordry. Austin: University of Texas Press, 1981.

Gaster, Theodor. "Myth and Story." In *Sacred Narrative: Readings in the Theory of Myth,* edited by Alan Dundes. Los Angeles: University of California Press, 1984.

Geertz, Clifford. *Local Knowledge.* New York: Basic Books, 1983.

Gibson, Clare. *Sacred Symbols.* Edison, NJ: Chartwell Books, 2002.

Gilbert-Rolfe, Jeremy. *Beauty and the Contemporary Sublime.* New York: Allworth Press, 1999.

Harris, Michael. "Beyond Aesthetics: Visual Activism in Ile-Ife." In *The Yoruba Artist: New Theoretical Perspectives on African Arts,* edited by Rowland Abiodun, Henry J. Drewal, and John Pemberton III. Washington DC: Smithsonian Institution, 1994.

Heller, Sophia. *The Absence of Myth.* Albany: State University of New York Press, 2006.

Henry, Ann. "Memories of Minshall." *The Guardian,* 10 February 2005.

Hernandez, Michael D., Jr., and Linda M. Smith. *Behind the Masks.* Carbondale: University Museum, Southern Illinois University Carbondale, 2005.

Holm, Bill. *Spirit and Ancestor: A Century of Northwest Coast Indian Art at the Burke Museum.* Seattle: University of Washington Press, 1987.

Holý, Ladislav. *Masks and Figures from Eastern and Southern Africa.* Prague: Drury House, 1967.

Houston, Jean. *The Search for the Beloved.* New York: Putnam, 1997.

http://www.aasen.dk/motiv_dellarte-uk.html

http://www.caribvoice.org/Profiles/minshall.htm

http://www.casadelacuesta.com/

http://www.centerfordesigninnovation.org/htm

http://www.dallasnews.com/sharedcontent/dws/dn/opinion/columnists/rdreher/stories/033008dnedidreher.1597db91.html

http://www.dougcurranphotos.com/htm/nyau_04.htm

http://movies.nytimes.com/2009/11/13/movies/13fantastic.html?emc=eta

http://translate.google.com/translate?hl=en&sl=it&u=http://www.exibart.com/profilo/eventiV2.asp%3Fidelemento%3D20856&ei=fVolSsq0ENSEtwfm6YzfBg&sa=X&oi=translate&resnum=6&ct=result&prev=/search%3Fq%3DMuseo%2BInternazionale%2BDella%2BMaschera%26hl%3Den%26sa%3DG

https://sites.google.com/site/mythandtheatre/Home/summer -vol-1number-2/the-mask-of-sedna html

Izzo, David Garrett. *The Influence of Mysticism on 20th Century British and American Literature.* Jefferson, NC: McFarland, 2009.

James, Thurston. *The Prop Builder's Mask Making Handbook.* White Hall, VA: Betterway Publications, 1990.

Jenkins, Ronald Scott. *Acrobats of the Soul: Comedy and Virtuosity in Contemporary American Theatre.* New York: Theatre Communications Group, 1988.

_____. *Subversive Laughter: The Liberating Power of Comedy.* New York: Macmillan International, 1994.

Jennings, Sue. *Art Therapy and Dramatherapy.* London: Jessica Kingsley Publishers, 1993.

Kam, Garrett. *Ramayana.* Singapore: Tien Wah Press, 2000.

Kane, Leslie. "Reflections of the Past in *True West* and *A Lie of the Mind.*" In *The Cambridge Companion to Sam Shepard,* edited by Matthew Roudané. Cambridge: Cambridge University Press, 2002.

Kasfir, Sidney. "Elephant Women, Furious and Majestic." *African Arts* 31, no. 2 (winter 1998).

Kermode, Frank, and John Hollander. *The Oxford Anthology of English Literature,* vol. II. London: Oxford University Press, 1973.

Kerrigan, Dylan, and Nicholas Laughlin. "Bikinis, Beads, Braids." *Caribbean Beat* 65. 2004. http://www.meppublishers.com/online/caribbean-beat/archive/article.php?issue=65&id=cb65-1-64.

Kirk, Ruth. *The Wisdom of the Elders: Native Traditions on the Northwest Coast.* Vancouver/Toronto: Douglas & McIntyre, 1986.

Laver, James. *Costume in the Theatre.* New York: Hill and Wang, 1964.

LeVasseur, Bill, and Heidi LeVasseur. *La Casa de la Cuesta.* n.d. http://www.casadelacuesta.com.

Lévi-Strauss, Claude. *The Way of the Masks.* Vancouver/Toronto: Douglas & McIntyre, 1975.

LoCicero, Don. *Superheroes and Gods.* Jefferson, NC: McFarland, 2008.

Lommel, Andreas. *Masks: Their Meaning and Function.* New York/Toronto: McGraw-Hill, 1970.

Luciano, Eleonora. *The Mask of Comedy: The Art of Italian Commedia.* Louisville, KY: JB Speed Art Museum, 1990.

Mackey-Kallis, Susan. *The Hero and the Perennial Journey Home in American Film.* Philadelphia: University of Pennsylvania Press, 2001.

Macnair, Peter, Robert Joseph, and Bruce Grenville. *Down from the Shimmering Sky: Masks of the Northwest Coast.* Seattle: University of Washington Press, 1998.
Makin, Susan. *A Consumer's Guide to Art Therapy.* Springfield, IL: Charles Thomas Publisher, 1994.
Martin, Sergio. *Dario Fo: The Theatre of the Eye.* Florence, Italy: S.E.S. s.r.l., 1984.
Mason, David A. *Spirit of the Mountains: Korea's San-Shin and Traditions of Mountain Worship.* Elizabeth, NJ: Hollym International Corporation, 1999.
Masterpieces from the muse du quai Branly Collections. Paris: Musée du quai Branly, 2006.
Matthews, Glenna. "Forging a Cosmopolitan Civic Culture: The Regional Identity of San Francisco and Northern California." In *Many Wests—Place, Culture, and Regional Identity,* edited by Michael C. Steiner and David M. Wrobel. Lawrence: University Press of Kansas, 1997.
Mauldin, Barbara. *Carnival!* Seattle: University of Washington Press, 2004.
_____. *Tigers, Devils, and the Dance of Life, Masks of Mexico.* Santa Fe: Museum of New Mexico Press, 1999.
Molinowski, Bronislaw. "The Role of Myth in Life." In *Sacred Narrative: Readings in the Theory of Myth,* edited by Alan Dundes. Los Angeles: University of California Press, 1984.
Morita, Toshiro. *Kumadori.* Tokyo: JICC, 1985.
Napier, David. *Masks: Transformation and Paradox.* Berkeley: University of California Press, 1987.
Naversen, Ron. "Learning to Carve Masks in Bali." *Theatre Design & Technology* 40, no. 1 (2004): 38–43.
Nelson, Victoria. *The Secret Life of Puppets.* Cambridge, MA: Harvard University Press, 2001.
Nunley, John. *Masks: Faces of Culture.* New York: Harry N. Abrams, 1999.
_____, and Judith Bettelheim. *Caribbean Festival Arts: Each and Every Bit of Difference.* Seattle: University of Washington Press and the Saint Louis Art Museum, 1988.
Ott, Martin. *African Theology in Images.* Zomba, Malawi: Kachere Publications, 2000.
Ottenberg, Simon. *Masked Rituals of Afikpo: The Context of an African Art.* Seattle: University of Washington Press, 1975.
Pernet, Henry. "The Ritual Mask and Its Wearer." *Ritual Masks, Deceptions and Revelations.* Columbia: University of South Carolina Press, 1992.
Pirsig, Robert. *Zen and the Art of Motorcycle Maintenance.* New York: Bantam Books, 1974.
Raine, Lauren. "The Mask of Sedna." *Coreopsis: A Journal of Myth and Theatre* 1, no. 1 (2009). https://sites.google.com/site/mythandtheatre/Home/summer -vol-1number-2/the-mask-of-sedna html.
Ray, Dorothy Jean. *Eskimo Masks: Art and Ceremony.* Seattle: University of Washington Press, 1967.
Riggio, Milla. "Geraldo Andrew Vieira: Making Mas." *The Drama Review* 42, no. 3 (1998).
_____. "Play Mas—Play Me, Play We." In *Carnival: Culture in Action,* edited by Milla Riggio. New York: Routledge, 2004.
_____, and Richard Schechner. "Peter Minshall: A Voice to Add to the Sound of the Universe." In *Carnival: Culture in Action—The Trinidad Experience,* edited by Milla Riggio. New York: Routledge, 2004.
Roudané, Matthew. *The Cambridge Companion to Sam Shepard.* Cambridge: Cambridge University Press, 2002.
Savella, Alessandro. *The Carnival of Venice.* Milan: Amilcare Pizzi S.p.A. Cinisello B., Silvana Editoriale, 1984.
Scott, A. O. "Fantastic Mr. Fox." *The New York Times.* 15 November 2009. http://movies.nytimes.com/2009/11/13/movies/13fantastic.html?emc=eta.
Segy, Ladislas. *African Sculpture Speaks.* New York: Lawrence Hill, 1952.
Sendak, Maurice, and Gross, Terry. "Looking Back on Wild Things with Maurice Sendak." *Fresh Air with Terri Gross.* 1986. Interview rebroadcast October 23, 2009. Interview reproduced with the permission of WHYY, Inc.
Shearar, Cheryl. *Understanding Northwest Coast Art: A Guide to Crests, Beings and Symbols.* Toronto: Douglas & McIntyre Washington, 2000.
Simmons, Gene. *Kiss and Make-Up.* New York: Crown, 2001.
Slattum, Judy. *Masks of Bali: Spirits of an Ancient Drama.* San Francisco: Chronicle Books, 1992.
Smith, Susan. *Masks in the Modern Drama.* Berkeley: University of California Press, 1984.
Sorell, Walter. *The Other Face: The Mask in the Arts.* New York: Bobbs-Merrill, 1973.
Stoner, Megan. "The Lion, the Witch, and the War Scenes: How Narnia Went from Allegory to Action Flick." In *Fantasy Fiction Into Film Essays,* edited by Leslie Stratyner and James R. Keller. Jefferson, NC: McFarland, 2007.
Stratyner, Leslie, and James R. Keller. *Fantasy Fiction into Film.* Jefferson, NC: McFarland, 2007.
Tancons, Claire. *Lighting the Shadow: Trinidad in and out of Light.* Caribbean Contemporary Arts Exhibit. 7 October–4 November 2004.
Taymor, Julie, and Alexis Green. *The Lion King: Pride Rock on Broadway.* New York: Hyperion, 1997.
Telotte, J. P. *Replications.* Urbana: University of Illinois Press, 1995.
Terme, Abano. *Dario Fo: Masks, Puppets, and Men Paintings.* 2005. http://translate.google.com/translate?hl=en&sl=it&u=http://www.exibart.com/profilo/eventiV2.asp%3Fidelemento%3D20856&ei=fVolSsq0ENSEtwfm6YzfBg&sa=X&oi=translate&resnum=6&ct=result&prev=/search%3Fq%3DMuseo%2BInternazionale%2BDella%2BMaschera%26hl%3Den%26sa%3DG.
Teuten, Timothy. *A Collector's Guide to Masks.* Secaucus, NJ: Wellfleet Books, 1990.
Thornburg, Mary K. Patterson. *The Monster in the Mirror: Gender and Sentimental/Gothic Myth in Frankenstein.* Ann Arbor: University of Michigan Research Press, 1987.
Tseëlon, Efrat. *Masquerade and Identities.* London: Routledge, 2001.
Webster's New Collegiate Dictionary. Springfield, MA: G. & C. Merriam, 1980.
Whitten, Dorothea S., and Norman E. Whitten, Jr.

Imagery and Creativity: Ethoaesthetics and Art Worlds in the Americas. Tucson: University of Arizona Press, 1993.
Wilsher, Toby. *The Mask Handbook: A Practical Guide*. New York: Routledge, 2007.
Worley, Alec. *Empires of the Imagination*. Jefferson, NC: McFarland, 2005.
Wyatt, Gary. *Mythic Beings: Spirit Art of the Northwest Coast*. Vancouver/Toronto: Douglas and McIntyre, 1999.
_____. *Spirit Faces: Contemporary Masks of the Northwest Coast*. Vancouver/Toronto: Douglas and McIntyre, 1994.
Yarrow, Ralph, and Franc Chamberlain. *Jacques Lecoq and the British Theatre*. New York: Routledge, 2002.
Yoshida, Kenji. "Masks and Secrecy among the Chewa." *African Arts* 26, no. 2 (1993).
"Your Brain on Jazz: Creativity Soars when Inhibition Takes 5." *News & Record* (Greensboro). 11 March 2008.

Interviews

Abrantes, Samuel. Interview with the author. 9 December 2005.
Adebisi, Agbedi. Interview with the author. 29 July 2006.
Adeoloa, Kowale. Interview with the author. 29 July 2006.
Ajala, Sangodare Gbadegesin. Interview with the author. 30 July 2006.
Ajani, Adigun. Interviews with the author. 29 July–7 August 2006.
Akangbe Ogun, Kasali. Interview with the author. 30 July 2006.
Alström, Torbjörn. Interviews with the author. 30 May through 5 June 2002.
Álvarez, Alicia Martínez. Interview with the author. 6 July 2009.
Anom, I. Bagus. Interview with the author. 6 February 2003.
Besson, Gérard. Interview with the author. 6 July 2005.
Boucher, Claude. Interview with the author. 24 July 2006.
Castillo, Juan Horta. Interview with the author. 29 October 2004.
Chavez, Manuel. Interview with the author. 2 July 2009.
Clemdore, Sheldon. Interview with the author. 10 July 2005.
Cook, Xstine. Interview with the author. 17 April 2003.
Dada, Gabriel. Interview with the author. 6, August 2006.
Dawig, I. Wayan. Interview with the author. 1 February 2003.
Delgado, Antonio. Interview with the author. 5 July 2009.
Dibo, Ivete. Interview with the author. 12 December 2005.
Donvieve. Interview with the author. 15 March 2003.
Faust, Rob. Interviews with the author. 27 April–28 April 2008.
Fava, Antonio. Interview with the author. 31 May 2002.
Fonseca, Venicio. Interview with the author. 11 December 2005.
Griffith, Marlon. Interview with the author. 9 July 2005.
Horta, Manuel Abeiro. Interview with the author. 6 July 2009.
Iwasaki, Kyoun. Interview with the author. 5 July 2003.
Kim, Dong-Pyo. Interview with the author. 12 March 2003.
LeVasseur, Bill. Interviews with the author. 29 June–7 July 2009.
Marrs, Bruce. Interviews with the author. 17 March 2003, 9 July 2003, 18 November 2003, 15 March 2002.
May, Phil. Interview with the author. 3 July 2009.
Muyaes, Karima. Interview with the author. 5 July 2009.
Meyer, Michael. Interviews with the author. 7 August 2008, 10 July 2008.
Newman. Interview with the author. 16 September 2001.
Ogunyemi, Agibike. Interview with the author. 31 July 2006.
Ojeyemi, Ojetunji. Interview with the author. 2 August 2006.
Osunyemi, Oyabo. Interview with the author. 4 August 2006.
Perusquia, Dalio Angel. Interview with the author. 1 July 2009.
Rabiu, Abesu. Interview with the author. 3 August 2006.
Radtke, Joyce. Interview with the author. 16 March 2003.
Raine, Lauren. Interview with the author. 26 July 2002.
Reece, Victor. Interview with the author. 28 July 2002.
Rufus, Olowolafe. Interview with the author. 5 August 2006.
Sartori, Donato. Interviews with the author. 1 June 2002, 21 June 2006.
Sheldon, Clemdore. Interview with the author. 10 July 2005.
Suryasa, I. Made. Interview with the author. 9 February 2003.
Taiwo, Olurotimi. Interview with the author. 5 August.
Vieira, Geraldo. Interview with the author. 10 July 2005.
Vieira, Geraldo, Jr. Interview with the author. 10 July 2005.
Wren, Jim. Interview with the author. 25 June 2008.
Yoshikawa, Touryu. Interview with the author. 6 July 2003.

Correspondence

Alström, Torbjörn. Letters to the author. 27 July 2001, 30 August. 2009.
Cook, Xstine. Email communication with the author. 20 May 2009, 26 May 2009.
Curran, Douglas. Email communication with the author. 21 May 2009.
Duddleston, Ed. Phone interview with the author. 28 August 2003.

Faust, Rob. Email to the author. 27 June 2008.
Hamm, Kate. Phone interview with the author. 6 September 2003.
Lee, Sangdae. Letter to the author. 13 August 2009.
LeVasseur, Bill. Letter to the author. 20 July 2009.
Marrs, Bruce. Letters to the author. 18 November 2001, 4 September 2002.
Naversen, Ron. Frequent correspondence with the author. 2009.
Phillips, Sandy. Phone interview with the author. 2 September 2003.
Piizzi, Paola. Letter to the author. 17 September 2009.
Raine, Lauren. Letters to the author. 27 June 2008.
Reece, Victor. Phone interview with the author. 28 July 2001.
Schirle, Joan. Frequent correspondence with the author. 2001–2009.
Zaslove, Arne. Phone interview with the author. 6 July 2006.
_____. Letters to the author. 12 June 2009, 22 June 2009, 18 September 2009, 21 September 2009, and 22 June 2009.

Index

Numbers in ***bold italics*** indicate pages with photographs.***1A***, ***1B*** etc. indicate the first section of color plates and ***2A***, ***2B*** etc. indicate the second.